Oat Protein

Oat Protein

Processing, Function, and Applications

Xinzhong Hu

College of Food Engineering and Nutritional Science
Shaanxi Normal University
Xi'an, Shaanxi, China

Hamad Rafique

College of Food Engineering and Nutritional Science
Shaanxi Normal University
Xi'an, Shaanxi, China

Tian Ren

College of Food Engineering and Nutritional Science
Shaanxi Normal University
Xi'an, Shaanxi, China

WILEY

This edition first published 2026

Xinzhong Hu and Hamad Rafique contributed equally to this work and share first authorship.

Registered Offices

John Wiley & Sons, Inc., 111 River Street, Hoboken, NJ 07030, USA
John Wiley & Sons Ltd, New Era House, 8 Oldlands Way, Bognor Regis, West Sussex, PO22 9NQ, UK

For details of our global editorial offices, customer services, and more information about Wiley products visit us at http://www.wiley.com.

The manufacturer's authorized representative according to the EU General Product Safety Regulation is Wiley-VCH GmbH, Boschstr. 12, 69469 Weinheim, Germany, e-mail: Product_Safety@wiley.com.

Wiley also publishes its books in a variety of electronic formats and by print-on-demand. Some content that appears in standard print versions of this book may not be available in other formats.

Library of Congress Cataloging-in-Publication Data has been applied for:

Print ISBN: 9781394369492
ePDF ISBN: 9781394369515
ePUB ISBN: 9781394369508
oBook ISBN: 9781394369522

Cover Design: Wiley
Cover Images: Jianliang Xu/stock.adobe.com, Nitr/Shutterstock, Bluesuntnt/Shutterstock

Contents

Preface *xi*

1 Introduction to Oat Protein *1*
1.1 The Rise of Plant-based Proteins *1*
1.1.1 The Importance of Plant-based Protein for Human Health *1*
1.1.2 Comparative Analysis of Plant-based and Animal-based Proteins *3*
1.2 Historical and Current Significance of Oat Protein *5*
1.2.1 The Historical Significance of Oats and Oat Protein *5*
1.2.1.1 The Health Benefits of Oat for Human Being *5*
1.2.1.2 The Health Benefits of Oat for Animal Husbandry *6*
1.2.2 The Current Significance of Oats and Oat Protein *7*
1.2.2.1 The Utilization of Oats and Oat Protein *7*
1.2.2.2 The Unique Characteristic of Oat Protein *9*
1.2.2.3 Low Allergenicity Profile Relative to Other Gluten-containing Grains *10*
1.3 Scope and Objectives of the Book *12*
1.3.1 Scope of This Book *12*
1.3.2 Objectives of This Book *13*
References *14*

2 Significance of Oat Protein over Cereal and Legumes *17*
2.1 Introduction *17*
2.2 Distribution of Protein and Other Components in Hulled and Naked Oats *17*
2.3 Comparison of Protein and Other Components with Common Cereals *20*
2.4 Comparison of Oat Protein with Common Pseudocereals *22*
2.5 Comparison of Oat Protein with Legumes *23*
2.6 Challenges of Incorporating Legume and Pulses in Food Applications *25*
2.6.1 Allergenicity *25*
2.6.2 Digestibility *25*
2.6.3 Beany Flavour *26*
2.6.4 Texture *26*
Summary *27*
References *27*

3 Chemical Composition and Structural Characteristics of Oat Protein *35*
3.1 Amino Acid Profile of Oat Protein *35*
3.2 Nutritional Quality Evaluation of Oat Protein *37*
3.3 Regulatory and Physiological Functions of Amino Acids *38*
3.3.1 Branched Chain Amino Acids *38*
3.3.2 Arginine *40*
3.3.3 Aspartic Acid *40*
3.4 Classification of Oat Protein *41*
3.4.1 Globulins *41*
3.4.2 Prolamins *42*
3.4.3 Albumins *43*
3.4.4 Glutelin *43*
3.5 Molecular and Structural Features of Oat Protein *43*
3.5.1 Primary Structure of Oat Protein *43*
3.5.2 Secondary and Tertiary Structure of Oat Protein *45*
3.5.3 Quaternary Structure of Oat Protein *47*
Summary *48*
References *49*

4 Extraction and Purification Technologies of Oat Protein *57*
4.1 Introduction *57*
4.2 Defatting of Oat Flour *58*
4.3 Liquid-assisted Protein Extraction *59*
4.4 Protein Extraction with Dry Fractionation Method *61*
4.5 Advanced Protein Extraction Methods *62*
4.5.1 Deep Eutectic Protein Extraction *62*
4.5.2 Ultrasonic-assisted Protein Extraction *63*
4.5.3 Enzyme-assisted Extraction *64*
4.5.4 Pulsed Electric Field *65*
4.5.5 Extraction with Combined Techniques *66*
4.6 Existing Challenges in Protein Extraction *67*
4.7 Future Perspective for Industrial Scale Protein Extraction *68*
References *68*

5 Physical and Chemical Processing of Oat Protein *75*
5.1 Introduction *75*
5.2 Physical Processing of Protein *75*
5.2.1 Thermal Processing *76*
5.2.2 High-pressure Processing *77*
5.2.2.1 High Hydrostatic Pressure *77*
5.2.2.2 Dynamic High-pressure Fluidization *78*
5.2.3 Extrusion Processing *79*
5.2.4 Cold Plasma Processing *80*
5.3 Chemical Processing of Protein *81*

5.3.1 Glycation *81*
5.3.2 Acylation *83*
5.3.3 Deamidation *84*
5.3.4 pH Shifting *85*
5.4 Biological Processing of Protein *86*
5.4.1 Enzymatic Processing *86*
5.4.2 Fermentation Processing *87*
5.5 Effect of Processing on Functional and Physicochemical Characteristics of Oat Proteins *88*
5.5.1 Texturization Characteristics *88*
5.5.2 Oat Dough Characteristics: High Hardness and Low Elasticity *91*
5.5.3 Emulsifying Foaming Characteristics *92*
5.5.4 Protein Conversion Coefficient *93*
5.5.5 High Lipase Activity *94*
Summary *96*
References *96*

6 Functional Properties of Oat Protein *107*
6.1 The Importance of Functionality in Food Applications *107*
6.1.1 Defining Functional Properties *107*
6.1.2 Why Oat Protein's Functionality Matters *108*
6.1.3 Benchmarking Against the Competition *108*
6.2 Solubility and pH Stability *109*
6.2.1 The Fundamental Role of Solubility in Oat Protein Functionality *109*
6.2.2 Modification Strategies for Enhanced Solubility *111*
6.2.3 Characterization Techniques *112*
6.3 Emulsification and Foaming Capacity *112*
6.3.1 Fundamental Principles of Interfacial Activity *112*
6.3.2 Oat Protein as an Emulsifier *112*
6.3.3 Foaming Behaviour and Stabilization Mechanisms *113*
6.3.4 Oat Protein as a Foaming Agent *114*
6.3.5 Practical Applications *115*
6.4 Gelation and Texturization *116*
6.4.1 Molecular Basis of Oat Protein Gelation *116*
6.4.2 Factors Influencing Gel Properties *116*
6.4.3 Comparative Analysis with Other Plant Proteins *117*
6.4.4 Industrial Applications *118*
6.5 Interactions with Polysaccharides *119*
6.5.1 Unique Synergistic Effects with Polysaccharides *119*
6.5.2 Precision Modulation of Functional Properties *120*
6.5.3 Environmental Factors Governing Interaction Behaviour *122*
6.5.4 Applications in Food System *122*
6.6 Conclusion and Future Perspectives *123*
References *125*

7 Applications, Product Development and Regulations *129*
7.1 Food Industry Applications *129*
7.1.1 Plant-based Dairy Alternatives *129*
7.1.2 Meat Analogues and Structured Products *131*
7.1.3 Bakery and Confectionery Applications *133*
7.1.4 Beverages and Emulsions *135*
7.1.5 Infant Formula and Clinical Nutrition *137*
7.1.6 Cosmetic and Pharmaceutical Uses *138*
7.2 Product Development Strategies *139*
7.2.1 Formulation Design Principles *139*
7.2.2 Processing Technology Integration *139*
7.2.3 Clean Label *140*
7.3 Global Regulatory Framework *141*
7.3.1 Safety Assessment and Approval Processes *141*
7.3.2 Labelling Requirements *141*
7.3.3 Regional Regulatory Variations *142*
7.4 Commercialization and Market Implementation *143*
7.4.1 Scale-up Challenges *143*
7.4.2 Consumer Acceptance and Market Positioning *144*
7.5 Case Studies in Product Development *145*
7.5.1 Successful Commercial Products Analysis *145*
7.5.2 Development Process Documentation *146*
7.6 Future Trends and Innovation Opportunities *147*
7.6.1 Emerging Applications *147*
7.6.2 Technological Advancements *149*
7.6.3 Market Evolution and Growth Projections *150*
References *152*

8 Nutritional and Health Aspects of Oat Proteins *157*
8.1 Introduction *157*
8.2 Potential of Oat Protein as a Part of Daily Nutrition *158*
8.3 Role in Chronic Disease Prevention *159*
8.3.1 Oat Protein in Prevention of Oxidative Stress *161*
8.3.2 Oat Protein in Prevention of Diabetes *163*
8.3.3 Oat Protein in Prevention of Hypertension *164*
8.3.4 Oat Protein in Immune Function *166*
8.3.5 Oat Protein in Hypoxia *166*
8.3.6 Oat Protein in Fatigue Prevention *167*
8.3.7 Oat Protein in Anti-thrombotic Function *167*
8.3.8 Oat Protein in Cholesterol Management *168*
8.3.9 Oat Protein in Preventing Cancer *169*
8.3.10 Oat Protein in Neuroprotective Function *170*
8.3.11 Role of Oat Protein in Coeliac Disease *170*
Summary *171*
References *172*

9 Future Perspective of Oat Protein *181*
9.1 Sustainability: Carbon Footprint Comparison with Animal Proteins *181*
9.2 Emerging Technologies *183*
9.2.1 High-protein Oat Varieties Breeding *184*
9.2.2 Oat Protein Polymerization *185*
9.2.2.1 Oat Protein Form Polymers with Other Components During the Extrusion Process *185*
9.2.2.2 High Pressure Can Change the Oat Protein Molecular Weight *185*
9.2.3 Enzymatic Hydrolysis Technology Can Increase the Protein Functions *186*
9.2.4 Oat Protein Non-food Utilization *186*
9.3 Challenges in Scaling and Commercialization *187*
9.3.1 Raw Material Supply and Quality Control *187*
9.3.2 Processing Technology Bottleneck *188*
9.3.3 Market and Brand Challenges *188*
9.3.4 Policy Requirement *189*
9.4 Consumer Perception and Market Trend *190*
9.4.1 Fitness and Athletic Populations *190*
9.4.2 Chronic Disease Management *190*
9.4.3 Metabolic Regulation and Wheat Protein Allergy Groups *191*
9.4.4 Special Physiological Stages *191*
9.4.5 Cosmetic Applications *191*
References *192*

Index *195*

Preface

Oat protein represents a strategic resource in the realm of whole grains and serves as a core driver of the future food revolution. As a benchmark crop in the whole grain sector, the physiological benefits of oats' soluble dietary fibre, particularly β-glucan, have been widely recognized by the global scientific community, solidifying oats' reputation as a symbol of healthy food. However, the unique value of oats extends far beyond this.

Oats boast a protein content significantly higher than that of traditional grains. Their amino acid profile combines the strengths of both grains and legumes, featuring a high proportion of branched-chain amino acids, which support muscle synthesis and metabolic regulation. Additionally, their lysine content approaches that of soybeans, addressing a key limitation of grain proteins, while their gluten-free nature offers a safe alternative for individuals with allergies. These attributes position oat protein as an ideal plant-based protein, distinguished by its nutritional density, digestibility and biological safety. Nevertheless, systematic research into its health mechanisms and ecological value remains an area requiring further exploration.

From laboratory research to industrial production, oat protein is paving an innovative path for the food industry. Its processing properties are redefining the boundaries of food innovation. Oat protein's thermal stability and water-holding capacity make it an excellent ingredient for baking, extrusion-based products and high-moisture foods, while its low allergenicity unlocks high-value markets, including infant formula and specialized medical nutrition. Through physical shearing or enzymatic hydrolysis, oat protein can form stable gels and emulsions, providing essential structural support for plant-based dairy alternatives, meal replacement powders and similar products. Notably, its synergistic interaction with β-glucan enhances satiety and modulates gut microbiota, propelling the evolution of functional foods towards precision nutrition. These technological advancements not only elevate the value of oat protein but also inject new vitality into the traditional cereal processing industry.

As a strategic choice for the future, oat protein is poised to redefine its global value. Aligned with the rising global trend towards plant-based diets and the imperative of carbon neutrality, the ecological and health benefits of oat protein are transitioning from a regional resource to a global strategic asset. Ongoing molecular and clinical research is uncovering its potential in addressing metabolic syndrome, muscle atrophy and other conditions, paving the way for personalized nutrition solutions. By leveraging cutting-edge technologies such as fermentation engineering and molecular modification, challenges related to protein solubility and flavour are being overcome, enabling the development of premium, consumer-friendly products. Capitalizing on the low-carbon footprint of oat cultivation, a sustainable supply chain—from farm to fork—can be established, positioning oat protein as a key alternative to animal proteins. This initiative also contributes to global food security and climate governance. If current research and application barriers are overcome, oat protein will not only serve as an innovative food ingredient but also emerge as a pivotal force in transforming human nutrition paradigms and fostering ecological balance.

Xi'an, China
March, 2026

Xinzhong Hu
Hamad Rafique
Tian Ren

1

Introduction to Oat Protein

Oats are widely regarded as one of the most nutritious cereals, boasting a protein content of 12–20%, which is significantly higher than that of other major cereals such as rice (7–10%), wheat (11–15%) and millet (7–11%). Oat protein (OP) contains a relatively higher proportion of essential amino acids, including lysine, valine, isoleucine, methionine, histidine and threonine, which enhances its nutritional value compared to many other grains. Additionally, OP is rich in branched-chain amino acids (BCAAs) that play crucial physiological roles in energy production, muscle growth and recovery. Furthermore, the amino acid composition of OP aligns with the FAO's recommended nutritional requirements for adults, except for methionine.

Beyond its nutritional benefits, OP exhibits higher consumer acceptability in comparison to other plant-based proteins, such as pea, lupin and soy proteins. Notably, the carbon footprint of OP is more than 50% lower than that of dairy proteins. Food products enriched with OP can significantly reduce greenhouse gas emissions and land use when used as substituted for animal-based proteins. For example, oat-based beverages emit 16–41% fewer greenhouse gas compared to cow's milk. Moreover, OP is less allergenic than other plant proteins, including soy and pea proteins, which makes it an ideal ingredient for the expanding meat alternative market.

OP also possesses considerable potential as a functional food ingredient due to its wide range health-protective properties, including antioxidant, antidiabetic, heart-friendly and neuroprotective effects. In terms of physicochemical attributes, OP is characterized by moderate water solubility, favourable emulsifying capacity and a balanced hydrophobic-hydrophilic characteristic, rendering it suitable for diverse food formulations. However, its functional properties can be further enhanced through processing techniques like enzymatic hydrolysis and ultrasonication, thereby expanding its potential industrial applications.

1.1 The Rise of Plant-based Proteins

1.1.1 The Importance of Plant-based Protein for Human Health

Proteins function as essential structural and functional components of body cells, participating in critical biological functions such as intercellular signalling, systemic coordination, immune cell production and function, tissue repair and hormonal regulation of physiological processes [1]. These macromolecules are indispensable for human growth, development and the maintenance of normal physiological functions [2, 3]. For healthy adults weighing approximately 60 kg with moderate physical activity levels, daily protein intake should constitute 10–15% of total energy intake, equivalent to 1.2–1.5 g/kg body weight. Specific population requirements are as follows: older adults (> 65 years): 1.5–1.8 g/kg/day; vegetarians: 1.7–2.0 g/kg/day; postoperative recovery patients: 1.8–2.2 g/kg/day.

According to the 2022 China Food and Nutrition Development Report, the average daily energy intake of Chinese residents in 2020 was 3,328.9 kcal, and the average daily protein consumption was 105.4 g. The proportion of protein in energy intake was approximately 12.7%, with 46.3 g of plant-based protein and 38.6 g of animal-based protein per day. Currently, both the average daily energy supply and protein supply per capita exceed the 2020 recommended daily intake targets set in the China Food and Nutrition Development Outline (2014) (2,200–2,300 kcal, 78 g). The average per-capita daily protein supply in China is lower than in Portugal and the United States (115.0–117.7 g) but is relatively close to that of most developed countries (104.2–109.7 g) and higher than that of South Korea, Japan, South Africa and India (64.9–99.0 g). Overall, the energy and protein supply for Chinese residents is above the world average, indicating a need to optimize protein intake through dietary modification [2–4].

Approximately 30–50% of daily protein requirements for healthy adults are typically met through animal and soy-derived products (e.g., meat, eggs, dairy and soy), while the remaining 50–70% derives from cereals, pulses and other plant-based foods [4]. Although cereals contain only ~10% protein by weight, their high consumption as dietary staples establishes them as a significant protein source. Proteins are catabolized into amino acids, yielding approximately 4 kcal per gram. While plant proteins may have suboptimal amino acid profiles, their consumption confers substantial health benefits.

First, Healthier Ageing: Middle-aged adults with higher plant-protein intake show a 46% greater probability of healthy ageing compared to low consumers. Conversely, each 3% increase in energy intake from animal proteins corresponds to a 6% reduction in healthy ageing probability.

Second, Disease Prevention: Elevated plant-protein intake correlates with reduced incidence of chronic diseases (e.g., cardiovascular conditions) and lower all-cause mortality.

Third, Metabolic Advantages: Plant proteins contain no cholesterol, have significantly lower saturated fat, and are accompanied by abundant dietary fibre—critical for cardiometabolic health [5, 6].

Sustainability and Health Are the Key Drivers of Behavioural Change and Consumer Choice: Sustainability and health have emerged as pivotal factors driving behavioural change and consumer decision-making. Growing awareness of the environmental and health benefits of plant-based dairy products is catalyzing shifts in consumer behaviour. Compared to animal-based dairy alternatives, plant-based options exhibit a significantly lower environmental footprint, including reduced greenhouse gas emissions, land utilization and water consumption [5, 6].

Consumer insights reveal that the plant-based category is experiencing a transformative shift towards more conscious dietary patterns. Approximately 60% of consumers in the United States report adopting healthier lifestyles and diets, while 43% indicate increased purchase of sustainable products compared to three years ago [5, 6].

Chinese Enduring Tradition with Plant-based Proteins: China has a rich history spanning more than 2,000 years of edible plant protein consumption, with recorded evidence of tofu production dating back to the Han Dynasty. This long-standing tradition of predominantly soybean-based protein intake has shaped the dietary philosophy of 'grains as the foundation of nourishment', wherein daily plant protein consumption is primarily derived from foods such as tofu and soy milk.

Over time, the diversity of plant-based protein foods in China has steadily expanded, now encompassing a wide range of modern processed products. Traditional soy-based foods include tofu, dried tofu and bean curd cream, while plant-based beverages consist of soy milk, walnut milk, almond milk and other nut-based drinks. The modern processed food category comprises plant-based meats, protein powders and meal-replacement products [7, 8].

Asian Dominance in the Plant-based Dairy Market: Asia constitutes the world's largest market for plant-based dairy products, primarily driven by the traditionally high consumption of soy-based beverages, which account for more than half of the region's plant-based milk sector. According to consumer insights, 'new-generation plant-based milk' products—such as those similar to Oatly's formulations—have achieved a 16% market penetration rate in China. This category has undergone rapid expansion, with approximately 45% of consumers adopting these products within the past year, propelled by increasing coffee consumption, shifting dietary habits and global trends towards sustainability and nutrition [9].

Euromonitor data reveal that the retail value of Asia's plant-based dairy industry (excluding soy beverages in China) reached approximately US$8 billion in 2020, accounting for 4.7% of the total dairy market. Moderate growth is expected through 2025. China's plant-based dairy market is projected to double by 2025, partially driven by the emergence of innovative brands such as Oatly. The nutritional advantages of plant-based dairy alternatives include the presence of dietary fibre (notably β-glucan in oat milk), beneficial unsaturated fats, and the absence of lactose-related dietary concerns. These combined nutritional and environmental benefits have made plant-based dairy products an increasingly attractive choice among consumers, highlighting the substantial and growing global demand for sustainable dairy alternatives [9, 10].

1.1.2 Comparative Analysis of Plant-based and Animal-based Proteins

Exogenous protein sources are generally classified into two primary categories: plant-based and animal-based proteins. Plant-derived proteins include cereals, pulses or legumes, seeds, nuts and their processed products, whereas animal-derived proteins comprise dairy products, meat and meat derivatives, poultry, eggs and seafood [5, 6].

Nutritional and Functional Characteristics. Plant-based foods constitute a cost-effective and abundant source of protein for human consumption. The majority of plant-derived proteins are concentrated in seeds and grains, commonly classified as cereals or legumes (including oilseed legumes). A notable characteristic of plant proteins, such as OP, is their complete absence of cholesterol. Typically, plant-based foods contain protein, starch, lipids, soluble and insoluble dietary fibres and non-starch polysaccharides.

In contrast, animal-derived proteins generally exhibit superior nutritional profiles. They possess higher digestibility, enhanced nutrient bioavailability, and provide all essential amino acids in optimal proportions, while remaining free from anti-nutritional factors (Table 1.1). These features render animal proteins more anabolic, thereby making them more effective in supporting tissue growth and maintaining skeletal muscle mass compared with equivalent quantities of plant proteins.

On a per-weight or per-energy basis, animal protein sources deliver significantly higher levels of six essential micronutrients—vitamin A, riboflavin (B2), vitamin B12, iron, calcium and zinc—along with generally superior digestibility and bioavailability relative to plant-based alternatives.

Table 1.1 Comparison between animal and plant-based proteins.

Classification	Animal-based proteins	Plant-based proteins
Digestible	Animal proteins are primarily dominated by casein, which is easily broken down by digestive enzymes, with a biological utilization rate of over 90%	Plant proteins are typically surrounded by cellulose and contain anti-nutritional factors such as dietary fibre, phytic acid and protease inhibitors, making them less digestible (60–90% digestibility) than animal proteins
Protein types	Mainly consist of myoplasmic proteins, matrix proteins and myofibrillar proteins, with myofibrillar proteins forming the basis of the fibrous structure, which is difficult to replace or mimic by other proteins	Mostly storage proteins, including albumin, globulin, prolamin and glutelin, with their composition varying significantly depending on the plant source
Protein structure	Typically spherical, with symmetrical molecules that offer good solubility and are predominantly α-helix	Usually fibrous in shape, with symmetric molecules that are mostly insoluble in water, predominantly β-fold
Combined nutrition	Rich in vitamin B12, vitamin D, heme iron, zinc, but contains higher amounts of saturated fatty acids	Rich in magnesium, dietary folate and vitamin A, with higher amounts of MUFA and PUFA, especially omega-3 fatty acids
Cholesterol	High natural cholesterol levels	Low levels of dietary cholesterol
Fibre	Lacks fibre	Contains higher amounts of both soluble and insoluble fibre, including prebiotics
Processing effect	Processed meat products may contain carcinogens	Processed products may loss some nutritional value
Cost	High	Low
Health effect	May increase the risk of heart disease, cancer, diabetes, high cholesterol, weight gain	May reduce the risk factors for all of the above non-communicable diseases
Water requirement (m^3/t)	Milk: 1020; eggs: 3265; chicken: 4325; pork: 5988; lamb: 10415; beef: 15415	Soybean: 2145; corn: 1222; oat: 1788; wheat: 1827

Processing Considerations. Many animal-derived protein products undergo high-temperature processing to produce value-added items. However, excessive heat treatment (e.g., 115 °C for 20–180 minutes) can cause amino acid racemization in poultry proteins, substantially reducing protein quality as assessed by digestibility [5, 6].

Environmental and Resource Implications. The production of plant proteins offers considerable advantages in terms of environmental sustainability and resource efficiency. Compared with animal protein production, cultivating plant proteins requires significantly less fertilizer, fewer pesticides and reduced water input, while generating lower waste and greenhouse gas emissions.

For example, producing 1 kg of beef protein demands approximately 18 times more land, 10 times more water, 9 times more fuel, 12 times more fertilizer and 10 times more pesticide than producing an equivalent quantity of protein from kidney beans. Beef production also generates 5–6 times more manure per kilogram of protein than chicken or egg production. The carbon footprint of beef protein production (~36 kg CO_2/kg protein) is nearly 15 times higher than that of plant protein (~2.5 kg CO_2/kg protein). Similarly, producing pea protein requires only about one-sixth of the water needed for whey protein production.

Notably, animal agriculture occupies 77% of global agricultural land yet contributes only 18% of the world's caloric intake. In contrast, plant protein crops demonstrate 4- to 25-fold higher productivity per unit area [5, 6].

1.2 Historical and Current Significance of Oat Protein

1.2.1 The Historical Significance of Oats and Oat Protein

1.2.1.1 The Health Benefits of Oat for Human Being

Archaeological evidence indicates that oats (*Avena sativa*) were first cultivated as a cold-tolerant forage crop around 2000 BCE [11, 12]. During the Roman era, approximately 90% of the oat harvest was allocated to feeding war horses. Today, oats are primarily utilized for feed/straw (two-thirds) and human consumption (one-third). Their relatively high fat content (≈6.7%) provided livestock with essential energy to withstand cold climates, thereby supporting the demands of military campaigns [13].

1.2.1.1.1 Nutritional and Historical Significance

OP is a high-quality plant-based protein source (≈14% protein), with 36.45% comprising essential amino acids, including 7.12% lysine, effectively compensating for the amino acid deficiencies commonly observed in cereal proteins. During World War II, Northern Europe relied on oats as a protein supplement to alleviate meat shortages. Similarly, China's Yi people traditionally consumed roasted oat flour as a portable, energy-dense food during travel [13].

1.2.1.1.2 Medicinal and Modern Health Benefits

The *Compendium of Materia Medica* (1578) and *Complete Treatise on Agricultural Administration* (1639) both documented oats' benefits for spleen health and tuberculosis treatment. Later, Western medicine recognized their cholesterol-lowering properties, culminating in FDA certification as a functional food in 1997. A 2021 study demonstrated that daily intake of 30 g reduces LDL cholesterol by 12.8% [11]. This effect is primarily attributed to β-glucan, which forms a gel-like complex with proteins, slows gastric emptying and supports glycaemic control in diabetes management.

1.2.1.1.3 *Global Consumption Patterns*

Ancient Roman physician Claudius Galenus noted the dietary use of oats. Regions with high oat consumption (e.g., Scotland, Slavic Highlands and Sherpa communities) exhibit better overall health and disease resistance. Sherpas, for instance, primarily consume fried oats, which serve as a staple food for Himalayan climbers [14].

1.2.1.1.4 *Cultural and Culinary Context*

The origin of traditional oat-based foods such as 'Wowo' remains uncertain, though folklore links them to historical figures including Han Dynasty Chancellor Cao Cao and Genghis Khan. In major oat-producing regions (e.g., Shanxi, Inner Mongolia), oat-based foods are celebrated for their high caloric and protein content, though they are less digestible, making them ideal for heavy labourers. A local saying reflects this: '40 miles of oat flour sustain like 30 miles of millet cake; 20 miles of buckwheat noodles leave one famished' [11, 13].

1.2.1.1.5 *Oat Milk and Innovative Products*

Oat milk, a plant-based beverage derived from oats, retains β-glucan (1.2 g/100 mL) and dietary fibre through enzymatic processing, mitigating nutrient loss associated with traditional methods [9, 10]. Another innovation, Pulled Oats® (Finland), employs thermal processing to replicate meat's fibrous texture, providing a sustainable, high-protein alternative enriched with β-glucan and fibre.

1.2.1.2 The Health Benefits of Oat for Animal Husbandry

The initial oat varieties cultivated in Europe and North America differed from those in China, resulting in divergent uses and perceptions of the crop [11, 15]. Europe and North America primarily grew hulled oats, whose tough hulls rendered them unsuitable for human consumption under early processing methods. Consequently, oats were predominantly utilized as livestock feed. Observing that animals fed oats exhibited enhanced muscular strength, endurance and sustained energy, Europeans and North Americans initially adopted oats as premium feed for warhorses [11, 15].

1.2.1.2.1 *Nutritional Composition of Oat Grass*

Oat grass exhibits crude protein content ranging from 7 to 18% [11, 15]. Within this fraction, neutral detergent insoluble protein constitutes 21–25%, acid detergent insoluble protein 9–19% and soluble protein 26–46%. Notably, non-protein nitrogen accounts for 66–82% of the soluble protein fraction, with moderately degradable true protein representing the largest proportion. No significant difference in crude protein content exists between hulled and naked oat varieties [11, 15].

1.2.1.2.2 *Feeding Effects on Livestock*

Research on oat grass utilization, primarily as hay and silage, demonstrates substantial benefits for cattle, sheep and rabbits. A study conducted by China Agricultural University's Forage Processing and Utilization Team showed that replacing corn straw silage with oat silage in beef cattle diets significantly improved production performance. The oat silage group exhibited a 39.8% increase in daily weight gain (from 2.46 to 3.44 kg) and a 38.4% improvement in feed conversion efficiency, reducing feed costs per kilogram of weight gain by 13.9% [15–21].

For sheep, including 25% oat hay in mixed roughage optimizes growth performance and immune function. In aquaculture, supplementing 5% oat bran improves Nile tilapia growth while alleviating copper ion-induced stress on intestinal health [15].

1.2.1.2.3 Oat Hay Benefits for Tibetan Livestock

With a crude protein content of 10.6%, oat hay serves as an essential winter supplement for yaks and Tibetan sheep on the Qinghai-Tibet Plateau. Studies confirm its superior nutritional value and palatability compared with natural forage in the yellowing stage. Supplementation significantly increases weight gain (yaks: 8.4 ± 0.76 kg; Tibetan sheep: 7.9 ± 0.73 kg, $p < 0.05$) and enhances nitrogen utilization. Oat hay also improves production performance and product quality in horses, sheep and dairy cows [15].

1.2.1.2.4 Oat Silage Advantages for Dairy Cows

Oat silage (5.9–12.2% crude protein) enhances dairy cow productivity, increasing milk fat percentage, total fat and protein content. Replacing 22.7% of corn silage with oat silage improves dry matter intake and milk yield. Feeding oat hay during the dry period reduces artificial delivery rates and postpartum ketosis incidence, while improving overall health and milk quality. Total protein intake increases by 6%, further boosting milk production [21–23].

1.2.1.2.5 Oat Straw Characteristics and Limitations

Oat straw typically contains 2–9% low-quality protein deficient in essential amino acids. While its protein, fat and digestible fibre content surpasses that of wheat, barley and corn straw, its high crude fibre and low energy density limit its suitability for pigs and chickens. However, crushed oat straw can help prevent gastric ulcers in pigs [15].

Oats have historically been regarded as the premier feed for horses and have evolved into a crucial crop for feeding horses, pigs, cattle and poultry. Whole oats, crushed oats, oat flour and bran are suitable for feeding young and fattening animals. Oat hay can be processed into various feed forms, including green feed, hay, silage, grass pellets and grass cakes, and can be combined with leguminous crops to produce compound feed. In the Northern Hemisphere, oat hay is commonly used as a winter feed for livestock [15, 24, 25].

1.2.2 The Current Significance of Oats and Oat Protein

1.2.2.1 The Utilization of Oats and Oat Protein

1.2.2.1.1 Global Oat Production and China's Role

In 2023, oats ranked as the world's eighth-largest cereal crop by production volume, following maize, wheat, rice, soybeans, barley (including naked barley), sorghum and millet. Global oat output reached 26.335 million tons, with approximately 70% designated for forage and 8.5 million tons for human consumption [26]. As the centre of origin for hulless oats (*Avena nuda*), China is the world's sixth-largest producer and consumer of oats, with a cultivation area of approximately 667,000 hectares (≈10 million mu) and an annual production of around 850,000 tons. China contributes 2.5% of global oat output while representing only 0.1% of domestic grain production, prioritizing human consumption supplemented by forage use. Despite exceeding the domestic output of buckwheat (*Fagopyrum* spp.), Job's tears (*Coix lacryma-jobi*), and quinoa (*Chenopodium quinoa*), China's share in global production of these minor grains remains substantially lower than that of oats (Table 1.2).

According to USDA data, global oat production remained relatively stable at ~23 million tons until 2023, when it declined to 19.432 million tons due to climatic factors—a reduction of approximately 6 million tons from 2022, resulting in a modest increase in international oat prices. The EU maintained stable production, increasing from 7.524 to 7.754 million tons, consistently holding over 30% of the global market share. Russia experienced a notable decline, with production decreasing from 4.527 to 3 million tons, reducing its global share by 7.24% points. Canadian production remained stable at ~3.358 million tons, as did Australia at approximately 1.5 million tons.

The global oat utilization market is highly diversified, with animal feed (48.3%), food and beverages (43%) and personal care/cosmetics (5.5%) representing the main sectors. The EU has consistently dominated consumption, accounting for approximately 30% of global demand over the past decade, driven by traditional oat consumption habits and a well-established processing industry. In contrast, Russia's share of global oat consumption has steadily declined from 21.10% in 2015 to 12.29% in 2024.

According to the China Rural Statistical Yearbook, China's oat cultivation area increased for five consecutive years from 2019 to 2023, expanding from 7.68 million to 8.32 million hectare. This growth reflects rising domestic demand for oat-based health foods and industrial applications.

Table 1.2 Cereal crop production shares (global and China).

Crop	Global production (1000 tons)	China production (1000 tons)	Global share (%)	China grain share (%)
Maize	1,163,497	277,203	23.825	40.377
Wheat	808,442	137,720	17.035	20.060
Rice	776,461	208,490	26.851	30.368
Soybeans	348,856.4	20,283.5	5.814	2.954
Barley	154,877	1,960	1.266	0.285
Sorghum	57,582	2,969.9	5.157	0.432
Millet	30,860	2,806.5	9.094	0.409
Oats	26,385	600	2.274	0.087
Buckwheat	2,235	506	22.639	0.074
Job's tears	444.7	145	32.606	0.021
Quinoa	159	37.5	23.585	0.005

Data Sources: FAO STAT (2023) for global cereal data; China National Bureau of Statistics (2023) for Chinese grain data. Job's Tears global/China and Quinoa China data sourced from Industry reports/web sources. Data of barley includes qingke (hulless highland barley); data of millet includes Encompasses foxtail millet, proso millet and broomcorn millet; data of oats includes naked oats predominant in China.

1.2.2.1.2 Nutritional Advantages of OP

Oats contain among the highest protein levels of major cereals, providing 1.6–2.3 times the protein density of wheat and rice. OP represents a nutritionally advanced plant-based protein source with structural similarities to legume proteins but with distinct advantages: it lacks beany off-flavours, contains negligible gluten (<20 ppm in purified forms), and possesses a high proportion of BCAAs at 18–22% of total amino acids—surpassing most plant proteins in muscle-supportive potential. Globally, textured OP products have gained considerable traction in European markets. In contrast, OP utilization in China remains underdeveloped, constrained by limited raw material availability, technical processing barriers and minimal commercialization [13].

1.2.2.1.3 Global Oat Product Classification

From an international perspective, oat-based products can be broadly categorized into four sectors:

Daily Food Products: Steel-cut oats, oat-based baked goods, oat milk, oat-derived alcoholic beverages and oat cream.
Nutritional and Health Products: High-β-glucan oat flour, instant oat beverages and high-purity OP powders.
Pharmaceutical Raw Materials: Bioactive oat extracts, including oat saponins, polyphenols and anti-inflammatory alkaloid preparations.
Industrial Applications: Cosmetic and pet care raw materials such as colloidal oats, oat oil and oat-based animal feed [26].

In China, oat products are similarly classified into four corresponding categories, though the specific product types and processing forms differ markedly:

Daily Food Products: Oat debraned rice, oat flakes and composite flour products (e.g., multigrain noodles, steamed buns, crispy rice).
Nutrition and Health Products: Oat medicinal porridge, oat-based beverages and OP powder.
Medicinal Raw Materials: Oat-derived β-glucan and polyphenol extracts.
Industrial Applications: Skincare raw materials including oat colloids and oat peptides.

1.2.2.2 The Unique Characteristic of Oat Protein

1.2.2.2.1 Protein Content in Oat

Oat grains contain 12–20% protein, substantially higher than staple cereals such as wheat (11–15%), rice (7–10%) and maize (7–12%). Chinese naked oats (*A. nuda*) exhibit an average protein content of 14.94%, with nearly half of all varieties exceeding 15%. In contrast, hulled oats (*A. sativa*), which are more widely cultivated internationally, average 11.77% protein, with most cultivars ranging between 10 and 15% [27].

1.2.2.2.2 Composition of OP

Oat protein is composed of four principal fractions: globulins (70–80%), albumins (1–12%), prolamins (4–15%) and glutenins ($\leq$ 10%) [28]. Globulin, the predominant storage protein in oats, is salt-soluble and structurally comparable to the 11S globulin (glycinin) of soy protein. It consists of three subunits (12S, 7S and 3S), with a molecular weight (MW) of 54–60 kDa. The 12S subunit comprises acidic (A, 32 kDa) and basic (B, 22 kDa) polypeptides, while the 7S subunit contains polypeptides of 55–65 kDa and the 3S subunit consists of two polypeptides (15 and 21 kDa).

The water-soluble albumin fraction (MW: 19–21 kDa) contains enzymes involved in the plant's metabolic and defence systems. The alcohol-soluble prolamin fraction (known as avenin, MW: 20–40 kDa) shares structural similarities with sulphur-rich subunits of wheat (α- and γ-gliadins), rye (γ-secalins) and barley (B-hordeins). Although deficient in proline and glutamine, avenins serve a storage role functionally analogous to glutenins in wheat. The minor glutenin fraction comprises heterogeneous polypeptides with MW ranging from 10 to 90 kDa [28].

1.2.2.2.3 Nutritional Superiority of OP

Oat protein demonstrates a protein efficiency ratio (PER) exceeding 2.0, markedly higher than that of wheat and maize (both < 1.5), indicating superior biological utilization in humans [29]. It also contains higher concentrations of essential amino acids, particularly lysine, valine, isoleucine, threonine, histidine and methionine, than other cereal proteins. Among its fractions, globulins possess the highest levels of both essential amino acids (e.g., lysine, valine, phenylalanine, histidine) and non-essential amino acids (e.g., arginine, glutamic acid).

Furthermore, the amino acid composition of OP closely aligns with human nutritional requirements, effectively supporting growth and development. Consumer sensory evaluations have consistently shown that oat protein exhibits superior flavour acceptability compared with other plant-based proteins such as pea, lupin and soy [29].

1.2.2.3 Low Allergenicity Profile Relative to Other Gluten-containing Grains

Gluten proteins, which constitute 80–85% of the total protein content in wheat, rye, barley and their hybrid varieties, frequently trigger adverse immune reactions, including coeliac disease, non-coeliac gluten sensitivity and wheat allergy. Coeliac disease—a non-IgE-mediated autoimmune disorder—is induced by gliadin-triggered Th2 lymphocyte activation in genetically susceptible individuals (e.g., carriers of HLA-DQ2/DQ8 genes). Symptoms, including bloating, abdominal pain, diarrhoea and flatulence, typically manifest within hours to days after gluten ingestion. In contrast, wheat allergy arises when allergens bind to high-affinity, allergen-specific IgE receptors on effector cells (primarily mast cells and basophils), leading to acute reactions such as urticaria, angioedema, asthma, allergic rhinitis, abdominal pain and vomiting within 1–3 hours of exposure; severe cases may progress to anaphylactic shock and, in rare instances, fatality.

Oats have attracted attention as a functional cereal crop due not only to their nutritional benefits but also to their relatively low allergenic potential compared with wheat, barley and rye. While all cereals contain storage proteins—some of which are immunogenic—oats are considered safer for individuals with wheat allergy or gluten-related disorders. Unlike wheat, where gliadins and glutenins form a complex gluten matrix capable of triggering severe allergic and autoimmune reactions, OPs (primarily avenins) account for only 10–15% of total OP and exhibit markedly lower immunogenicity [30].

Multiple clinical and in vitro studies have demonstrated that oat consumption is generally safe for most individuals with coeliac disease and does not elicit the same immune response as gluten from wheat, rye or barley. For example, Comino et al. [30] found that while some oat cultivars contain avenin sequences capable of activating coeliac-related T cells, their immunogenic potential is cultivar-dependent and significantly weaker than wheat gliadins, suggesting that carefully selected oat varieties can be safely incorporated into gluten-free diets [31]. Similarly, Arentz-Hansen et al. reported that only a subset of coeliac patients exhibited T-cell reactivity to avenin peptides, further supporting the low immunogenicity of oats [31]. In contrast, wheat contains a broad spectrum of immunoreactive peptides affecting nearly all coeliac patients [32].

Regarding IgE-mediated food allergies, OPs are less likely to provoke allergic reactions than wheat. A large-scale European study found that the prevalence of oat-specific IgE was substantially lower (0.1–0.2%) compared with wheat (0.4–0.5%) [33]. While oat allergy does occur, it is relatively rare and is often observed in individuals with multiple food allergies or in occupational settings (e.g., bakers exposed to oat dust) [34]. A study in children with wheat allergy reported a 33.3% cross-reactivity rate with oats, significantly lower than the 60% observed with barley, indicating that oats may represent a safer alternative for wheat-allergic individuals, although individual tolerance assessment remains essential [35].

However, gluten contamination in oats remains a concern. Some gluten detection kits may overestimate gluten content due to cross-reactivity, highlighting the need for accurate testing methods to ensure the safety of oat-based products for gluten-sensitive individuals [30]. The primary oat allergens—lipid transfer proteins (LTPs), serpins and avenins—exhibit low sensitization rates in the general population. Additionally, oats are widely incorporated into dermatological formulations (e.g., colloidal oatmeal) for sensitive skin, owing to their anti-inflammatory and soothing properties, which would be unlikely if oats were a major allergen.

Recent studies continue to support the notion that oats generally possess lower allergenic potential compared to other cereals, such as wheat, barley and rye. Nevertheless, variations in individual responses and differences among oat cultivars necessitate careful evaluation.

A pivotal study involving 73 HLA-DQ2.5-positive coeliac disease patients assessed the in vivo T-cell response to avenin peptides following oat consumption. Only 8% exhibited avenin-specific T-cell responses, indicating that the majority of coeliac patients tolerate oats without immunogenic activation. Notably, barley ingestion elicited a more robust T-cell response, further emphasizing oats' comparatively lower immunogenicity [36].

Another study analyzing avenin sequences from different oat varieties revealed significant differences in their potential to activate immune responses. Some cultivars contained avenin peptides with higher immunotoxic potential, whereas others were deemed safe for coeliac patients. This variability underscores the importance of selecting appropriate oat cultivars for individuals with gluten sensitivities [37].

Oats represent a compelling alternative to wheat and other gluten-containing grains, particularly as a source of plant-based protein. OP isolate contains a well-balanced amino acid profile with relatively high lysine content, rendering it nutritionally superior to many other cereal proteins [38].

Due to their mild immunogenicity, OPs are increasingly explored as a hypoallergenic alternative in novel plant-based foods. Their low prolamin content, combined with evidence of minimal T-cell activation and IgE response, positions OP as a promising candidate for hypoallergenic food products.

Additionally, OPs exhibit excellent functional properties, including water-holding capacity, emulsification and solubility, supporting their application in diverse food systems.

These properties often surpass those of other plant proteins, such as wheat gluten or barley protein, which are less well tolerated by sensitive individuals [30, 32].

In conclusion, evidence indicates that oats and OPs are generally well tolerated and exhibit significantly lower allergenic potential compared to other major cereals. Their limited content of immunogenic prolamins, low prevalence of IgE sensitization and demonstrated safety in gluten-free diets (when properly sourced) support the use of oats as a safer and nutritionally advantageous option.

OPs, owing to their functional properties and low allergenicity, offer substantial potential as an alternative protein source in hypoallergenic and gluten-free food formulations, addressing the growing consumer demand for safe and plant-based protein products [39, 40].

1.3 Scope and Objectives of the Book

1.3.1 Scope of This Book

Oats are widely regarded as one of the most nutritious cereals, characterized by a high protein content. OPs contain a comparatively higher proportion of essential amino acids, including lysine, valine, isoleucine, methionine, histidine and threonine, which contribute to their nutritional superiority over many other grains. The abundant presence of BCAAs plays a crucial role in physiological processes, including energy production, muscle growth and recovery. Furthermore, the amino acid composition closely aligns with the Food and Agriculture Organization's (FAO) recommended nutritional requirements for adults, with the exception of methionine. Beyond their favourable nutritional profile, OPs demonstrate higher consumer acceptability compared to other plant-based proteins, such as pea, lupin and soy. Additionally, OP exhibits a carbon footprint more than 50% lower than that of dairy proteins.

Food products enriched with OP have the potential to mitigate greenhouse gas emissions and reduce land use when substituting animal-based proteins. For example, oat-based beverages generate 16–41% fewer greenhouse gas emissions compared with cow's milk. Moreover, OP is less allergenic than other plant proteins, including soy and pea, positioning it as a promising ingredient for the meat alternative market.

OP also confers diverse health-protective effects, including antioxidant, antidiabetic, cardioprotective and neuroprotective properties, thereby establishing its value as a functional food ingredient. In terms of physicochemical attributes, OP demonstrates moderate water solubility, favourable emulsifying properties and balanced hydrophobic–hydrophilic characteristics, rendering it suitable for a wide range of food formulations. However, its functional properties can be further enhanced through processing techniques such as enzymatic hydrolysis and ultrasonication, thereby improving its industrial applicability.

This book positions oats as a cornerstone of the plant-based revolution, emphasizing their role as a nutritionally balanced, whole-grain resource capable of addressing global food security challenges. While oats are often celebrated for their heart-healthy β-glucans and fibre, this work shifts the focus to their underappreciated protein fraction—a hypoallergenic, gluten-free ingredient with remarkable functional versatility.

Bridging the gap between academia and industry, the book synthesizes cutting-edge research on OP's unique chemistry, from amino acid composition and interactions with β-glucans to advanced extraction techniques that overcome historical challenges such as lipid co-isolation. It also explores functional properties critical for modern food innovation, including emulsification in dairy alternatives, gelation in plant-based meats and texturization in gluten-free baked goods.

Furthermore, the book examines the nutritional benefits of OP, including the generation of bioactive peptides and their potential role in mitigating chronic diseases. Unlike existing literature, which primarily focuses on oats' carbohydrates or offers broad surveys of plant proteins, this interdisciplinary volume uniquely positions OP as a sustainable and scalable solution for 21st-century food systems. It integrates sustainability metrics, such as carbon footprint comparisons, with real-world case studies on oat milk, vegan cheeses and biodegradable materials.

By uniting fundamental science, applied technology and market-driven insights, the book enables researchers, product developers and policymakers to elevate OP from an overlooked by-product to a mainstream, environmentally sustainable food ingredient. This transformation heralds a new era of nutritionally dense, ethically produced and consumer-centric foods, poised to make a lasting impact on global health and sustainability.

Current literature either focuses narrowly on the functionality of oat β-glucans or addresses OP only as a minor subtopic. This book addresses a critical gap by providing the first comprehensive resource dedicated to the chemistry, functionality and applications of OP.

Targeted Value for Key Stakeholders:

For Researchers: A definitive reference on OP's structural properties, extraction challenges and health benefits, supported by over 600 peer-reviewed studies.

For Industry Professionals: Practical strategies for incorporating OP into product development, including solutions to overcome gelation challenges in vegan cheeses.

For Policymakers: Data-driven insights into OP's role in sustainable food systems, aligned with the United Nations Sustainable Development Goals (SDGs).

For Educators: A valuable textbook for graduate courses in plant protein science, featuring diagrams, case studies and discussion questions.

In summary, this book is urgently needed to unlock OP's potential as a nutritionally balanced, environmentally sustainable and functionally versatile ingredient. By translating cutting-edge research into real-world applications, it empowers stakeholders across academia, industry and policy to advance OP from a niche ingredient to a mainstream staple, thereby contributing to human health, food security and global sustainability.

1.3.2 Objectives of This Book

Growing awareness of the environmental footprint of animal protein production has prompted consumers to shift towards plant-based sources to satisfy their demand for high-protein and protein-enriched foods, favouring these sustainable alternatives. Cereals remain a globally important dietary protein source, with oats distinguished by their higher protein content, unsaturated fatty acids, soluble fibre and antioxidant compounds compared to Triticeae cereals such as wheat and barley. The unique protein composition of oats is gluten-free, making them a safe food ingredient for most individuals with coeliac disease.

Oats rank as the seventh most abundant cereal crop produced worldwide. However, they are considered a minor cereal grain, as production volumes lag significantly behind those of maize, rice and wheat, contributing less than 1% of global cereal production. Oat production began declining in the latter half of the 20th century, driven by farm mechanization, reduced demand for horse feed and the replacement of oats with soy as the primary protein source for livestock.

Today, approximately 75% of oats continue to be used as animal feed, although food utilization has increased as the health-promoting properties of oats for human consumption have gained wider recognition. Traditionally, oats are consumed in the form of oat flour or flakes, but industrial-scale OP ingredients have only recently been developed. Modern fractionation technologies allow β-glucan extraction from oat grains while simultaneously yielding concentrated protein fractions as a by-product, providing the food industry with a novel, high-quality plant protein source.

Oats are predominantly a crop of northern latitudes, thriving under moderate temperatures and long photoperiods. Major oat-producing countries include Russia, Canada, Poland and the Nordic nations. Oats exhibit strong resilience, tolerating drought conditions and acidic soils, and are generally more resistant to plant diseases than other cereals. They also demonstrate competitive growth against weeds, reducing the need for agrochemical and fertilizer inputs, which translates to lower production costs and environmental impact. Oats are well-suited for organic farming systems. Under European conditions, oat yields average 3.5 t/ha, and with 12–15% protein content in whole grain (including hulls), this corresponds to a protein yield of approximately 0.4–0.75 t/ha. While oilseeds such as rapeseed and sunflower offer comparable protein yields, legumes can achieve up to 1.2 t/ha. Breeding strategies aimed at increasing oat grain yield, analogous to those implemented in wheat, could substantially enhance oat productivity and protein output.

References

1 X. Z. Hu, Y. M. Wei, and C. Z. Ren, 'Oat Quality and Processing', Beijing: Science Press, 2009. [In Chinese].

2 Chinese Nutrition Society, 'Scientific Research Report on the Dietary Guidelines for Chinese Residents 2021', 2022. [In Chinese].

3 Chinese Nutrition Society, 'Dietary Guidelines for Chinese Residents', 2022. [In Chinese].

4 Institute of Food and Nutrition Development, Ministry of Agriculture and Rural Affairs, 'China Food and Nutrition Development Report 2022', 2022. [In Chinese].

5 R. N. Sudarshan, P. D. W. Janitha, and S. Laurie. 'Sustainable Protein Sources,' Academic Press, 2017.

6 M. Annamalai, L. T. Lim, and A. Amanat, 'Plant Protein Foods', Springer, 2022.

7 H. W. Francis and J. W. Peter, 'Oats Chemistry and Technology', AACC International Inc., 2011.

8 Y. F. Chu, 'Oats Nutrition and Technology', John Wiley & Sons, Ltd, 2017.

9 White Book of China Oat Milk Industry, 2021. https://www.doc88.com/p-67816055511478.html [In Chinese].
10 White Book of China Oat Milk Industry, 2023. https://ifnd.caas.cn/xwzx/kyjz/b25a427ad1004d85a472cd8bbba940bd.htm [In Chinese].
11 C. Z. Ren and Y. G. Hu, 'China Oat', China Agriculture Press, 2013. [In Chinese].
12 Y. Y. Peng et al., 'Reference genome assemblies reveal the origin and evolution of allohexaploid oat', *Nat. Genet.*, vol. 54, pp. 1248–1258, 2022.
13 X. Z. Hu and C. Z. Ren, 'Oat Processing and Function', Beijing: Science Press, 2016. [In Chinese].
14 G.A. Batalova and C. Z. Ren, 'Use of Oats in the Food, Medicine and Cosmetic', Shaanxi Press, 2011.
15 F. Y. Yang, 'Research Progress on Forage Production, Processing and Utilization in China', Springer, 2022.
16 X. Wang, H. Liu, Y. Wang, Y. Lin, K. Ni, and F. Yang, 'Effects of lactic acid bacteria and cellulase additives on the fermentation quality, antioxidant activity, and metabolic profile of oat silage', *Bioresour. Bioprocess.*, vol. 11, no. 1, p. 92, 2024.
17 X. M. Li et al., 'Impacts of low temperature and ensiling period on the bacterial community of oat silage by SMRT', *Microorganisms*, vol. 9, p. 274, 2021.
18 L. Y. Feng, 'Comprehensive Evaluation of Nutritional Value of Paper Mulberry, Alfalfa and Oats,' Shaanxi: Northwest A&F University, 2021. [In Chinese].
19 M. M. Chen, 'Analysis of Genetic and Nutrition Value of Oat Germplasm Resources', Jilin: Northwest Normal University, 2024. [In Chinese].
20 N. N. Liu et al., 'Application of the Cornell Net Carbohydrate and Protein System to evaluate the quality of early and late maturing oats', *Pratacult. Sci.*, vol. 37, no. 10, pp. 2049–2056, 2020. [In Chinese].
21 C. Z. Guo et al., 'Effects of oat bran addition on the growth Performance and intestinal health of Nile tilapia (*Oreochromis niloticus*) exposed to copper ions', *Aquac. Nutr.*, vol. 2023, p. 5329546, 2023.
22 A. Rebole, J. Trevino, C. Barro, C. Alzueta, and R. Caballero, 'Chemical changes associated with the field drying of oat forage', *Field Crop. Res.*, vol. 47, no. 2, pp. 221–226, 1996.
23 J. C. Trevino, C. Centeno, L. T. Ortiz, and R. Caballero, 'Changes in the non-structural carbohydrates associated with the field drying of oat forage', *J. Sci. Food Agric.*, vol. 67, no. 3, pp. 393–397, 1995.
24 M. T. Harper, J. Oh, F. Giallongo, J. C. Lopes, G. Roth, and A. N. Hristovet, 'Effects of feeding sorghum and oat silages on feed intake, milk production and composition, and enteric methane production in lactating dairy cows', *J. Anim. Sci.*, vol. 94, no. 5, p. 689, 2016.
25 M. H. Li et al., 'Effects of oat hay feeding during the dry period on postpartum production performance in dairy cows', *China Dairy Cattle*, vol. 7, pp. 11–14, 2016. [In Chinese].
26 X. Z. Hu and C. Z. Ren, 'China Oat Industry Report (2016–2020)', Shaanxi Press, 2021. [In Chinese].
27 X. Wang, Y. Lei, H. Rafique, L. Zou, and X. Z. Hu, 'Effect of stir-frying on physicochemical and functional properties of oat protein isolates', *Foods*, vol. 12, no. 14, p. 2670, 2023.
28 T. He, J. Wang, and X. Hu. 'Effect of heat treatment on the structure and digestion properties of oat globulin', *Cereal Chem.*, vol. 98, no. 3, pp. 740–748, 2021.

29 H. Rafique et al., 'Dietary-nutraceutical properties of oat protein and peptides', *Front. Nutr.*, vol. 9, p. 950400, 2022.

30 I. Comino et al., 'Diversity in oat potential immunogenicity: basis for the selection of oat varieties with no toxicity in coeliac disease', *Gut*, vol. 64, no. 6, pp. 930–938, 2011.

31 H. Arentz-Hansen et al., 'The molecular basis for oat intolerance in patients with celiac disease', *PLoS Med.*, vol. 1, no. 1, p. e17, 2004.

32 EFSA Panel on Dietetic Products, Nutrition and Allergies (NDA), 'Scientific opinion on the safety of oats for individuals with coeliac disease', *EFSA J.*, vol. 12, no. 4, p. 3691, 2014.

33 C. Bindslev-Jensen et al., 'Standardization of food challenges in patients with immediate reactions to foods-position paper from the EAACI', *Allergy*, vol. 61, no. 5, pp. 690–697, 2006.

34 E. Gómez Torrijos, L. Moreno Lozano, and R. Garcia Rodriguez, 'Occupational allergic respiratory disease and eosinophilic esophagitis by wheat flour in a baker', *Arch. Bronconeumol.*, vol. 55, no. 10, pp. 541–542, 2019.

35 W. Srisuwatchari, S. Piboonpocanun, U. Wangthan, O. Jirapongsananuruk, N. Visitsunthorn, and P. Pacharn, 'Clinical and in vitro cross-reactivity of cereal grains in children with IgE-mediated wheat allergy', *Allergol. Immunopathol.*, vol. 48, no. 6, pp. 589–596, 2020.

36 M. Y. Hardy et al., 'Ingestion of oats and barley in patients with celiac disease mobilizes cross-reactive T cells activated by avenin peptides and immuno-dominant hordein peptides', *J. Autoimmun.*, vol. 56, pp. 56–65, 2015.

37 J. Gil-Humanes et al., 'Molecular and immunological characterization of gluten proteins isolated from oat cultivars that differ in toxicity for celiac disease', *PLoS One*, vol. 7, no. 12, p. e52649, 2012.

38 X. Huang, H. Ahola, M. Daly, C. Nitride, E.C. Mills, and T. Sontag-Strohm, 'Quantification of barley contaminants in gluten-free oats by four gluten ELISA kits', *J. Agric. Food Chem.*, vol. 70, no. 7, pp. 2366–2373, 2022.

39 Y. T. Xiang, X. L. Wang, X. Z. Hu, C. Z. Ren, L. C. Guo, and L. Li, 'Study on lipase activity differences among oat varieties and predictive modeling for high-quality varieties with low lipase activity', *Sci. Agric. Sin.*, vol. 55, no. 21, pp. 4104–4117, 2022. [In Chinese].

40 Y. T. Xiang, L. Zou, R. Dong, X. Wang, and X. Hu, 'Enzymatic characteristics and potential natural inhibitors of oat lipase', *J. Cereal Sci.*, vol. 114, p. 103794, 2023.

2

Significance of Oat Protein over Cereal and Legumes

2.1 Introduction

Oats are among the most nutritious cereal grains and rank as fifth most widely consumed crop globally, with an annual production of approximately 23 million tons. Oat grains are typically categorized into two types: naked oats (*Avena nuda L.*) and hulled oats (*Avena sativa L.*). The cultivation of oats occurs globally, with leading producers including the United States, Canada, Russia and European union. China is also among the significant contributors to global production. Oats are notable for their relatively higher protein content and significant level of lipids, as well as various bioactive compounds including beta-glucan, phenolic compounds, avenanthramides and flavonoids.

2.2 Distribution of Protein and Other Components in Hulled and Naked Oats

Food experts and nutritionist have highlighted the significance of oats owing to their diverse nutritional profile. Starch as the main caloric nutrient, comprising up to 66% (Table 2.1), while protein make up to 24% [1]. Globulins are the main storage proteins in oats, comprising 70–80% of the overall protein content. Prolamines (avenins) constitute 10–15%, whereas albumins, mainly consisting of enzymes, represent 9–20% of total proteins [2]. The lipid content of oats exceeds 10%, with approximately 40% comprising triglycerides, predominantly consisting of two unsaturated fatty acids (linoleic and oleic acids) and one saturated fatty acid (palmitic acid) [3]. Research has focused on non-caloric nutrients, especially soluble fibre components such as β-glucan and phenolic compounds like avenanthramides (AVNs) [3]. Oat β-glucan is a polysaccharide made up of D-glucose monomers connected (1–3) and (1–4) β-glycosidase bonds. The concentration is mainly found in the endosperm cell wall, ranging from 2 to 7%, primarily influenced by genotype [4]. Oat β-glucan has been extensively researched for its significant physiological effects in humans. It decreases plasma levels of total and low-density lipoproteins (LDL) cholesterol, and increases high-density lipoproteins (HDL)

Table 2.1 Comparison of chemical composition of naked and hulled oats.

Chemical composition (%)	Naked oats	Hulled oats
Carbohydrates	72.07 ± 1.55	67.84 ± 1.23
Crude protein	14.34 ± 1.67	11.5 ± 1.32
Lipids	8.36 ± 0.77	4.79 ± 0.6
Crude fibre	3.23 ± 0.60	13.5 ± 1.68
Crude ash	2.0 ± 0.21	2.28 ± 0.20

Source: Ref. [6] with permission of Elsevier.

Table 2.2 Content of polyphenols, avenanthramides and β-glucan in naked and hulled oats (dry matter).

Components	Naked oats	Hulled oats
Polyphenols (g_{CAE} /kg DM)		
Free—Polyphenols	0.94 ± 0.19	0.81 ± 0.09
Bound—Polyphenols	1.14 ± 0.21	1.13 ± 0.22
Total—Polyphenols	2.09 ± 0.36	1.93 ± 0.27
AVNs (mg $_{FAE}$ /kg DM)		
2c—AVNs	94 ± 78	28 ± 38
2p—AVNs	72 ± 57	24 ± 23
2f—AVNs	83 ± 66	33 ± 31
Total—AVNs	294 ± 194	85 ± 89
***β*-glucan** (g/100 g DM)	3.44 ± 0.38	3.29 ± 0.63

Source: Ref. [3] with permission of Elsevier.

cholesterol, improves postprandial satiety, reduces hunger, modulates postprandial glycaemic and insulin responses, elevates blood immunoglobulin levels and prevents cancer [5].

The main phenolic compounds in oats include ferulic acid, p-coumaric acid, caffeic acid, vanillic acid, hydroxybenzoic acids and their derivatives [7]. Phenols exist in both free and bound forms (Table 2.2). Among the free polyphenols, AVNs play a crucial role owing to their physiological importance. First identified in oats by Collins (1889), they predominantly occur in the bran fraction [8]. AVNs represent a category of alkaloids characterized by an anthranilic acid derivative linked to a hydroxycinnamic acid derivative, which are found exclusively in oats. Various AVNs varieties have been identified, with 2p, 2c and 2f being the most prominent. The numeral 2 represents 5-hydroxy-anthranilic acid, while the letters p, c and refer to p-coumaric, caffeic and ferulic acid moieties, respectively [9]. Oat AVNs exhibit antioxidant activity that is 10_3- times greater than that of other phenolic compounds, such as vanillin ferulic acid, caffeic acid and p-coumaric acid, with from 2c showing the highest in vitro antioxidant capacity compared to forms 2p and 2f [10]. In humans, their bioavailability is higher than that observed in rats [11]. At the physiological level, both in vivo, AVNs exhibit anti-inflammatory, vasodilatory, cytoprotective and anti-pruritic properties. In vitro studies revealed the anti-proliferative effects of AVNs on various colon cancer cell lines [12].

Compared to hulled oats and other cereal, naked oats grain contains a high content of protein and lipids, and a lower fibre content. Mainly, the defining attribute of protein is its comparatively higher amino acid composition, which has significant nutritional value. Similarly, higher lipid content serves as an excellent source of important unsaturated fatty acids. It has been previously demonstrated that naked oat cultivars had a superior nutritive protein value compared to other cereal, however, lysine remains the limiting amino acid [6]. A comprehensive overview of naked and hulled oats nutrition value is provided in Table 2.3, the information of this table is collected from a previous reference [6].

Table 2.3 Comparison of amino acids composition of naked and hulled oats.

Amino acids	Naked oats	Hulled oats
Essential Amino acids		
Lysine	2.76	2.73
Methionine + Cystine	3.66	4.08
Cystine	2.40	2.74
Threonine	2.59	2.46
Isoleucine	2.49	2.32
Tryptophan	1.18	1.15
Valine	3.31	3.20
Leucine	5.25	5.26
Histidine	1.76	1.74
Phenylalanine	5.92	5.88
Tyrosine	2.35	2.26
Non-essential Amino acids		
Arginine	5.32	5.79
Aspartic Acid	7.02	7.37
Serine	3.38	3.86
Glutamic Acid	18.24	19.12
Proline	4.01	4.54
Glycine	3.93	3.81
Alanine	3.72	3.59

Source: Ref. [6] with permission of Elsevier

2.3 Comparison of Protein and Other Components with Common Cereals

Compared to other cereals such as wheat, barley, rice, millet, sorghum and corn, oats hold particular significance due to their superior protein content (Table 2.4). A number of methods have been established to assess the quality of dietary protein over time. The protein efficiency ratio (PER), protein digestibility corrected amino acids score (PDCAAS), and digestible indispensable amino acid score (DIAAS) have been established to assess protein quality. These techniques evaluate whether a food qualifies as a 'source of protein' excellent or exceptional in America [13]. The protein rating method in Canada utilizes the PER to assess protein content claims by monitoring rat weight gain over a specific period after protein consumption [14]. PDCAAS, a prevalent method for evaluating dietary protein quality, employs digestibility obtained from rat bioassays and the limiting amino acid score. The expert committee on protein evaluation in human nutrition recommended DIASS as a substitute for PDCAAS after critiques of its implementation. DIAAS, the most recent protein quality evaluation instrument, is not used to validate protein content assertions in any jurisdiction [15]. In vitro methods for PDCCAAS and DIAAS assessments are being explored as rapid, economical alternatives to animal testing that adhere to protein dietary guidelines. Identifying protein-dense sources and innovating processing, techniques to enhance the nutritional quality of cereals are challenges in plant protein research [16].

Oat protein has reported a PDCAAS ranging from 0.41 to 0.60, with lysine identified as the limiting amino acid (Table 2.5). This value is even higher than the PDCAAS of wheat protein (0.37–0.54) and almond protein (0.32–0.34) [17, 18], but lower than that of pea proteins (0.73–0.89) and soy protein (0.9–0.93), respectively [17, 19]. In contrast

Table 2.4 Comparison of protein contents among cereals.

Cereals	Protein (%)	Fractions	References
Oat	15–20	Globulins, albumins, prolamins, glutenins	[20, 21]
Wheat	11–15	Glutenins, gliadins, globulins, albumins	[22, 23]
Barley	10–16	Globulins, prolamins, glutelin, albumins	[20]
Rice	7–10	Glutelin, globulins, prolamins	[24]
Millet	7–13	Glutelins, prolamins, globulins, albumins	[25]
Sorghum	6–18	Prolamins, glutelin, globulins	[26]
Maize	7–12	Prolamins, albumins, globulins, glutelin	[22, 27, 28]
Rye	6.5–14.5	Albumin, globulins, prolamins, glutelins	[29, 30]
Quinoa	14–20	Globulins, albumins, chenoprotein	[22, 31]
Buckwheat	9–15	Albumins, globulins, prolamins, glutelins	[22, 32]
Amaranth	15-16	Albumins, globulins, prolamins, glutelin-like	[22, 33]
Pea	20–25	Globulins, albumins, prolamins, glutelin	[34, 35]
Soybean	40	Globulins, albumins, glutelin, prolamins	[36, 37]
Mung bean	20–31	Globulins, albumins, glutelin, prolamins	[38]

Table 2.5 Protein quality comparison of oat and other cereal and legumes.

Protein	Limiting amino acid (s)	Digestibility (%)	PDCAAS	References
Oat	Met	90.3–94.2	0.41–0.64	[21]
Wheat	Lys, Thr, SAA	72.7–85.3	0.525	[19, 39]
Barley	Lys	76–83	0.46–0.50	[37]
Rye	Lys	75–82	0.54–0.63	[16]
Rice	Lys	73–79	0.4–0.5	[40, 41]
Maze	Lys, Trp	67.36–87.5	0.43–0.53	[42]
Buckwheat	Lys	90	0.54	[43, 44]
Sorghum	Lys	88–92	0.47–55	[16]
Millet	Lys	81–90	0.42–60	[16]
Amaranth	Trp	76–82	0.64	[43, 45, 45]
Quinoa	Met, Ile	76.3–80.5	0.68	[43, 47]
Pea	SAA, Trp	83–90	0.66–0.91	[37]
Soybean	SAA	95–98	0.92–1.0	[37]
Chickpea	Arg, Asp	63–79	0.78–0.84	[48, 49]
Mung bean	Met, Cys, Trp	64.14–77	0.7–0.78	[38, 50]

to oat proteins, pulse proteins, such as lentils and pea proteins, are rich in lysine but limited in sulphur-containing amino acids, making them complimentary offer opportunities for developing plant-based protein blends with improved nutritional quality. Such combinations could enhance PDCAAS values, potentially approaching that of cow's milk (PDCAAS = 1), and serve as promising ingredients for plant-based alternatives.

The metabolic response of a protein is defined by its amino acid composition, digestibility and the absorption efficiency of resulting amino acids and peptides. The measures of digestibility indicate the degree to which protein is absorbed, thereby affecting dietary protein requirements. Several factors including protein structure, processing and antinutritional compounds affect protein digestibility [16]. However, modifying these parameters can improve the overall digestibility of proteins. Any of plant protein can lack essential amino acids (EAAs) and may possess antinutritional characteristics. For example, cereals contain reduced concentrations of lysin, whereas legumes are limiting in sulphur-containing amino acids particularly methionine and cysteine. The collective intake of these foods can improve the availability of limiting amino acids that meets amino acids requirements. Plant protein sources are improved by the inclusion of fibres, oligosaccharides and both polyunsaturated and monounsaturated fatty acids.

Protein quality is often evaluated according to its digestibility and EAA composition. The amino acid composition is crucial for evaluating the nutritional value of proteins, and many methods are available to analyze the extent to which protein fulfil human amino acid requirements. Diverse dietary proteins exhibit varying abilities to meet IAA and nitrogen needs, and the consumption of those rich in nutritional density and IAA is associated with improved overall diet quality and nutrient adequacy. The bioavailability and digestibility of amino acids is influenced by host characteristics, including age, physiological condition and health status, as well as by the dietary matrix, which encompasses lipids, carbohydrates and antinutritional factors. Plant-based proteins sources, such as grains and legumes, often have worse protein quality and amino acid scores (AASs) due to insufficient EAA content, which may be as low as 90%, and are commonly categorized as 'incomplete'. The scores are influenced by genetic, environmental variables and cognitive processes [16]. Optimizing the efficacy of plant protein sources to meet protein needs requires assessing the contribution of each source. Increased consumption of plant protein sources can enhance IAA intake, and different plant sources can synergistically complement each other (for example, combining legumes and cereals within a single day) to provide complementary amino acid profile. Varied dietary proteins are essential for meeting IAA requirements. The PDCAAS of a specific protein source is crucial for evaluating its quality, although it is of less importance when the diet comprises proteins from many sources. Flexitarian diets, including both plant and animal proteins, are beneficial. Integrated several protein sources with distinct amino acid profiles improves the quality of a protein-dense diet [16].

However, an increase in plant-based protein intake raises concerns about antinutritional factor such as enzyme inhibitors, phenolic chemicals and phytates. While these compounds may impede nutrient absorption, they might also provide health benefits, and food processing can reduce their concentrations, thereby influencing amino acid bioavailability. The availability of lysine may decrease due to Millard reactions during heat processing, hence impacting protein synthesis.

2.4 Comparison of Oat Protein with Common Pseudocereals

Wheat, rice and maize are each reported to have a worldwide output of 778, 787.3 and 1150 million metric tons, respectively. When compared to these grains, the worldwide output of buckwheat, quinoa and chia seeds was anywhere between 0.175 and 3.97 million metric tons, which is nearly 500–4500 times lower than the production of theses grains. Wheat, rice and maize are all farmed on a worldwide scale, but the cultivation of pseudo cereals is centred mostly in the region where they originated (e.g., Latin America). As an instance, it was estimated that the bulk of quinoa was produced in the countries of Peru (0.106 million metric tons), Bolivia (0.0388 million metric tons), and Ecuador (0.001482 million metric tons) [44]. The cultivation of amaranth, on the other hand was reported to take place in a number of nations, including Nepal, China, Mexico, Indonesia, Central America, India, Malaysia, South America and Southern and Eastern Africa [44]. On the other hand, The Food and Agriculture Organization did not record the production statistics of amaranth and as a result, none of those data were accessible for comparison. In spite of low production quantities, the compound annual growth rate (CAGR) for pseudo cereals anywhere in the world is nearly 1.5–2.1 times higher than the CAGR for cereal grains, which ranges from 3.01 to 7.15%. Pseudo cereals in comparison to cereal grains have a more diverse composition and greater number of health advantages, which means that they have a good commercial potential [44].

Pseudo cereal grains are edible seeds from dicotyledonous species, recognized from their resemblance and high starch content identical to true cereals, which are monocotyledons of the Poaceae family [51]. Pseudo cereals represent a promising category of crops for future, attributed to their significant genetic variability, which facilitate adaptation to a range of environments, from tropical to temperate climates [52, 53]. 'Sub-exploited foods' might be defined as foods that were supplanted by more effective foods in the world's diet throughout 20th century. Pseudo cereals and their components such as protein can be utilized for diverse innovative food applications including the production of products for individuals with gluten intolerance, the substitution of animal derived proteins and the development of novel food packaging materials and edible, biodegradable containers [54].

The protein concentration of pseudo cereals ranges from 10 to 20%. The nutritional content of pseudo cereals protein is much superior to that of cereals and some legumes. Amaranth has elevated level of lysine, arginine, tryptophan and sulphur containing amino acid. The lysine concentration in amaranth is double that of wheat and thrice that of maize. The nutritional value is much higher as compared to barely, maize and wheat [54]. Buckwheat exhibits high protein quality, with a biological value exceeding 90%, likely attributable to its elevated level of EAAs and sulphur containing amino acids [55]. The chemical composition of buckwheat is similar to that of cereals, characterized by low lysine content, while proline and glutamic acid constitute approximately 50% of the total amino. In addition, chia seeds have greater level of aspartic acid, arginine and glutamic acid then the majority of cereal grains. The protein in quinoa seeds is abundant in EAAs, particularly methionine, threonine and lysine that are often the limiting amino acids in various cereal grains [54].

The most important component of a protein is an EAA, which must be supplied from food as humans are unable to synthesize it. Thus, compared to the other amino, the EAAs are more important for development and upkeep of metabolic functions. Furthermore, a third category exists termed 'conditionally essential' amino acid. These amino acids cannot be synthesized by the body under physiological and pathological conditions, making their intake essential in such circumstances [56]. The amino acid scores of pseudocereals are nearly equivalent to the essential amino acid index (EAAI) values for amaranth, buckwheat and quinoa. Among pseudocereals, buckwheat and chia are notable for their high content of EAA. Chia seeds, in particular, contain a higher concentration of aromatic amino acids compared with other pseudocereals.

Digestibility is a critical factor in determining the nutritional value of protein. The PDCAAS is estimated to assess protein quality in human nutrition across various life stages [56]; EAA content can be estimated. The in vitro protein digestibility (IVPD) of pseudo cereals is generally high exceeding 70%, except for chia seeds that exhibit a lower IVPD value of approximately 50%. This review presents a comparative analysis of the characteristics of amaranth, buckwheat, quinoa, chia, wattle and album proteins grounded in current research findings. Additionally, it highlights various protein isolation techniques, amino acid composition and the evaluation of protein quality in all pseudocereals [54].

2.5 Comparison of Oat Protein with Legumes

Legume proteins play a critical function among plant proteins because of their balanced and full amino acid composition. Soy and pea proteins have PDCAAS of 1.0 and 0.89, respectively, similar to high quality proteins such as eggs and milk. Other legume proteins often have lower values, mostly ranging from 0.5 to 0.7. Furthermore, legume proteins demonstrate enhanced functionality, such as solubility, foaming capability and water and oil retention, providing a strong foundation for their widespread use in the food industry [57]. Besides their beneficial nutritional and functional properties, legume properties have potential for sustainability. Data suggests that each 100 g of legume protein produces around 90% less greenhouse gas emission than the same weight of cow protein. Substituting beef with legumes in the US diet might provide emissions reductions of 46–74%, freeing over 40% of agricultural land resources [57]. However, unpleasant beany flavour, and possible allergic reactions. These difficulties have considerably hindered the extensive use of bean proteins un the food industry.

Integrating chickpeas and oats as sources of plant-based proteins offers several advantages. Investigating several innovative plant protein sources might improve nutritional quality. Pulses, such as peas and chickpeas, provide comparable protein quality with cereal proteins like oats [58]. Pulses provide acceptable amounts of lysine and leucine; however, they are deficient in sulphur containing amino acids, namely methionine and cystine. Cereal proteins, despite their deficiency in sulphur containing amino acids, namely methionine and cysteine. Cereal proteins, despite their deficiency in lysine, have somewhat elevated concentrations of sulphur containing amino acids compared to pea and chickpea proteins [59]. The use of oats as a cereal protein source is particularly advantageous due to its high lysine content compared to other cereals.

Peas, chickpeas and oats have unique nutritional compositions and are excluded from the 'Big Nine' allergens. Furthermore, they are non-GMO crops that have several agronomic benefits [60–62]; United States Department of Agriculture: Food Safety & Inspection Service, 2024). Incorporating chickpea and oat proteins into plant protein sources improves economic stability and ecological resilience by alleviating food system stress and consumer demand across various protein.

Furthermore, oats and chickpeas are recognized and familiar to consumers. Oats have traditionally been a key ingredient in household, used in multiple products, such as oats milk, which has experienced significant growth in popularity in recent years [63, 64]. Chickpeas are among the most widely consumed legumes worldwide, with US consumption showing a steady increase in recent decades [65]. The utilization of chickpeas and oats as protein sources demonstrates significant advantages, as indicated by project market value of US$13.3 billion and US$75.8 million for the years 2032 and 2022, respectively [66]. Expanding the plant protein market to include chickpea and oat protein ingredients offer a promising strategy, though it is accompanied by specific challenges.

The current utilization of novel plant proteins in food is constrained by their inferior functional properties compared to soy protein, along with gaps in fundamental knowledge. The utilization of pea protein is on the rise; nonetheless functional challenges persist, including restricted solubility, gelation and emulsification characteristics [67]. Extensive research on pea proteins has enable the successful development of various pea proteins ingredient and products. In contrast, studies on chickpea protein are scarce, with most literature focusing on finding associated with proteins isolates produced via alkaline extraction and isoelectric precipitation (AE-IEP) methods the use of elevated alkalinity in chickpea protein extraction altered the protein's structural characteristics, subsequently resulting in reduced functional performance. The findings and limited research regarding the development and scalability of chick pea protein extraction have led to the commercial unavailability of chickpea proteins isolates (CPI).

Similar to limited research on chickpea protein, there is a lack of studies addressing the practicality and scalability of oat protein isolate (OPI) synthesis. As a result, OPI is not available for commercial use. Oat protein concentrate (OPC), obtained through dry fractionation, is available in the market [68]. OPC exhibits limited solubility and reduced foaming and emulsification properties compared to other plant proteins, which hinder its application in food products. The development of scalable method for producing a functional oat protein component is essential.

A recent study demonstrated the effective scaling of pea protein isolate (PPI) synthesis via AE-IEP, with protein solubilization and extraction performed under moderate alkaline condition (pH 7.5) [69]. The produced PPI preserved its protein structural integrity and demonstrated improved functional properties compared to a commercially produced PPI [69]. The result indicates that similar AE-IEP conditions can be utilized to improve the production of ChPI and OPI. No studies have been identified regarding the scalability of ChPI or OPI extraction under moderate AE-IEP conditions. This knowledge is essential for the development of nutritionally and functionally diverse plant protein ingredients, aiding food manufactures in selecting protein components for various applications.

2.6 Challenges of Incorporating Legume and Pulses in Food Applications

2.6.1 Allergenicity

The development of legume protein products has been hindered by the well-established serious issue of allergenicity, particularly with regard to soy proteins. The first documented human allergic response to soy occurred in 1934 [70]. Subsequently, soy was identified as none of the top eight allergens, which collectively account for 90% of all allergic reactions. Additionally, soy has been found in at least 16 allergens [71]. Nearly all allergic reactions to soy are attributed to protein mediated factors, primarily β-conglycinin and glycinin. Soy allergy typically induces mild symptoms; however, it can also lead to severe reactions, such as small intestinal colitis, eczema or other IgE-mediated clinical manifestations and pathologies [72]. Studies indicates that soy protein has a significantly elevated concentration threshold for eliciting allergic reactions, approximately 100 times higher than other allergens, suggesting a relatively low incidence of such reactions. With other legume proteins are generally less allergic than soy proteins, they still contain allergens to varying extents. Prolamin and 7S globulin in lentil protein, 7S globulin and 11S globulin in chickpea, as well as prolamin and 7S globulin in mung bean, are identified as significant allergenic proteins [73]. Pea protein is widely regarded as a hypoallergenic food source, resulting in its extensive marketing under the 'hypoallergenic' label. Pea protein allergies are well documented in the literature. Vicilin, convicilin and non-specific lipid transfer protein (nsLTP) are identified as significant allergens. The allergenicity of legume proteins is prevalent and represents a significant safety concern that necessitates ongoing research.

2.6.2 Digestibility

In addition to the nutrient composition of proteins, protein digestibility serves as a critical factor in assessing their adequacy for human nutritional needs. In the context of plant-based food product serving as substitute for animal proteins, comparing their digestibility to that of animal proteins is particularly significant. The digestibility of legume proteins is generally lower than that of animal proteins, a difference attributed to structural variations and the presence of antinutrients in legumes, including phytic acid, trypsin inhibitors and lectins [74]. Alongside the comparison of the proteins, it is crucial to also compared the plant-based foods in which they are processed. Researcher conducted a comparison of plant-based beef and traditional beef using an in vitro simulated stomach and intestine. The study revealed that plant-based beef exhibits a higher digestion rate in the stomach, whereas its digestion in the intestine occurred at a slower rate compared to beef. This discrepancy may arise from the differencing structures of the two, with plant-based beef consisting of globular proteins and traditional beef comprising fibrous proteins. Plant-based meat releases a greater quantity of bioactive peptides during digestion. In comparison to animal proteins, soy proteins exhibit greater advantages relative to other plant proteins. Soy protein (95%) exhibits greater digestibility than wheat protein (91%) [75]. Furthermore, variations in legume protein types may result in differencing digestibility levels, with the digestibility ranking of common legume protein being soy, lentil, chickpea and common beans [76]. The high digestibility of soy protein is attributed to minimal β -sheet structure, which negatively correlates with the digestibility of legume proteins [77]. Overall, while legume proteins exhibit superior digestibility relative to other plant proteins, notable differences remain when compared to animal proteins, both in terms of protein structure and the resultants product.

2.6.3 Beany Flavour

The development of legume proteins and relative derivatives has been hindered by the common issues of beany flavour. The characteristic beany flavour of legume proteins arises from derivatives of polyunsaturated fatty acid, which are catalyzed by lipoxygenase to yield hydroperoxide derivatives. These compounds are subsequently degraded into volatile substances such as alcohols, aldehydes, ketones, acids and amines [78]. These volatile compounds encompass fatty alcohols, fatty aldehydes, fatty ketones, furans and their derivatives, as well as over 20 aromatic compounds [79]. Volatiles typically exhibit very low threshold, often within the range of parts per million (ppm) or parts per billion (ppb). For instance, (Z)-3 Hexenal, a significant contributor to the beany flavour in soy, has a threshold of 0,00012 ppb. The beany flavour of legume proteins poses a significant challenge to their application in the food industry, particularly within plant-based products. Legume proteins, primarily derived from soy and pea, are the predominant proteins in plant-based meat product. However, they often impart an undesirable beany flavour that negatively impacts consumer acceptance of these products. Likewise, a significant issue with plant-based dairy products derived from legume proteins is the present of beany flavour, exemplified by soy milk, here the primary source of off-flavour is the endogenous enzyme lipoxygenase [80].

2.6.4 Texture

The texture of plant-based foods serves as a critical indicator of consumer acceptance, particularly for plant-based meat products, which are anticipated to have a texture comparable to that of meat. Nevertheless, the texture and mouthfeel of existing plant-based meat products remain inferior to that of traditional meat. The texture of plant-based meat is typically characterized by fibre degree, tensile strength, hardness, elasticity, juiciness and tenderness [81]. the fibre degree is regarded as the most significant metric, typically represented by the ratio of vertical to parallel shear directions measured by the texture analyzer in conjunction with microscopic observation. In comparison to the plant-based meat, animal meat exhibits a more aligned fibre orientation, a denser and more compact structure, as well as a layered architecture [82]. The fibre structure of real meat contributes to its high-water holding capacity, leading to notable juiciness and tenderness [83]. In addition to machine assessment, sensory evaluation offers a direct measure of consumer acceptability. The texture of plant-based meat is evaluated through human oral processing and perception. The initial perception of hardness occurs in the mouth, and as the physical state of plant-based meat alters, the release of water or oil contributed to its overall juiciness and tenderness [84]. A previous study conducted sensory evaluations of plant-based meat and beef using 20 trained personnel. Their findings indicated that although plant-based meat exhibited greater hardness, its overall acceptability was comparable to that of beef, with similar characteristics in elasticity and chewiness. Furthermore, plant based dairy products are frequently contrasted with animal dairy. The distribution of dispersed-phase protein, lipids, starch and other particles in continuous phase water may result in undesirable textures, including chalkiness and grittiness in plant-based dairy products [85]. Additionally, plant-based yogurts have been characterized by a thin watery mouthfeel. Likewise, the texture of plant-based fats derived from legume proteins, encompassing lubricity and friction characteristics, may vary from that of animal fats [86]. The absence of pertinent studies has led to an evaluation of plant-based fats that lacks systematic and thorough analysis.

Summary

Oat protein stands out over other cereal and many legume proteins because it has a more balanced amino acid profile, especially higher lysine, better digestibility and a globulin-rich structure that provides superior solubility and functional properties. It is naturally gluten-free, has a mild flavour, and produces bioactive peptides with antioxidant, antihypertensive and neuroprotective effects. These nutritional and functional advantages make oat protein highly suitable for modern plant-based, health-focused and functional food applications.

References

1 R. Singh, S. De, and A. Belkheir, '*Avena sativa* (oat), a potential neutraceutical and therapeutic agent: an overview', *Crit. Rev. Food Sci. Nutr.*, vol. 53, no. 2, pp. 126–144, 2013, https://doi.org/10.1080/10408398.2010.526725.

2 C. Klose and E. K. Arendt, 'Proteins in oats; their synthesis and changes during germination: a review', *Crit. Rev. Food Sci. Nutr.*, vol. 52, no. 7, pp. 629–639, 2012, https://doi.org/10.1080/10408398.2010.504902.

3 E. Antonini, F. Lombardi, M. Alfieri, G. Diamantini, R. Redaelli, and P. Ninfali, 'Nutritional characterization of naked and dehulled oat cultivar samples at harvest and after storage', *J. Cereal Sci.*, vol. 72, pp. 46–53, 2016, https://doi.org/10.1016/j.jcs.2016.09.016.
4 R. Redaelli et al., 'Genetic and environmental variability in total and soluble β-glucan in European oat genotypes', *J. Cereal Sci.*, vol. 57, no. 2, pp. 193–199, 2013, https://doi.org/10.1016/j.jcs.2012.09.003.
5 C. Daou and H. Zhang, 'Oat beta-glucan: its role in health promotion and prevention of diseases', *Compr. Rev. Food Sci. Food Saf.*, vol. 11, no. 4, pp. 355–365, 2012, https://doi.org/10.1111/j.1541-4337.2012.00189.x.
6 W. Biel, K. Bobko, and R. Maciorowski, 'Chemical composition and nutritive value of husked and naked oats grain', *J. Cereal Sci.*, vol. 49, no. 3, pp. 413–418, 2009, https://doi.org/10.1016/j.jcs.2009.01.009.
7 V. Verardo, C. Serea, R. Segal, and M. F. Caboni, 'Free and bound minor polar compounds in oats: different extraction methods and analytical determinations', *J. Cereal Sci.*, vol. 54, no. 2, pp. 211–217, 2011, https://doi.org/10.1016/j.jcs.2011.05.005.
8 C. L. Emmons, D. M. Peterson, and G. L. Paul, 'Antioxidant capacity of oat (*Avena sativa* L.) extracts. 2. In vitro antioxidant activity and contents of phenolic and tocol antioxidants', *J. Agric. Food Chem.*, vol. 47, no. 12, pp. 4894–4898, 1999, https://doi.org/10.1021/jf990530i.
9 K. Bratt et al., 'Avenanthramides in oats (*Avena sativa* L.) and structure–antioxidant activity relationships', *J. Agric. Food Chem.*, vol. 51, no. 3, pp. 594–600, 2003, https://doi.org/10.1021/jf020544f.
10 D. M. Peterson, M. J. Hahn, and C. L. Emmons, 'Oat avenanthramides exhibit antioxidant activities in vitro', *Food Chem.*, vol. 79, no. 4, pp. 473–478, 2002, https://doi.org/10.1016/S0308-8146(02)00219-4.
11 R. T. Koenig, J. R. Dickman, M. L. Wise, and L. L. Ji, 'Avenanthramides are bioavailable and accumulate in hepatic, cardiac, and skeletal muscle tissue following oral gavage in rats', *J. Agric. Food Chem.*, vol. 59, no. 12, pp. 6438–6443, 2011, https://doi.org/10.1021/jf2002427.
12 M. Meydani, 'Potential health benefits of avenanthramides of oats', *Nutr. Rev.*, vol. 67, no. 12, pp. 731–735, 2009, https://doi.org/10.1111/j.1753-4887.2009.00256.x.
13 C. P. F. Marinangeli and J. D. House, 'Potential impact of the digestible indispensable amino acid score as a measure of protein quality on dietary regulations and health', *Nutr. Rev.*, vol. 75, no. 8, pp. 658–667, 2017, https://doi.org/10.1093/nutrit/nux025.
14 Canadian Food Inspection Agency, 'Reasonable Daily Intake for Various Foods (Schedule K)', 2021.
15 FAO/WHO, 'Dietary Protein Quality Evaluation in Human Nutrition: Report of an FAO Expert Consultation', 2013.
16 A. G. A. Sá and J. D. House, 'Protein quality of cereals: digestibility determination and processing impacts', *J. Cereal Sci.*, vol. 117, p. 103892, 2024, https://doi.org/10.1016/j.jcs.2024.103892.
17 K. F. Michaelsen et al., 'Choice of foods and ingredients for moderately malnourished children 6 months to 5 years of age', *Food Nutr. Bull.*, vol. 30, no. 3_suppl3, pp. S343–S404, 2009, https://doi.org/10.1177/15648265090303S303.

18 S. Ahrens, M. Venkatachalam, A. M. Mistry, K. Lapsley, and S. K. Sathe, 'Almond (*Prunus dulcis* L.) protein quality', *Plant Foods Hum. Nutr.*, vol. 60, no. 3, pp. 123–128, 2005, https://doi.org/10.1007/s11130-005-6840-2.

19 S. M. Rutherfurd, A. C. Fanning, B. J. Miller, and P. J. Moughan, 'Protein digestibility-corrected amino acid scores and digestible indispensable amino acid scores differentially describe protein quality in growing male rats', *J. Nutr.*, vol. 145, no. 2, pp. 372–379, 2015, https://doi.org/10.3945/jn.114.195438.

20 J. McLauchlan, A. I. I. Tyler, B. Chakrabarti, C. Orfila, and A. Sarkar, 'Oat protein: review of structure-function synergies with other plant proteins', *Food Hydrocoll.*, vol. 154, p. 110139, 2024, https://doi.org/10.1016/j.foodhyd.2024.110139.

21 L. Kumar, R. Sehrawat, and Y. Kong, 'Oat proteins: a perspective on functional properties', *LWT*, vol. 152, p. 112307, 2021, https://doi.org/10.1016/j.lwt.2021.112307.

22 F. Boukid, S. Folloni, S. Sforza, E. Vittadini, and B. Prandi, 'Current trends in ancient grains-based foodstuffs: insights into nutritional aspects and technological applications', *Compr. Rev. Food Sci. Food Saf.*, vol. 17, no. 1, pp. 123–136, 2018, https://doi.org/10.1111/1541-4337.12315.

23 S. Gammoh et al., 'Functional and bioactive properties of wheat protein fractions: impact of digestive enzymes on antioxidant, α-amylase, and angiotensin-converting enzyme inhibition potential', *Molecules*, vol. 28, no. 16, p. 6012, 2023, https://doi.org/10.3390/molecules28166012.

24 A. N. Beloshapka, P. R. Buff, G. C. Fahey, and K. S. Swanson, 'Compositional analysis of whole grains, processed grains, grain co-products, and other carbohydrate sources with applicability to pet animal nutrition', *Foods*, vol. 5, no. 2, p. 23, 2016, https://doi.org/10.3390/foods5020023.

25 N. Sachdev, S. Goomer, L. R. Singh, V. M. Pathak, D. Aggarwal, and R. K. Chowhan, 'Current status of millet seed proteins and its applications: a comprehensive review', *Appl. Food Res.*, vol. 3, no. 1, p. 100288, 2023, https://doi.org/10.1016/j.afres.2023.100288.

26 R. Xiao et al., 'Enzymatic production and physicochemical and functional properties of sorghum protein isolates', *Int. J. Biol. Macromol.*, vol. 283, p. 137421, 2024, https://doi.org/10.1016/j.ijbiomac.2024.137421.

27 D. Ignjatovic-Micic, J. Vancetovic, D. Trbovic, Z. Dumanovic, M. Kostadinovic, and S. Bozinovic, 'Grain nutrient composition of maize (*Zea mays* L.) drought-tolerant populations', *J. Agric. Food Chem.*, vol. 63, no. 4, pp. 1251–1260, 2015, https://doi.org/10.1021/jf504301u.

28 M. Ortiz-Martinez, J. T. Otero-Pappatheodorou, S. O. Serna-Saldívar, and S. García-Lara, 'Antioxidant activity and characterization of protein fractions and hydrolysates from normal and quality protein maize kernels', *J. Cereal Sci.*, vol. 76, pp. 85–91, 2017, https://doi.org/10.1016/j.jcs.2017.05.021.

29 E. K. Arendt and E. Zannini, 'Rye', In: Cereal Grains for the Food and Beverage Industries, Elsevier, pp. 220–243e, 2013, https://doi.org/10.1533/9780857098924.220.

30 E. Schall, V. É. Budai, B. Czipó, E. Jaksics, A. Farkas, and S. Tömösközi, 'Protein composition of rye varieties and a commercial mixture from an industrial mill', *J. Cereal Sci.*, vol. 122, p. 104110, 2025, https://doi.org/10.1016/j.jcs.2025.104110.

31 S. Wang, S. Miao, and D.-W. Sun, 'Modifying structural and techno-functional properties of quinoa proteins through extraction techniques and modification methods', *Trends Food Sci. Technol.*, vol. 143, p. 104285, 2024, https://doi.org/10.1016/j.tifs.2023.104285.

32 F. Zhu, 'Buckwheat proteins and peptides: biological functions and food applications', *Trends Food Sci. Technol.*, vol. 110, pp. 155–167, 2021, https://doi.org/10.1016/j.tifs.2021.01.081.

33 M. Malik et al., 'Nutritional composition, functionality, and processing technologies for amaranth', *J. Food Process. Preserv.*, vol. 2023, pp. 1–24, 2023, https://doi.org/10.1155/2023/1753029.

34 R. Kornet, J. Yang, P. Venema, E. van der Linden, and L. M. C. Sagis, 'Optimizing pea protein fractionation to yield protein fractions with a high foaming and emulsifying capacity', *Food Hydrocoll.*, vol. 126, p. 107456, 2022, https://doi.org/10.1016/j.foodhyd.2021.107456.

35 Y. Shen, S. Hong, and Y. Li, 'Pea protein composition, functionality, modification, and food applications: a review', *Adv. Food Nutr. Res.*, vol. 101, pp. 71–127, 2022, https://doi.org/10.1016/bs.afnr.2022.02.002.

36 L. Zheng, J. M. Regenstein, L. Zhou, and Z. Wang, 'Soy protein isolates: a review of their composition, aggregation, and gelation', *Compr. Rev. Food Sci. Food Saf.*, vol. 21, no. 2, pp. 1940–1957, 2022, https://doi.org/10.1111/1541-4337.12925.

37 P. Qin, T. Wang, and Y. Luo, 'A review on plant-based proteins from soybean: health benefits and soy product development', *J. Agric. Food Res.*, vol. 7, p. 100265, 2022, https://doi.org/10.1016/j.jafr.2021.100265.

38 Z. Yi-Shen, S. Shuai, and R. FitzGerald, 'Mung bean proteins and peptides: nutritional, functional and bioactive properties', *Food Nutr. Res.*, vol. 62, 2018, https://doi.org/10.29219/fnr.v62.1290.

39 X. Jiang, J. Tian, Z. Hao, and W. Zhang, 'Protein content and amino acid composition in grains of wheat-related species', *Agric. Sci. China*, vol. 7, no. 3, pp. 272–279, 2008, https://doi.org/10.1016/S1671-2927(08)60066-8.

40 K. Liu, J. Zheng, and F. Chen, 'Effect of domestic cooking on rice protein digestibility', *Food Sci. Nutr.*, vol. 7, no. 2, pp. 608–616, 2019, https://doi.org/10.1002/fsn3.884.

41 S. M. Phillips, 'The impact of protein quality on the promotion of resistance exercise-induced changes in muscle mass', *Nutr. Metab. (Lond).*, vol. 13, no. 1, p. 64, 2016, https://doi.org/10.1186/s12986-016-0124-8.

42 M. Garrido-Balam, L. Chel-Guerrero, S. Gallegos-Tintoré, A. Castellanos-Ruelas, W. Rodriguez-Canto, and D. Betancur-Ancona, 'Nutritional characterization of quality protein maize (QPM) (*Zea mays* L.) protein concentrates', *Food and Humanity*, vol. 1, pp. 1250–1255, 2023, https://doi.org/10.1016/j.foohum.2023.09.022.

43 Y. Zeng, E. Chen, X. Zhang, D. Li, Q. Wang, and Y. Sun, 'Nutritional value and physicochemical characteristics of alternative protein for meat and dairy—a review', *Foods*, vol. 11, no. 21, p. 3326, 2022, https://doi.org/10.3390/foods11213326.

44 A. Nandan et al., 'Nutritional and functional perspectives of pseudocereals', *Food Chem.*, vol. 448, p. 139072, 2024, https://doi.org/10.1016/j.foodchem.2024.139072.

45 V. Rao and A. Poonia, 'Protein characteristics, amino acid profile, health benefits and methods of extraction and isolation of proteins from some pseudocereals—a review', *Food Prod. Process. Nutr.*, vol. 5, no. 1, p. 37, 2023, https://doi.org/10.1186/s43014-023-00154-z.

46 X. Zhang, J. Shi, Y. Fu, T. Zhang, L. Jiang, and X. Sui, 'Structural, nutritional, and functional properties of amaranth protein and its application in the food industry: a review', *Sustain. Food Proteins*, vol. 1, no. 1, pp. 45–55, 2023, https://doi.org/10.1002/sfp2.1002.

47 S. A. Elsohaimy, T. M. Refaay, and M. A. M. Zaytoun, 'Physicochemical and functional properties of quinoa protein isolate', *Ann. Agric. Sci.*, vol. 60, no. 2, pp. 297–305, 2015, https://doi.org/10.1016/j.aoas.2015.10.007.

48 N. Begum, Q. U. Khan, L. G. Liu, W. Li, D. Liu, and I. U. Haq, 'Nutritional composition, health benefits and bio-active compounds of chickpea (*Cicer arietinum* L.)', *Front. Nutr.*, vol. 10, 2023, https://doi.org/10.3389/fnut.2023.1218468.

49 M. G. Nosworthy et al., 'Thermal processing methods differentially affect the protein quality of chickpea (*Cicer arietinum*)', *Food Sci. Nutr.*, vol. 8, no. 6, pp. 2950–2958, 2020, https://doi.org/10.1002/fsn3.1597.

50 Q. Feng et al., 'Mung bean protein as an emerging source of plant protein: a review on production methods, functional properties, modifications and its potential applications', *J. Sci. Food Agric.*, vol. 104, no. 5, pp. 2561–2573, 2024, https://doi.org/10.1002/jsfa.13107.

51 L. Alvarez-Jubete, E. K. Arendt, and E. Gallagher, 'Nutritive value of pseudocereals and their increasing use as functional gluten-free ingredients', *Trends Food Sci. Technol.*, vol. 21, no. 2, pp. 106–113, 2010, https://doi.org/10.1016/j.tifs.2009.10.014.

52 D. C. Joshi et al., 'From zero to hero: the past, present and future of grain amaranth breeding', *Theor. Appl. Genet.*, vol. 131, no. 9, pp. 1807–1823, 2018, https://doi.org/10.1007/s00122-018-3138-y.

53 D. C. Joshi et al., 'Revisiting the versatile buckwheat: reinvigorating genetic gains through integrated breeding and genomics approach', *Planta*, vol. 250, no. 3, pp. 783–801, 2019, https://doi.org/10.1007/s00425-018-03080-4.

54 A. M. Malik and A. Singh, 'Pseudocereals proteins- a comprehensive review on its isolation, composition and quality evaluation techniques', *Food Chem. Adv.*, vol. 1, p. 100001, 2022, https://doi.org/10.1016/j.focha.2021.100001.

55 O. Sytar, M. Brestic, M. Zivcak, and L.-S. Phan Tran, 'The contribution of buckwheat genetic resources to health and dietary diversity', *Curr. Genomics*, vol. 17, no. 3, pp. 193–206, 2016, https://doi.org/10.2174/1389202917666160202215425.

56 WHO, 'Protein and Amino Acid Requirements in Human Nutrition', 2007.

57 X. Zhang et al., 'Legumes as an alternative protein source in plant-based foods: applications, challenges, and strategies', *Curr. Res. Food Sci.*, vol. 9, p. 100876, 2024, https://doi.org/10.1016/j.crfs.2024.100876.

58 J. Boye, F. Zare, and A. Pletch, 'Pulse proteins: processing, characterization, functional properties and applications in food and feed', *Food Res. Int.*, vol. 43, no. 2, pp. 414–431, 2010, https://doi.org/10.1016/j.foodres.2009.09.003.

59 I. Joye, 'Protein digestibility of cereal products', *Foods*, vol. 8, no. 6, p. 199, 2019, https://doi.org/10.3390/foods8060199.

60 H. Harwatt, J. Sabaté, G. Eshel, S. Soret, and W. Ripple, 'Substituting beans for beef as a contribution toward US climate change targets', *Clim. Change*, vol. 143, no. 1–2, pp. 261–270, 2017, https://doi.org/10.1007/s10584-017-1969-1.

61 R. Menon, T. Gonzalez, M. Ferruzzi, E. Jackson, D. Winderl, and J. Watson, 'Oats—from farm to fork', *Adv. Food Nutr. Res.*, pp. 1–55, 2016, https://doi.org/10.1016/bs.afnr.2015.12.001.

62 M. E. Nelson, M. W. Hamm, F. B. Hu, S. A. Abrams, and T. S. Griffin, 'Alignment of healthy dietary patterns and environmental sustainability: a systematic review', *Adv. Nutr.*, vol. 7, no. 6, pp. 1005–1025, 2016, https://doi.org/10.3945/an.116.012567.

63 Mordor Intelligence, 'Protein Ingredients Market Size, Growth & Industry Analysis', 2025.

64 J. L. M. Son, 'An Analysis of U.S. Dairy and Non-Dairy Milk Demand', 2023.

65 C. D. Rehm, S. R. Goltz, J. A. Katcher, L. L. Guarneiri, M. R. Dicklin, and K. C. Maki, 'Trends and patterns of chickpea consumption among United States adults: analyses of National Health and Nutrition Examination Survey data', *J. Nutr.*, vol. 153, no. 5, pp. 1567–1576, 2023, https://doi.org/10.1016/j.tjnut.2023.03.029.

66 Future Market Insights, 'Chickpea Protein Market', 2023.

67 F. Bu, G. Nayak, P. Bruggeman, G. Annor, and B. P. Ismail, 'Impact of plasma reactive species on the structure and functionality of pea protein isolate', *Food Chem.*, vol. 371, p. 131135, 2022, https://doi.org/10.1016/j.foodchem.2021.131135.

68 J. Spaen and J. V. C. Silva, 'Oat proteins: review of extraction methods and techno-functionality for liquid and semi-solid applications', *LWT*, vol. 147, p. 111478, 2021, https://doi.org/10.1016/j.lwt.2021.111478.

69 L. Hansen, F. Bu, and B. P. Ismail, 'Structure-function guided extraction and scale-up of pea protein isolate production', *Foods*, vol. 11, no. 23, p. 3773, 2022, https://doi.org/10.3390/foods11233773.

70 W. W. Duke, "Soy bean as a possible important source of allergy," *J Allergy (Cairo)*, vol. 5, no. 3, pp. 300–302, Mar. 1934, doi: 10.1016/S0021-8707(34)90228-8.

71 P. Meinlschmidt, D. Sussmann, U. Schweiggert-Weisz, and P. Eisner, 'Enzymatic treatment of soy protein isolates: effects on the potential allergenicity, technofunctionality, and sensory properties', *Food Sci. Nutr.*, vol. 4, no. 1, pp. 11–23, 2016, https://doi.org/10.1002/fsn3.253.

72 F.-G. Chizoba Ekezie, J.-H. Cheng, and D.-W. Sun, 'Effects of nonthermal food processing technologies on food allergens: a review of recent research advances', *Trends Food Sci. Technol.*, vol. 74, pp. 12–25, 2018, https://doi.org/10.1016/j.tifs.2018.01.007.

73 X. Zhang, T. Zhang, Y. Zhao, L. Jiang, and X. Sui, 'Structural, extraction and safety aspects of novel alternative proteins from different sources', *Food Chem.*, vol. 436, p. 137712, 2024, https://doi.org/10.1016/j.foodchem.2023.137712.

74 M. Z. Mulla, P. Subramanian, and B. N. Dar, 'Functionalization of legume proteins using high pressure processing: effect on technofunctional properties and digestibility of legume proteins', *LWT*, vol. 158, p. 113106, 2022, https://doi.org/10.1016/j.lwt.2022.113106.

75 G. Schaafsma, "The Protein Digestibility–Corrected Amino Acid Score," *J Nutr*, vol. 130, no. 7, pp. 1865S-1867S, Jul. 2000, doi: 10.1093/jn/130.7.1865S.

76 I. C. Ohanenye et al., 'Legume seed protein digestibility as influenced by traditional and emerging physical processing technologies', *Foods*, vol. 11, no. 15, p. 2299, 2022, https://doi.org/10.3390/foods11152299.

77 M. Carbonaro, P. Maselli, and A. Nucara, 'Structural aspects of legume proteins and nutraceutical properties', *Food Res. Int.*, vol. 76, pp. 19–30, 2015, https://doi.org/10.1016/j.foodres.2014.11.007.

78 B. Wang et al., 'Insights into formation, detection and removal of the beany flavor in soybean protein', *Trends Food Sci. Technol.*, vol. 112, pp. 336–347, 2021, https://doi.org/10.1016/j.tifs.2021.04.018.

79 W. S. U. Roland, L. Pouvreau, J. Curran, F. van de Velde, and P. M. T. de Kok, 'Flavor aspects of pulse ingredients', *Cereal Chem.*, vol. 94, no. 1, pp. 58–65, 2017, https://doi.org/10.1094/CCHEM-06-16-0161-FI.

80 C. M. Duarte et al., 'Use of European pulses to produce functional beverages – from chickpea and lupin as dairy alternatives', *J. Funct. Foods*, vol. 98, p. 105287, 2022, https://doi.org/10.1016/j.jff.2022.105287.

81 X. Zhang et al., 'The texture of plant protein-based meat analogs by high moisture extrusion: a review', *J. Texture Stud.*, vol. 54, no. 3, pp. 351–364, 2023, https://doi.org/10.1111/jtxs.12697.

82 X. Zhang, Y. Zhao, T. Zhang, Y. Zhang, L. Jiang, and X. Sui, 'Potential of hydrolyzed wheat protein in soy-based meat analogues: rheological, textural and functional properties', *Food Chem. X*, vol. 20, p. 100921, 2023, https://doi.org/10.1016/j.fochx.2023.100921.

83 D. Frank, Y. Oytam, J. Hughes, C. K. McDonnell, and R. Buckow, 'Sensory perceptions and new consumer attitudes to meat', In: New Aspects of Meat Quality, Elsevier, pp. 853–886, 2022, https://doi.org/10.1016/B978-0-323-85879-3.00016-7.

84 S. Cordelle, A. Redl, and P. Schlich, 'Sensory acceptability of new plant protein meat substitutes', *Food Qual. Prefer.*, vol. 98, p. 104508, 2022, https://doi.org/10.1016/j.foodqual.2021.104508.

85 R. Moss, J. LeBlanc, M. Gorman, C. Ritchie, L. Duizer, and M. B. McSweeney, 'A prospective review of the sensory properties of plant-based dairy and meat alternatives with a focus on texture', *Foods*, vol. 12, no. 8, p. 1709, 2023, https://doi.org/10.3390/foods12081709.

86 N. Nourmohammadi, L. Austin, and D. Chen, 'Protein-based fat replacers: a focus on fabrication methods and fat-mimic mechanisms', *Foods*, vol. 12, no. 5, p. 957, 2023, https://doi.org/10.3390/foods12050957.

3

Chemical Composition and Structural Characteristics of Oat Protein

Oat protein has gained growing attention in recent years due to its well-balanced amino acid profile, health-promoting properties and potential applications in the development of functional foods [1, 2]. Unlike many other cereal proteins, oat protein is characterized by a higher proportion of globulins and a relatively low content of prolamins, contributing to its superior nutritional quality [3]. Understanding the chemical composition and structural properties of oat proteins is essential for assessing their digestibility, bioavailability and techno-functional behaviour in food systems [4]. Moreover, detailed insights into protein classification and molecular structure allow better comparison with proteins from other plant sources, thereby informing strategies to enhance their application in food processing, nutrition and therapeutic product development [5]. This chapter presents a critical examination of the structural and compositional characteristics of oat proteins, providing a foundation for understanding their functional relevance in both nutritional science and industrial innovation.

3.1 Amino Acid Profile of Oat Protein

Proteins are essential for the development, maintenance and physiological functioning of the human body. Its nutritional quality is determined by its amino acid content, which should meet the established standards and matches the pattern required by human body [6], as well as by its digestibility and bioavailability. All amino acids are necessary for the development and functioning of muscles and organs [7, 8], as well as for the synthesis of enzymes, hormones and components of the immune system [9]. Generally, amino acids are categorized as essential amino acids (EAAs), and non-essential amino acids (NEAAs), depending on the body's, ability to produce specific amino acids. NEAAs can be synthesized by the human body, whereas EAAs cannot and must be obtained from dietary protein; therefore, adequate intake of EAAs is essential. Furthermore, some NEAAs, including Arg, Cys, Glu, Gly, Pro and Tyr, can become conditionally essential, particularly for preterm neonates [10]. In such instances, the body is unable to synthesize enough amounts of these amino acids, rendering them conditionally indispensable EAAs that must be obtained via dietary protein to offset inadequate production throughout certain life stages [10–12]. To satisfy metabolic demands and ensure the optimal functioning of body, sufficient protein intake is necessary to fulfil both total nitrogen and EAA requirements [12].

Oat protein possesses a balanced profile of both EAAs and NEAAs. In essence, the amino acids (AAs) composition of oat proteins varies among different fractions. In addition to containing the highest concentrations of EAAs like lysin, valine, phenylalanine and histidine, globulins also contain the highest concentration of NEAAs such as arginine and glutamic acid. These levels are notably higher compared to other fractions, like prolamin, albumins and glutelin [13]. Notably, the EAA globulins align with the FAO-recommended values for adults, except for methionine, which could be recognized as limited amino acid [14]. When assessing protein quality based on the ratio of EAAs to total AAs, both globulins (36%) and albumins (39%) surpass (36%) threshold, qualifying them as high-quality proteins. In contrast, the prolamin and glutelin fractions all below this standard and are therefore considered low-quality proteins [14]. The AAs composition within these fractions is influenced not only by the fractionation process but also by the specific oat variety, reflecting genetic differences and environmental factors. Moreover, the method of extraction, including variations in temperature, pH and solvents, has a substantial impact on the resulting AAs profile [15]. This information emphasizes the interplay between genetic, environmental and processing factors in determining the nutritional quality of oat protein fractions. Oat protein presents significant AAs profile, with a comparative overview provided in Table 3.1.

Oat protein comprises a substantial amount of branched-chain amino acids (Leucine, Isoleucine, Valine), which are essential for energy production and the upregulation of protein synthesis. This is particularly vital for older adults in the prevention or treatment of sarcopenia, as well as for athletes requiring improved muscle repair and increased muscle mass [16]. The microbiota of the large intestine is significant since it may metabolize any protein that arrives there, rendering it inaccessible to the host [17]. Furthermore, oat proteins are also rich in sulphur-containing AAs, such as methionine and cysteine, compared to legumes [18]. This unique composition makes oats an ideal complement legume

Table 3.1 Amino acids composition of oat protein (mg/100 mg) [20, 21].

Amino acid	Oat	FAO/WHO standard (adult)
EAA		
Leu	7.07	1.9
Ile	3.48	1.3
Val	4.77	1.3
Lys	3.46	1.6
Phe	5.23	1.9
Thr	2.65	0.9
His	2.13	1.6
Met	1.55	1.7
ΣEAA	30.34	

Amino acid	Oat	FAO/WHO standard (adult)
NEAA		
Ala	4.08	
Gly	3.75	
Arg	6.93	
Ser	5.12	
Glu	21.45	
Pro	4.08	
Cys	1.77	
Tyr	3.37	
Asp	6.10	
ΣNEAA	56.65	
ΣAA	86.99	
ΣEAA/ΣAA	34.87	

in protein blending strategies. By combining oat and legume proteins, the resulting blend achieves a higher overall protein quality, particularly due to enhanced lysine content, which is often limited in cereal proteins but abundant in legumes [19]. Such combinations effectively address the daily human requirement for EAA. Therefore, oat proteins are classified as high-quality proteins based on their EAA profile. The superior EAA ratio underscores the potential of oat proteins in formulating nutritionally balanced food products, especially after complement with legume proteins.

3.2 Nutritional Quality Evaluation of Oat Protein

Protein quality parameters determine the nutritional value of proteins by assessing the digestibility and availability of EAAs. The Protein Efficiency Ratio (PER), Biological Value (BV), Net Protein Utilization (NPU), Protein Digestibility-corrected Amino Acids Score (PDCAAS) and Digestible Indispensable Amino Acid Score (DIAAS) are WHO and FAO recommended methods and indices to assess the protein quality. It is important to acknowledge that each metric has its own set of benefits and drawbacks, and that there is no single universal solution. However, DIAAS is considered includes one of the superior protein quality evaluation techniques that evaluates amino acid composition and digestibility, enhancing the comprehension of protein source nutritional value and facilitating dietary recommendations and food product development [22]. The PDCAAS score for oat protein is moderate, ranging from 0.41 to 0.64, despite the fact that it has been shown to have high digestibility up to 90–94% [20]. Compared to other typical cereals, these two matrices are greater, whereas lower than most of legumes. Oat protein has a lower PDCAAS score than legumes do because it has a lower score for EAA (30.34), despite considering that its total AAS (86.99) is high [20, 21]. In addition, the protein equivalents of oats are larger than those of other cereals, which make it more suitable option and has potential to be effectively used by human body [23]. Because of its beneficial physiological and functional activities, as well as the fact that it is less allergenic than legumes, oat protein is attracting the attention of the community worldwide. Therefore, it is necessary to adjust the amino acid composition by boosting the EAAS of oat protein isolates (OPIs) via the use of effective and sustainable methods. This, in turn, will eventually lead to an increase in the usage of oat protein and market proportion.

3.3 Regulatory and Physiological Functions of Amino Acids

The quality of proteins is often debated, focusing mostly on the regulatory aspects of protein content claims and the physicochemical properties necessary for their incorporation into food systems. A significant amount of research has been undertaken on oat bioactive peptides, especially for the prevention of diabetes, hypertension and cardiovascular diseases among others [24]. Consequently, the separated amino acids get less attention in this context. Amino acids serve as both structural and energy sources during optimal cell development, differentiation and functionality.

They are essential for protein synthesis as monomer units and serve as substrates for biosynthetic processes. Amino acids metabolism abnormalities have been associated with the development of several illnesses. Protein or specific amino acids deficiency or altered metabolism is associated with the onset of metabolic disorders such as obesity, diabetes, along with neurological, immunological and cardiovascular issues [25]. This section focuses on the biological activity of certain amino acids found in oat proteins that are not linked to nutritional value. Oats possess a high concentration of EAAs, notably branched-chain amino acids (17.61% of total amino acid content) like leucine, isoleucine and valine. In addition to this, it also contains a significant quantity of NEAAs, such as arginine and aspartic acid (ASP), which are equally distributed within their protein composition (Figure 3.1). It is also essential to highlight that no regulatory agency presently allows health claims to be based on a single amino acid, despite the extensive research has been undertaken on the health benefits of individual amino acids [26, 27].

3.3.1 Branched Chain Amino Acids

Oat protein is significant source of branched-chain amino acids. Leucine, isoleucine and valine are classified as the three BCAAs, due to their aliphatic side chains with a branched carbon structure. Certain amino acids have long been acknowledged for their significant function in regulating health and metabolism. BCAAs exhibit lower solubility compared to other amino acids owing to their increased hydrophilicity. Their solubility fluctuates with pH due to electrostatic interactions with water molecules, being minimal in water at their isoelectric point (pI) [28, 29]. Conversely, it attains its zenith at pH values much above or below its pI [30]. This pH-dependent solubility is crucial for a wide variety of applications, including formulation, separation, and purification. The solubility of BCAAs may play a vital role in the formulation of powdered beverages, capsules and tablets. Moreover, BCAAs are utilized as dietary supplements, particularly by athletes. Recent research has focused on producing nanosuspensions or biopolymers to increase BCAA solubility, which impacts the

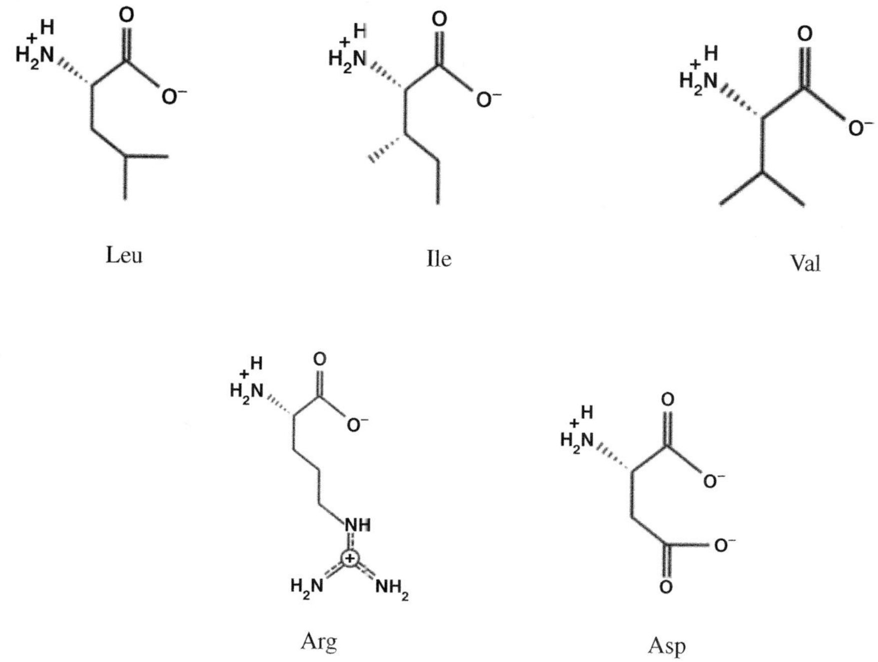

Figure 3.1 Amino acids structure with significant contribution in oat protein.

bioavailability of amino acids [31–33]. Similarly, these amino acids may be synthesized and ingested by biotechnological methods. The bioavailable derivatives of leucine and isoleucine, namely N-lactoyl derivatives and keto acids have been examined as substitutes in feed formulations for next-generation bioprocesses targeting monoclonal antibody production [34, 35]. To address solubility constraints, feeding procedures are devised that included dissolving leucine in ammonia solution and fermenting it with *Escherichia coli* [36]. This was executed to circumvent the constraints of solubility. Research indicated that individuals with obesity had elevated blood level of BCAAs [37]. In the last decades, it has been evident that plasma level of BCAAs in both animals and human are associated with obesity and insulin resistance [38–40].

Particularly, leucine constitutes 8.12% of total amino acid composition in oat protein. It is often present in high quality protein sources as one of the most prevalent amino acids. It is important in activation of the mammalian target of rapamycin (mTOR) signalling pathway, leading to enhanced protein synthesis in skeletal muscle, adipose tissue and placental cells [41, 42]. The amino acid leucine inhibits protein degradation while enhancing energy metabolism, including glucose absorption, mitochondrial biogenesis and fatty acid oxidation. This facilitates the generation of energy for protein synthesis [43]. Typically, over 80% of leucine is used in protein synthesis. The residual is transformed into protein ketoisocaproate (α-KIC) and β-hydroxy β-methybutyrate (β-HMB) inside the skeletal muscle [44, 45]. One potential possibility is that leucine metabolites influence diverse protein activities. The α-KIC and β-HMB are widely used dietary supplements for enhancing protein synthesis, inhibiting degradation and regulating energy balance in various *in vitro* and *in vivo* contexts [46]. Leucine and its metabolites have the capacity to significantly improve animal development and health.

3.3.2 Arginine

Oats are one of the foods that contain a substantial amount of arginine, comprising around 8% of the total amino acid profile [47]. Arginine (Arg) may display dual characteristics in many ways. Arg also contributes in promoting disorder owing to the hydrophobicity and charge of its side chain, facilitating protein folding via ionic and hydrogen bonding, as well as interactions with cations and positive ions. The methylation of histones, RNA-binding proteins and chaperones regulates several biological processes [48]. It has been reported that arginine is an abundant amino acid, ranking as the second most prevalent amino acid in protein–protein interactions following tryptophan, regarding amino acid composition [49]. Lysine is the amino acid most analogous to arginine regarding its structural connections. Moreover, it is the amino acid that most often substitutes arginine in the original sequence of proteins across many species [50]. Arginine maintains its protonated form at all physiologically relevant pH levels. Unlike lysine, arginine only acts as an H-donor, regardless of the environmental pH [51].

Arginine is a semi-essential amino acid that is necessary during injury, period of elevated stress and the body's development to its maximum potential. Arginine has the potential to alter cellular biochemical processes by converting into a variety of physiologically active compounds, in addition to serving as a substrate for protein synthesis [52]. Arginine is utilized in a multitude of metabolic processes to generate diverse array of physiologically active compounds, such as nitric oxide, agmatine, creatine phosphate, ornithine, polyamines and citrulline. Nitric oxide synthase and arginase, which are part of the urea cycle, are the two enzyme systems that are primarily responsible for regulating the availability of arginine. Arginine has a significant impact on a variety of physiological processes, such as the regulation of immune response, wound healing, blood vessels relaxation, hormone release, endothelial function and insulin sensitivity [52]. These effects of arginine are mediated by both nitric oxide dependent pathways. Because nitric oxide regulates a multitude of cellular activities, including the expression of adhesion molecules, platelet aggregation, leukocyte adhesion, among others. Furthermore, arginine has been associated with a variety of cellular and physiological effects, including its ability to influence the development of atherosclerotic cardiovascular disease and to enhance immunological function in both healthy and diseased individuals [52]. In conclusion, arginine is a biologically active dietary molecule that possesses a diverse array of pharmacological and physiological properties.

3.3.3 Aspartic Acid

Asp is an important component of protein synthesis and bodily functions, despite not being regarded as an EAA from nutritional perspective [53]. Asp contributes significantly to the total amino acid content of oat protein, accounting for 7.01%. The most common form of aspartate is L-aspartic acid (L-Asp), whereas D-aspartic acid (D-Asp) is present in much smaller amounts. Aspartate simultaneously exist in two distinct isoforms. Along with glutamic acid, the other dicarboxylic amino acid present in the body, ASP is transported through cell membrane by specific transporters [54]. At physiological pH, ASP has two carboxyl groups that are negatively charged. It serves as the substrate for the synthesis of proteins, nucleotides, asparagine, arginine and a number of other compounds involved in the growth of nervous tissue and neurotransmission. The purine–nucleotide cycle (PNC), the maltase–aspartate shuttle (MAS), neurotransmission and urea synthesis all depend critically on Asp. It also plays a significant role in the gluconeogenic process. One of the most distinctive functions of Asp is its role in brain development and hypothalamic function regulation [53].

3.4 Classification of Oat Protein

Oat protein primarily consists of globulins, prolamins, albumins and glutenin with approximate shares of (50–80, 4–15, 1–12, and > 10) percent of complete protein in respective manner [55]. A detailed overview of each fraction is discussed in this section.

3.4.1 Globulins

Globulins, the major fraction, are salt-soluble proteins comprising three subunits: 12S, 7S and 3S globulins. Among these, 12S globulin is the predominant form and is an oligomeric protein composed of six quaternary monomers subunits (54–60 kDa), structurally resembling soy 11S globulin [56, 57]. The 12S globulin contains two major subunits: the acidic A-subunit (33 kDa) and the basic B-subunit (22 kDa) [58]. The 7S globulins consist of polypeptides ranging from 55 to 65 kDa, while the 3S globulin fraction includes two polypeptides with molecular weight of approximately 15–21 kDa [55]. A meticulous analysis [59] of the genetic data derived from isolating cDNA clones encoding oat seed storage globulin mRNAs identifies the signal peptide cleavage site preceding the release of the 12S globulins, specifically occurring between the alanine residue at position 24 and the glutamine at position 25 of amino acids sequence. In addition, this helped to determine the site of the proteolytic cleavage that is responsible for the separation of the globulin into its acidic and basic subunits. This cleavage occurred between the asparagine at position 317 and the glycine at position 318 of sequence (Figure 3.2a). On the basis of these findings, the structure of oat globulin can be summarized as follows: a signal peptide consisting of 24 amino acids (Figure 3.2a, followed by an acidic polypeptide consisting of 293 amino acids, with a molecular weight of 33.1 kDa, and finally a basic polypeptide consisting of 201 amino acids with a molecular weight of 22.7 kDa. Cysteine residues, are located at position 121 and 324 and are considered important for the formation of interchain disulphide bonds in the native globulin. These residues are marked with a circle in Figure 3.2a. The α and β subunits are disulphide linked in the native globulin. Although the crystalline structure of 12S globulins has not yet been described, it is anticipated that the arrangement of subunits inside the hexamer is comparable to the structures of soy glycinin and other 11S globulins, which have been well-characterized [60]. Each subunit of normal 11S and 7S seed storage globulins is composed of two N-terminal and C-terminal domains that are quite identical to one another. These domains each feature an extended helix and a core β-barrel region.

Monocotyledonous (cereals, including oat) and dicotyledonous (legumes, including soy) seed globulins share structural domains throughout evolution [61]. After considering the crystalline structure of soy glycinin, oat globulin was anticipated to be a hexamer composed by two identical trimers (160 kDa each) that are hydrophobically face-to-face stacked [62]. Trimers are formed of three pairs of identical dimers with two unique polypeptides, α

(acidic, bigger) and β (basic, smaller), joined by a single disulphide bond (Figure 3.2b). The $\alpha - \beta$ dimer, with an estimated molecular mass of 54 kDa, is the fundamental unit in food processing. The results of our conducted SDS-page analysis represent the molecular weight distribution (Figure 3.2c). Additionally, oats include trace levels of 3S and 7S globulins, which are proteins that are thought to be similar to vicilin. 7S globulins are polypeptides with molecular weights ranging from 55 to 65 kDa, while the 3S fraction is composed of two polypeptides with molecular weights of around 15 and 21 kDa. The mobility of 3S and 7S globulins on sodium dodecyl sulphate–polyacrylamide gel electrophoresis (SDS–PAGE) was not changed by reducing agents, which suggests that there are no internal disulphide bonds [63]. There has been no research done on the functioning of individual oat 3S or 7S in food, and the structural role that these oats play in food and beverage is not well known.

3.4.2 Prolamins

Prolamins constitute the primary storage protein in several cereal grains, with the notable exceptions of rice and oat. In oats, prolamins (alcohol-soluble avenins) comprise a very small fractions of the overall protein composition, often ranging from 4 to 15% of total protein, and categorized into four subtypes: α-, β-, γ-, and -avenins. Avenins are isolated from

[Met–Ala–Thr–Thr–Ser–Phe–Pro–Ser–Val–Leu–Phe–Tyr–Ser–Cys–Ile–Phe–Leu–Leu–Tyr–Asn–Gly–Ser–Met–Ala–Gln]–[Leu–Phe–Gly–Gln–
Ser–Phe–Thr–Pro–Trp–Gln–Ser–Ser–Arg–Gln–Gly–Gly–Leu–Lys–Gly–Cys–Lys–Phe–Asp–Arg–Leu–Gln–Ala–Phe–Glu–Pro–Leu–Arg–Gln–Val–
Arg–Ser–Gln–Ala–Gly–Val–Thr–Glu–Tyr–Phe–Asp–Glu–Gln–Asn–Glu–Gln–Phe–Arg–**Cys**–Thr–Gly–Val–Phe–Val–Ile–Arg–Arg–Val–Ile–Glu–
Pro–Gln–Gly–Leu–Leu–Leu–Pro–Gln–Tyr–His–Asn–Ala–Pro–Gly–Leu–Val–Tyr–Ile–Leu–Gln–Gly–Arg–Gly–Tyr–Thr–Gly–Leu–Thr–Phe–Pro–
Gly–Cys–Pro–Ala–Thr–Phe–Gln–Gln–Gln–Phe–Gln–Pro–Phe–Asp–Gln–Ala–Gln–Asp–Gln–Ser–Gln–Ser–His–Leu–Lys–Asp–Glu–His–Gln–Arg–
Val–His–Arg–Phe–Lys–Gln–Gly–Asp–Val–Ile–Ala–Leu–Pro–Ala–Gly–Ile–Val–His–Trp–Gly–Tyr–Asn–Asp–Gly–Asp–Ala–Pro–Val–Val–Ala–Ile–
Tyr–Val–Phe–Asp–Val–Asn–Asn–Asn–Ala–Asn–Gln–Leu–Glu–Pro–Arg–Gln–Lys–Glu–Phe–Leu–Leu–Ala–Gly–Asn–Asn–Lys–Glu–Asp–Gln–
Gln–Phe–Gly–Gln–Asn–Ile–Phe–Ser–Gly–Phe–Asn–Ile–Gln–Leu–Leu–Ser–Glu–Ala–Leu–Gly–Ile–Ser–Gln–Gln–Ala–Ala–Gln–Arg–Ile–Gln–Ser–
Gln–Lys–Glu–Gln–Arg–Gly–Glu–Ile–Ile–Arg–Val–Thr–Gln–Ala–Leu–Gln–Phe–Leu–Lys–Pro–Thr–Met–Ser–Gln–Gln–Glu–Leu–Val–Glu–His–Gln–
Ala–Tyr–Gln–Pro–Ile–Gln–Ser–Gln–Glu–Gly–Gln–Ser–Thr–Gln–Tyr–Gln–Val–Gly–Gln–Ser–Thr–Gln–Tyr–Gln–Glu–Gly–Gln–Ser–Thr–Gln–Tyr–
Gln–Ala–Gly–Gln–Ser–Gln–Asp–Arg–Ser–Phe–Asn]–[Gly–Leu–Glu–Glu–Asn–Phe–**Cys**–Ser–Leu–Glu–Ala–Arg–Gln–Asn–Ile–Gly–Asn–Pro–Lys–
Arg–Ala–Asp–Thr–His–Asn–Pro–Arg–Ala–Gly–Arg–Ile–Thr–Arg–Leu–His–Gly–Gln–Asn–Phe–Pro–Ile–Leu–Asn–Leu–Val–Gln–Met–Ser–Ala–
Thr–Arg–Val–Asn–Leu–Tyr–Gln–Asn–Ala–Ile–Leu–Ser–Pro–Phe–Trp–Asn–Ile–Asn–Ala–His–Ser–Val–Val–Tyr–Met–Ile–Gln–Gly–His–Ala–Gln–
Val–Gln–Val–Asn–Asn–Asn–Gly–Gln–Thr–Val–Phe–Asn–Asp–Arg–Leu–Arg–Gln–Gly–Gln–Leu–Leu–Ile–Val–Pro–Gln–His–Tyr–Val–Val–Leu–
Lys–Lys–Ala–Glu–Arg–Glu–Gly–Cys–Gln–Tyr–Ile–Ser–Phe–Lys–Thr–Asn–Pro–Asn–Ser–Met–Val–Ser–His–Ile–Ala–Gly–Lys–Ser–Ser–Ile–Leu–
Arg–Ala–Leu–Pro–Val–Asp–Val–Leu–Ala–Asn–Ala–Tyr–Arg–Ile–Ser–Arg–Gln–Glu–Ala–Arg–Asn–Leu–Lys–Asn–Asn–Arg–Gly–Gln–Glu–Ser–
Gly–Val–Phe–Thr–Pro–Lys–Phe–Thr–Gln–Thr–Ser–Phe–Gln–Pro–Tyr–Pro–Glu–Gly–Glu–Asp–Glu–Ser–Ser–Leu–Thr–Asn–Lys–Ala–Ser–Glu]

(a)

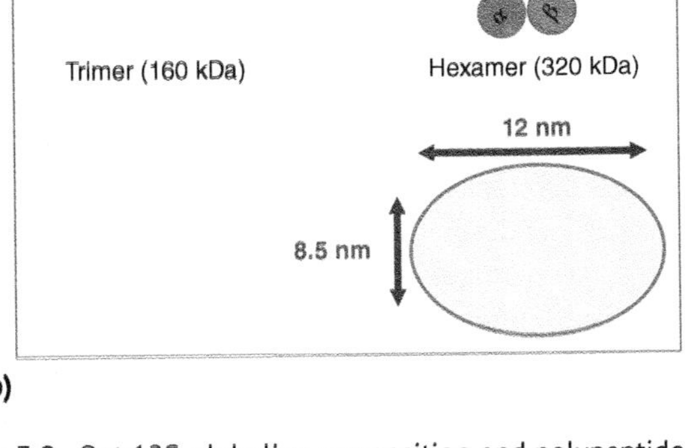

(b)

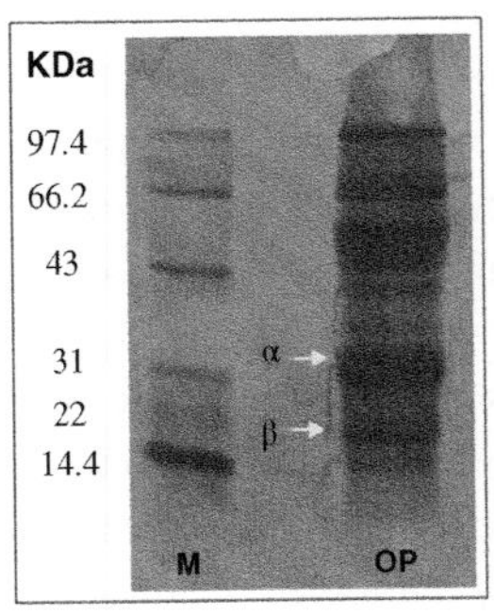

(c)

Figure 3.2 Oat 12S-globulins composition and polypeptide divisions in subunits.
Source: Ref. [4]

oats using ethanol, followed by precipitation with NaCl [64]. Prolamins in cereal grains mostly reside as monomers or low MW aggregates [65]. Oat prolamins have MW between 20 and 40 kDa and possess an pI ranging from pH 5.0 to pH 9.0. They share structural homology with the sulphur-rich α and γ-gliadins of wheat, β-hordeins of barley and γ-secalins of rye. Despite their functional similarity to wheat gluten in storage, avenins differ in amino acid composition being low in proline and glutamine [56–58]. Specifically, oat prolamins are characterized by elevated levels of BCAAs including leucine, valine and acidic amino acids such as ASP and glutamic acid, which enhance their unique nutritional profile.

3.4.3 Albumins

The albumin fraction accounts for 1–12% of oat protein, distinguished by its exceptional water solubility and restricted solubility at high salt concentrations, primarily enzymes related to protein quality and plant defence [13]. This fraction can be effectively extracted using dialysis of the salt extract from oat flour against water [66]. Generally, albumins are regarded as 2S oat proteins, characterized by their high content of EAAs such as cysteine and lysine [67, 68]. In contrast to globulins, albumins display a wider spectrum of charges during isoelectric focusing, with most components aggregating between pH 4.0 and 7.5. Research indicated that the albumin fraction consisted of separate bands with MW of 14–17 kDa, 20–27 kDa and 36–47 kDa [69]. Oat albumins, in contrast to globulins, have intrinsic fluorescence spectra with diminished peak intensities and extended peak wavelengths, indicating enhanced polarity and surface hydrophilicity. This discovery corroborates the findings from surface hydrophobicity investigations [70], further emphasizing the unique features of oat albumins.

3.4.4 Glutelin

Glutelin, also called residual proteins, is a mixture of tiny polypeptides, albumins, globulins and prolamins, consist of polypeptides with molecular wights ranging from 10 to 90 kDa [71]. In general, it is assumed that oats have a glutelin level of less than 10%, while the precise range is yet unclear. The efficacy of other fractions including albumins, globulins and prolamins extraction is directly correlated with its proportion [69]. Unlike other protein fractions, oat glutelin are not readily soluble, which makes its solubilization more challenging. Glutelin may be isolated when other fractions are completely dissolved in SDS and β-mercaptoethanol [71]. The aforementioned chemicals are employed to accomplish this effect. The isoelectric profile of oat glutelin may be separated into acidic (pH 4.5–6.5) and alkaline (pH 9.0–10), respectively [70].

3.5 Molecular and Structural Features of Oat Protein

3.5.1 Primary Structure of Oat Protein

The primary sequence of a protein serves as the fundamental template for its folding and conformation. Since the late 1970s, the sodium dodecyl sulphate–polyacrylamide gel electrophoresis (SDS–PAGE) has facilitated the separation, isolation and characterization of seed storage proteins from cereals and legumes [72–76]. This commonly employed acid hydrolysis techniques to determined amino acids composition typically expressed in molar percentage. In recent years, advance in genome sequencing have significantly enhanced our understanding of plant protein structures, shown by the publishing of the oat genome in 2022 [77]. This section utilizes amino acid composition analysis and sequence alignment comparisons to compare the structure of oat 12S globulin with rice glutelin and 11S legumins (pea legumin and soy glycinin). It is essential to recognize that 11S and 12S globulins are hexameric proteins that have experienced post-translational cleavage; yet, the structures used for alignment and amino acid comparisons refer to individual monomers consisting of α and β subunits prior to this cleavage [78].

The amino acids composition of a combination of α and β polypeptides found in the primary components of oat, pea, soy and rice proteins (Table 3.2). The data reveal a high content (> 24%) of amidic building blocks Gln/Glu and Asn/Asp, which is crucial feature of seed storage proteins. This is consistent with their biological role as a source of carbon and nitrogen that aids in the growth of seedlings after they have germinated [79, 80]. It is crucial to notice that Glu and Asp are shown with the composition values of Gln and Asp, respectively. This is because these two components cannot be distinguished by the acid hydrolysis approach. However, the analysis of cDNA clones encoding oat seed storage globulin indicates that in the natural oat protein state, uncharged Gln and Asn are more abundant than their charged counterparts, which might impact the solubility of oat storage protein. For instance, scientist report a Gln: Gln ratio of 2.5 : 1 and an Asn: Asp ratio of 2.3 : 1, resulting in expected mol% values of 15.2% Gln, 6.1% Glu, 6.9% Asn and 3.9% Asp

Table 3.2 Amino acid composition of α and β polypeptides in major fractions of proteins (mol%).

Amino acids	Oat	Rice	Soy	Pea
Ala	6.4	8.0	6.7	5.3
Gly	8.2	8.4	7.8	5.1
Leu	7.7	6.8	7.2	7.8
Ile	4.4	4.2	4.6	4.3
Val	5.8	6.2	5.6	4.5
Met	0.9	1.8	1.0	0.7
Phe	5.6	3.7	3.9	4.6
Pro	4.9	5.5	6.3	4.9
Ser	6.2	7.3	6.6	4.9
Thr	3.5	4.5	4.2	3.4
Cys	1.1	1.1	1.1	1.1
Tyr	3.5	3.2	2.5	3.2
Asp/Asn	9.9	10.0	11.8	12.2
Glu/Gln	21.4	14.6	18.8	19.7
Lys	2.6	4.4	4.1	5.0
Arg	6.4	8.7	5.9	9.2
His	2.0	2.6	1.8	2.7

[59, 75]. Another characteristic that is similar between the globulins of oat, soy, pea, is the quantity of sulphur that they contain. Cys and Met make up roughly (2 mol%) of the total [59, 75], while Cys residues have great relevance in the structural context as they play a critical role in the formation of disulphide bridges between α and β polypeptides. The Lys and Phe composition of oat globulins, on the other hand, is distinct from that of the other proteins. In oat globulin, Lys is present in lesser amounts (2.6 mol%), whereas Phe is present in higher concentration of (5.6 mol%).

As shown in Figure 3.3, the amino acids are distributed into three distinct categories: charged residues, polar and non-polar residues. A hydrophobic scale categorization was not employed due to concerns regarding its accuracy in the scientific literature, as it fluctuates based on environmental conditions and the initial materials utilized [81, 82]. When compared to non-polar residues, which are found in 43–52% of all proteins studied, charged amino acids are shown to be much less prevalent (11–17%). In terms of the proportion of the charged residues, oat had the lowest percentage (11%), with values that were closest to that soy (12%). On the other hand, pea legumin had the lowest composition of non-polar residues that was found overall (43%). Conversely, these values may fluctuate based on the kind of supply, and the observed variations among the studied proteins are minimal.

3.5.2 Secondary and Tertiary Structure of Oat Protein

Amino acid chains may be folded into α-helix, β-sheets or random coils by different non-covalent interactions, mostly hydrogen bonding. Research utilizing circular dichroism spectroscopy (CD), and Fourier-transform infrared spectroscopy (FTIR) to evaluate secondary

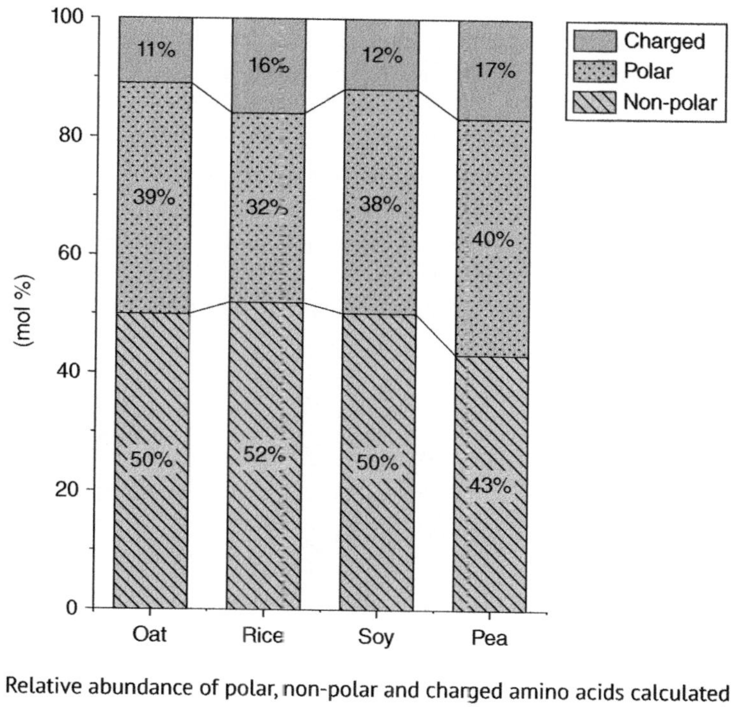

Figure 3.3 Relative abundance of polar, non-polar and charged amino acids calculated based on Table 3.2.

structure indicated that all examined proteins displayed a significant proportion (> 40%) of β-sheets and turns, with soy presenting the highest percentage at (63%) [60]. Relative to soy, the OPIs had roughly equivalent proportion of random coils (26%), and α-helix (29%). Rice glutelin had a superior α-helix content of 42%, whereas pea glutelin showed reduced concentration of 16% [60]. The secondary structure of oat globulin resembles that of seed proteins seen in rice and legumes. This information positioned the β-sheets confrontations as the most prominent characteristic in all discussed four protein structures.

Moreover, a significant lack of structural data exists for oat globulins and rice glutelin, even though secondary structure analysis of oat globulin is readily available. To compare the tertiary structures with a previously obtained 12S globulin monomer sequence, which included both subunits before post-translational cleavage, α-fold was employed to predict the tertiary structures based on the primary amino acid sequences [83, 84]. The folding algorithm accurately predicts a conserved jelly roll β-barrel in both proteins, indicating a high level of confidence in its predictions. The monomer structure illustrated in Figure 3.4 is represented by a circle adjacent to oat globulin. However, due to reduced confidence in the model, the terminal sequence at the protein's surface may provide limited information.

While knowledge about oats remains limited, recent years have seen scientists focus on the protein structures of legumes, including pea and soy. This phenomenon is likely attributable to the rising preference for plant proteins in comparison to meat. The XRD data of crystallized prolegumins and legumins indicate that the 11S monomer contains two elongated helical regions. Furthermore, two impeccably preserved jelly roll jars were found. Research indicates that these barrels are composed of eight β-strands arranged in four non-parallel sheets [85, 86]. Interestingly, the AlphaFold prediction for oats and rice reveals that all proteins are classified within the cuprin superfamily. A notable characteristic of this group is the presence of a highly conserved barrel region within the core proteins. Figure 3.4 illustrates the anticipated locations of these sections within oat 12S globulin. This resulted in the findings that all proteins examined exhibited identical secondary and tertiary molecular characteristics.

The hydrogen-bonded network of the β-strands in the jelly roll barrel sections is crucial for maintaining protein stability. It is evident that this network contributes to the resistance of proteins against degradation due to temperature, pH and non-specific proteolytic enzymes [87]. The conservation of amino acids in the production of the β-polypeptide (core) compared to the α-polypeptide (surface) in oat variants can be attributed to increased stability [76, 88]. It is also reported that the variance in the number of helices among 11S globulins

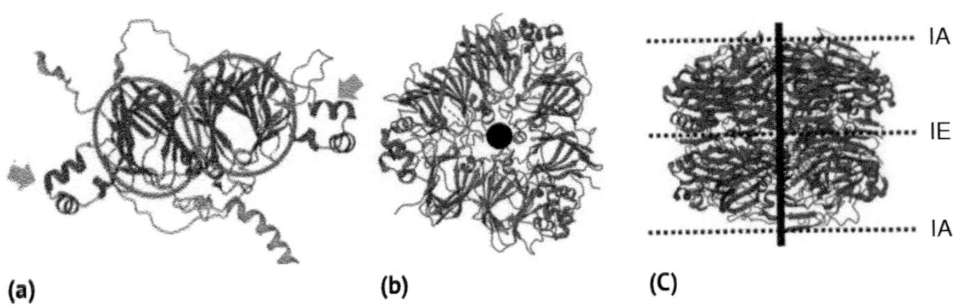

Figure 3.4 Tertiary and quaternary predicted structure of oat protein. (a) monomer; (b) trimer; (c) hexamer. *Source:* Ref. [60]

exceeds that of the number of β-strands [86]. This discovery provides further evidence that the jelly roll barrel, a structurally important component, is conserved across all oat species.

The AlphaFold model of the oat 12S globulin monomer can be validated through the superimposition of the soy 11S legumin monomer structure, derived from XRD, onto the predicted structure of the corresponding amino acids sequence (PDB identifier: P047776) illustrated in (Figure 3.5). The ChimeraX software facilitates the alignment of the structure, yielding a root mean square deviation (RMSD) value of 0.991 Å for all residue pairs. This indicates that the structure and the model align optimally. An RMSD value of 0 Å signifies that two protein structures are similar [89]. It is widely acknowledged that a comparison of two protein structures is valid when their RMSD value are 2.0 Å or lower. The regions exhibiting significant discrepancies between the predicted AlphaFold structure and the crystalline structure are indicated by spatially deviating and non-overlapping segments in the superimposed tertiary structure (Figure 3.5c). The XRD structure appropriately aligns with the predicted β subunit structure, which pertains to protein's core, including the extended helical region and jelly roll β-barrel. The terminals of the α subunit exhibited the greatest variation between the two structures, particularly at the C-terminus, which displayed the most significant differences. AlphaFold offers valuable insights into the core of the oat 12S globulin monomer (β subunit), indicating its advantages. The projected α subunit tertiary structure allows for limited inference of information, likely observable at the protein surface, in the absence of XRD data.

3.5.3 Quaternary Structure of Oat Protein

This section discusses the mechanism by which oat 12S globulin monomers get their folded confirmation in solution state. In 1978, Peterson presented a model for the self-assembly of oat 12 globulin, predicted based on molecular weight study of the protein and it was constituted via SDS-PAGE [74]. According to the 11S legumin model, the 12 S globulin has two subunits, α and β, presents in an equimolar ratio. It is suggesting that these subunits likely assemble into a compact hexameric structure stabilized by non-covalent interactions. The ratio of α and β subunits in 11S soy globulin may vary based on the individual soybean variety, and it is conceivable that this may also apply to oats [90].

The crystallographic characterization of oat globulins has so far been limited to the AlphaFold structure predicted for the monomeric form. The AlphaFold monomer suggests decreased model confidence in the C-terminal sequence of the α subunit, anticipated to be located on the protein's surface, as previously described. The commencement of trimer and hexamer stacking relies on post-translational cleavage, and the anticipated structure is

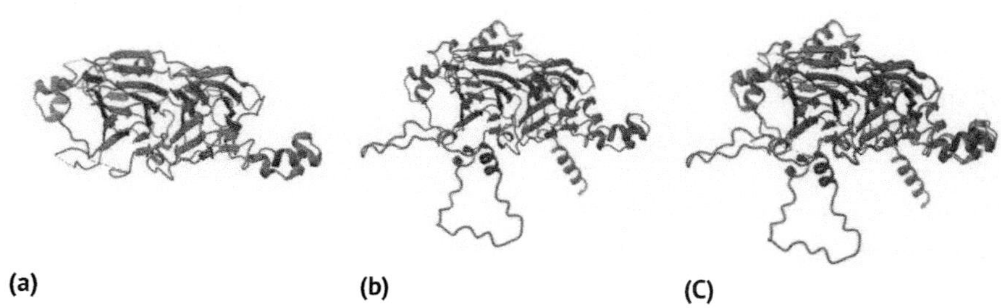

Figure 3.5 XRD crystallographic data to AlphaFold prediction for 11S soy globulin. (a) XRD crystallographic structure; (b) AlphaFold; (c) XRD structure + AlphaFold. *Source:* Ref. [60]

derived from monomeric sequence [91–94]. Due to the aforementioned reasons, replicating the stacking of monomers to synthesize the hexameric oat 12S globulin is challenging. To comprehend the synthesis mechanism of oat hexamer, researchers rely on XRD data acquired from legume timers and hexamers.

A model of 11S/12S globulin folding as established by XRD can be seen in Figure 3.5. In the first phase of this model, three monomeric subunits use electrostatic and hydrophobic interactions to form a trimer [85, 95]. Legume trimers are generally characterized by two distinct sides, IE and IA, exhibiting varying hydrophilic properties and curvatures [62]. Each monomer has an N-terminus located in the trimer's central cavity and a C-terminus situated on the outside [86]. Research using XRD on soy glycinin revealed that the formation of trimers results in neighbouring monomer units stacking in prolonged helical regions. Furthermore, the study emphasized the significance of non-specific hydrophobic contacts between two IE faces during the association of two trimers [85].

The second step of the self-assembly technique involves the simultaneous stacking of two trimmers. Laser light scattering tests indicate that oat globulin is expected to be arranged at 60 °angle, resulting in an oblate cylinder measuring 12 × 8.5 nm (Figure 3.2b) [75, 96]. Atomic force microscopy (AFM) provides measurements that were comparable to those acquired through alternative methods. The ellipsoidal OPI hexamer has a reported diameter of 12.1 nm [97]. Electron microscopy and small angle X-ray scattering (SAXS) provide evidence for these findings regarding legume proteins. The proteins under consideration exhibit dimensions ranging from 7.5 to 9 nm in height and from 10.4 to 12.6 nm in width [96, 98–100]. Following hexamerization, IA faces exhibit no interaction with IE faces, and IE faces do not preferentially stack with two comparable faces, as indicated by trimer dimensions in legumes. Researchers found that the combination of two trimers results in stronger connections at their IE faces, a phenomenon particularly observed in soy glycinin. This occurs due to the greater exposure of hydrophobic residues, which reduces curling of the IE faces.

Across several length scales, it has been shown that the structure of oat 12S globulin resembles that of 11S legumins and rice glutelin. At the amino acids sequence level, there is a higher degree of resemblance to rice; nonetheless, notable difference exists due to the extensive polymerization occurring in rice. It has been suggested that the quaternary structure of 12S globulin resembles that of legume storage proteins more than those of other cereals [1, 63, 74]. The exact quaternary structure configuration of oat 12S globulin, however, remains compared to those of legumes. Therefore, without precise structural information, it is challenging to precisely discuss about the features of oat protein quaternary structure.

Summary

In recent years, people have become more health-conscious and have transitioned from animal-based to plant-based alternatives. Oats, as a prominent and cost-effective source of high-quality protein, have garnered much attention among cereals. The protein in oats has a balanced profile, making it suitable for integration into various dietary systems. The amino acids contents of oats satisfy the nutritional standards for adults established by the FAO, making it a viable option for consumers. From the digestibility perspective, oat protein has a high score, categorizing it as one of the most favourable plant proteins. Although, this chapter provides fundamental information on oat protein in relation to legume proteins. The information about the precise quaternary structural configuration of oat 12S globulin is, however, lacking compared to that of legumes. Therefore, a comprehensive examination of the three-dimensional structure of oat 12S globulin is essential to validate existing protein structure predictions and to completely understand the structural characteristics of oat protein.

References

1 C. Klose and E. K. Arendt, 'Proteins in oats; their synthesis and changes during germination: a review', *Crit. Rev. Food Sci. Nutr.*, vol. 52, no. 7, pp. 629–639, 2012, https://doi.org/10.1080/10408398.2010.504902.

2 O. A. Sánchez-Velázquez et al., 'Impact of in vitro gastrointestinal digestion on peptide profile and bioactivity of cooked and non-cooked oat protein concentrates', *Curr. Res. Food Sci.*, vol. 4, pp. 93–104, 2021, https://doi.org/10.1016/j.crfs.2021.02.003.

3 S. Senarathna, R. Mel, and M. Malalgoda, 'Utilization of cereal-based protein ingredients in food applications', *J. Cereal Sci* , vol. 116, p. 103867, 2024, https://doi.org/10.1016/j.jcs.2024.103867.

4 R. Li, A. D. True, L. Sha, and Y. L. Xiong, 'Structure–functionality relationship and modification strategies of oat protein: challenges and opportunities', *Compr. Rev. Food Sci. Food Saf.*, vol. 24, no. 1, 2025, https://doi.org/10.1111/1541-4337.70091.

5 I. Joye, 'Protein digestibility of cereal products', *Foods*, vol. 8, no. 6, p. 199, 2019, https://doi.org/10.3390/foods8060199.

6 J. Boye, R. Wijesinha-Bettoni, and B. Burlingame, 'Protein quality evaluation twenty years after the introduction of the protein digestibility corrected amino acid score method', *Br. J. Nutr.*, vol. 108, no. S2, pp. S183–S211, 2012, https://doi.org/10.1017/S0007114512002309.

7 C. P. F. Marinangeli and J. D. House, 'Potential impact of the digestible indispensable amino acid score as a measure of protein quality on dietary regulations and health', *Nutr. Rev.*, vol. 75, no. 8, pp. 658–667, 2017, https://doi.org/10.1093/nutrit/nux025.

8 G. S. Gilani, C. Xiao, and N. Lee, 'Need for accurate and standardized determination of amino acids and bioactive peptides for evaluating protein quality and potential health effects of foods and dietary supplements', *J. AOAC Int.*, vol. 91, no. 4, pp. 894–900, 2008, https://doi.org/10.1093/jaoac/91.4.894.

9 G. Wu, 'Amino acids: metabolism, functions, and nutrition', *Amino Acids*, vol. 37, no. 1, pp. 1–17, 2009, https://doi.org/10.1007/s00726-009-0269-0.

10 EFSA Panel on Dietetic Products, Nutrition and Allergies (NDA), 'Scientific opinion on dietary reference values for protein', *EFSA J.*, vol. 10, no. 2, p. 2557, 2012, https://doi.org/10.2903/j.efsa.2012.2557.

11 'Institute of Medicine. Dietary Reference Intakes for Energy, Carbohydrate, Fiber, Fat, Fatty Acids, Cholesterol, Protein, and Amino Acids', Washington, D.C.: National Academies Press, 2005, https://doi.org/10.17226/10490.

12 S. Adhikari, M. Schop, I. J. M. de Boer, and T. Huppertz, 'Protein quality in perspective: a review of protein quality metrics and their applications', *Nutrients*, vol. 14, no. 5, p. 947, 2022, https://doi.org/10.3390/nu14050947.

13 X. Jing, C. Yang, and L. Zhang, 'Characterization and analysis of protein structures in oat bran', *J. Food Sci.*, vol. 81, no. 10, pp. C2337–C2343, 2016, https://doi.org/https://doi.org/10.1111/1750-3841.13445.

14 FAO, WHO, UNU, 'Protein and amino acid requirements in human nutrition', *World Health Organ. Tech. Rep. Ser.*, no. 935, p. 1, 2007, https://iris.who.int/handle/10665/43411.

15 O. V Kriger, E. V Kashirskikh, O. O. Babich, and S. Y. Noskova, 'Oat protein concentrate production', *Foods Raw Mater.*, vol. 6, no. 1, p. 47, 2018.

16 E. Blomstrand, J. Eliasson, H. K. Karlsson, and R. Köhnke, 'Branched-chain amino acids activate key enzymes in protein synthesis after physical exercise', *J. Nutr.*, vol. 136, no. 1, pp. S269–S273, 2006, https://doi.org/10.1093/jn/136.1.269S.

17 A. M. E. Hoogeveen, P. J. Moughan, E. S. de Haas, P. Blatchford, W. C. McNabb, and C. A. Montoya, 'Ileal and hindgut fermentation in the growing pig fed a human-type diet', *Br. J. Nutr.*, vol. 124, no. 6, pp. 567–576, 2020, https://doi.org/10.1017/S0007114520001385.

18 A. Bonke, S. Sieuwerts, and I. L. Petersen, 'Amino acid composition of novel plant drinks from oat, lentil and pea', *Foods*, vol. 9, no. 4, p. 429, 2020.

19 J. J. Abelilla, Y. Liu, and H. H. Stein, 'Digestible indispensable amino acid score (DIAAS) and protein digestibility corrected amino acid score (PDCAAS) in oat protein concentrate measured in 20- to 30-kilogram pigs', *J. Sci. Food Agric.*, vol. 98, no. 1, pp. 410–414, 2018.

20 L. Kumar, R. Sehrawat, and Y. Kong, 'Oat proteins: a perspective on functional properties', *LWT*, vol. 152, p. 112307, 2021, https://doi.org/10.1016/j.lwt.2021.112307.

21 F. Boukid, 'Oat proteins as emerging ingredients for food formulation: where we stand?' *Eur. Food Res. Technol.*, vol. 247, pp. 1–10, 2021.

22 P. J. Moughan and R. R. Wolfe, 'Determination of dietary amino acid digestibility in humans,' *J. Nutr.*, vol. 149, no. 12, pp. 2101–2109, 2019, https://doi.org/10.1093/jn/nxz211.

23 Y. Tang et al., 'Bioactive components and health functions of oat', *Food Rev. Int.*, vol. 39, no. 7, pp. 4545–4564, 2023, https://doi.org/10.1080/87559129.2022.2029477.

24 H. Rafique et al., 'Dietary-nutraceutical properties of oat protein and peptides', *Front. Nutr.*, vol. 9, pp. 1–14, 2022, https://doi.org/10.3389/fnut.2022.950400.

25 Z.-N. Ling, Y.-F. Jiang, J.-N. Ru, J.-H. Lu, B. Ding, and J. Wu, 'Amino acid metabolism in health and disease', *Signal Transduct. Target. Ther.*, vol. 8, no. 1, p. 345, 2023, https://doi.org/10.1038/s41392-023-01569-3.

26 A. Roberts, 'The safety and regulatory process for amino acids in Europe and the United States', *J. Nutr.*, vol. 146, no. 12, pp. 2635S–2642S, 2016, https://doi.org/10.3945/jn.116.234591.

27 E. Krasniqi, A. Boshnjaku, and L. Petrusevska Tozi, 'Approved health claims for amino acids in/as food supplements', *Maced. Pharm. Bull.*, vol. 62, no. 1, pp. 35–46, 2016, https://doi.org/10.33320/maced.pharm.bull.2016.62.01.003.

28 R. Carta and G. Tola, 'Solubilities of L-cystine, L-tyrosine, L-leucine, and glycine in aqueous solutions at various pHs and NaCl concentrations', *J. Chem. Eng. Data*, vol. 41, no. 3, pp. 414–417, 1996, https://doi.org/10.1021/je9501853.

29 A. A. Pradhan and J. H. Vera, 'Effect of acids and bases on the solubility of amino acids', *Fluid Phase Equilib.*, vol. 152, no. 1, pp. 121–132, 1998, https://doi.org/10.1016/S0378-3812(98)00387-2.

30 H.-C. Tseng, C.-Y. Lee, W.-L. Weng, and I.-M. Shiah, 'Solubilities of amino acids in water at various pH values under 298.15K', *Fluid Phase Equilib.*, vol. 285, no. 1–2, pp. 90–95, 2009, https://doi.org/10.1016/j.fluid.2009.07.017.

31 C. R. Hong, G. W. Lee, H.-D. Paik, P.-S. Chang, and S. J. Choi, 'Nanosuspended branched chain amino acids: the influence of stabilizers on their solubility and colloidal stability', *Food Sci. Biotechnol.*, vol. 26, no. 3, pp. 573–579, 2017, https://doi.org/10.1007/s10068-017-0100-8.

32 C. R. Hong, G. W. Lee, H.-D. Paik, P.-S. Chang, and S. J. Choi, 'Influence of lysolecithin and Tween 80 on the colloidal stability of branched chain amino acids in a nanosuspension system', *Food Chem.*, vol. 221, pp. 606–612, 2017, https://doi.org/10.1016/j.foodchem.2016.11.131.

33 C. R. Hong, G. W. Lee, H.-D. Paik, P.-S. Chang, and S. J. Choi, 'Influence of biopolymers on the solubility of branched-chain amino acids and stability of their solutions', *Food Chem.*, vol. 239, pp. 872–878, 2018, https://doi.org/10.1016/j.foodchem.2017.07.032.

34 C. Schmidt et al., 'Keto leucine and keto isoleucine are bioavailable precursors of their respective amino acids in cell culture media', *J. Biotechnol.*, vol. 321, pp. 1–12, 2020, https://doi.org/10.1016/j.jbiotec.2020.06.013.

35 C. Schmidt et al., 'Lactoyl leucine and isoleucine are bioavailable alternatives for canonical amino acids in cell culture media', *Biotechnol. Bioeng.*, vol. 118, no. 9, pp. 3395–3408, 2021, https://doi.org/10.1002/bit.27755.

36 B. Beckmann et al., 'An improved high cell density cultivation—iHCDC—strategy for leucine auxotrophic *Escherichia coli* K12 ER2507', *Eng. Life Sci.*, vol. 17, no. 8, pp. 857–864, 2017, https://doi.org/10.1002/elsc.201700054.

37 P. Felig, E. Marliss, and G. F. Cahill, 'Plasma amino acid levels and insulin secretion in obesity', *N. Engl. J. Med.*, vol. 281, no. 15, pp. 811–816, 1969, https://doi.org/10.1056/NEJM196910092811503.

38 C. J. Lynch and S. H. Adams, 'Branched-chain amino acids in metabolic signalling and insulin resistance', *Nat. Rev. Endocrinol.*, vol. 10, no. 12, pp. 723–736, 2014, https://doi.org/10.1038/nrendo.2014.171.

39 C. B. Newgard et al., 'A branched-chain amino acid-related metabolic signature that differentiates obese and lean humans and contributes to insulin resistance', *Cell Metab.*, vol. 9, no. 4, pp. 311–326, 2009, https://doi.org/10.1016/j.cmet.2009.02.002.

40 B. C. Batch et al., 'Branched chain amino acids are novel biomarkers for discrimination of metabolic wellness', *Metabolism*, vol. 62, no. 7, pp. 961–969, 2013, https://doi.org/10.1016/j.metabol.2013.01.007.

41 T. M. Filhiol, M. E. Johnstone, and M. B. Zemel, 'Effects of leucine on mitochondrial biogenesis and cell cycle in A-375 melanoma cells', *FASEB J.*, vol. 26, no. S1, 2012, https://doi.org/10.1096/fasebj.26.1_supplement.363.4.

42 F. Li, Y. Yin, B. Tan, X. Kong, and G. Wu, 'Leucine nutrition in animals and humans: mTOR signaling and beyond', *Amino Acids*, vol. 41, no. 5, pp. 1185–1193, 2011, https://doi.org/10.1007/s00726-011-0983-2.

43 X. Sun and M. B. Zemel, 'Leucine modulation of mitochondrial mass and oxygen consumption in skeletal muscle cells and adipocytes', *Nutr. Metab. (Lond).*, vol. 6, no. 1, p. 26, 2009, https://doi.org/10.1186/1743-7075-6-26.

44 A. Molfino, G. Gioia, F. Rossi Fanelli, and M. Muscaritoli, 'Beta-hydroxy-beta-methylbutyrate supplementation in health and disease: a systematic review of

randomized trials', *Amino Acids*, vol. 45, no. 6, pp. 1273–1292, 2013, https://doi.org/10.1007/s00726-013-1592-z.

45 M. Van Koevering and S. Nissen, 'Oxidation of leucine and alpha-ketoisocaproate to beta-hydroxy-beta-methylbutyrate in vivo', *Am. J. Physiol. Metab.*, vol. 262, no. 1, pp. E27–E31, 1992, https://doi.org/10.1152/ajpendo.1992.262.1.E27.

46 Y. Duan et al., 'The role of leucine and its metabolites in protein and energy metabolism', *Amino Acids*, vol. 48, no. 1, pp. 41–51, 2016, https://doi.org/10.1007/s00726-015-2067-1.

47 C. A. Fitch, G. Platzer, M. Okon, B. Garcia-Moreno E., and L. P. McIntosh, 'Arginine: its pKa value revisited', *Protein Sci.*, vol. 24, no. 5, pp. 752–761, 2015, https://doi.org/10.1002/pro.2647.

48 M. N. Gupta and V. N. Uversky, 'Biological importance of arginine: a comprehensive review of the roles in structure, disorder, and functionality of peptides and proteins', *Int. J. Biol. Macromol.*, vol. 257, p. 128646, 2024, https://doi.org/10.1016/j.ijbiomac.2023.128646.

49 A. X. Jones et al., 'Improving mass spectrometry analysis of protein structures with arginine-selective chemical cross-linkers', *Nat. Commun.*, vol. 10, no. 1, p. 3911, 2019, https://doi.org/10.1038/s41467-019-11917-z.

50 P. Gagneux, 'Protein structure and function', *J. Hered.*, vol. 95, no. 3, p. 274, 2004, https://doi.org/10.1093/jhered/esh040.

51 N. R. Seddon, 'Biochemistry (third edition)', *Biochem. Educ.*, vol. 16, no. 3, pp. 181–182, 1988, https://doi.org/10.1016/0307-4412(88)90210-5.

52 B. Tong and A. Barbul, 'Cellular and physiological effects of arginine', *Mini Rev. Med. Chem.*, vol. 4, no. 8, pp. 823–832, 2004, https://doi.org/10.2174/1389557043403305.

53 M. Holeček, 'Aspartic acid in health and disease', *Nutrients*, vol. 15, no. 18, p. 4023, 2023, https://doi.org/10.3390/nu15184023.

54 P. Kandasamy, G. Gyimesi, Y. Kanai, and M. A. Hediger, 'Amino acid transporters revisited: new views in health and disease', *Trends Biochem. Sci.*, vol. 43, no. 10, pp. 752–789, 2018, https://doi.org/10.1016/j.tibs.2018.05.003.

55 T. V. Nieto-Nieto, Y. X. Wang, L. Ozimek, and L. Chen, 'Inulin at low concentrations significantly improves the gelling properties of oat protein – a molecular mechanism study', *Food Hydrocoll.*, vol. 50, pp. 116–127, 2015, https://doi.org/10.1016/J.FOODHYD.2015.03.031.

56 O. Nivala, O. E. Mäkinen, K. Kruus, E. Nordlund, and D. Ercili-Cura, 'Structuring colloidal oat and faba bean protein particles via enzymatic modification', *Food Chem.*, vol. 231, pp. 87–95, 2017.

57 B. Zhang, X. Guo, K. Zhu, W. Peng, and H. Zhou, 'Improvement of emulsifying properties of oat protein isolate–dextran conjugates by glycation', *Carbohydr. Polym.*, vol. 127, pp. 168–175, 2015.

58 C. Yang, Y. Wang, and L. Chen, 'Fabrication, characterization and controlled release properties of oat protein gels with percolating structure induced by cold gelation', *Food Hydrocoll.*, vol. 62, pp. 21–34, 2017, https://doi.org/10.1016/J.FOODHYD.2016.07.023.

59 M. A. Shotwell, C. Afonso, E. Davies, R. S. Chesnut, and B. A. Larkins, 'Molecular characterization of oat seed globulins', *Plant Physiol.*, vol. 87, no. 3, pp. 698–704, 1988, https://doi.org/10.1104/pp.87.3.698.

60 J. McLauchlan, A. I. I. Tyler, B. Chakrabarti, C. Orfila, and A. Sarkar, 'Oat protein: review of structure-function synergies with other plant proteins', *Food Hydrocoll.*, vol. 154, p. 110139, 2024, https://doi.org/10.1016/j.foodhyd.2024.110139.

61 M. F. Marcone, Y. Kakuda, and R. Y. Yada, 'Salt-soluble seed globulins of dicotyledonous and monocotyledonous plants II. Structural characterization', *Food Chem.*, vol. 63, no. 2, pp. 265–274, 1998, https://doi.org/10.1016/S0308-8146(97)00159-3.

62 M. Adachi et al., 'Crystal structure of soybean 11S globulin: glycinin A3B4 homohexamer', *Proc. Natl. Acad. Sci.*, vol. 100, no. 12, pp. 7395–7400, 2003, https://doi.org/10.1073/pnas.0832158100.

63 S. R. Burgess, P. R. Shewry, G. J. Matlashewski, I. Altosaar, and B. J. Miflin, 'Characteristics of oat (*Avena sativa* L.) seed globulins', *J. Exp. Bot.*, vol. 34, no. 10, pp. 1320–1332, 1983, https://doi.org/10.1093/jxb/34.10.1320.

64 T. A. Egorov, A. K. Musolyamov, J. S. Andersen, and P. Roepstorff, 'The complete amino acid sequence and disulphide bond arrangement of oat alcohol-soluble avenin-3', *Eur. J. Biochem.*, vol. 224, no. 2, pp. 631–638, 1994, https://doi.org/10.1111/j.1432-1033.1994.00631.x.

65 B. Wang et al., 'Insights into formation, detection and removal of the beany flavor in soybean protein', *Trends Food Sci. Technol.*, vol. 112, pp. 336–347, 2021, https://doi.org/10.1016/j.tifs.2021.04.018.

66 Y. V. Wu, K. R. Sexson, J. F. Cavins, and G. E. Inglett, 'Oats and their dry-milled fractions. Protein isolation and properties of four varieties', *J. Agric. Food Chem.*, vol. 20, no. 4, pp. 757–761, 1972, https://doi.org/10.1021/jf60182a022.

67 P. R. Shewry and M. J. Pandya, 'The 2S albumin storage proteins', In: Seed Proteins (ed. P. R. Shewry and R. Casey), Dordrecht: Springer Netherlands, pp. 563–586, 1999.

68 R. J. Youle and A. H. C. Huang, 'Occurrence of low molecular weight and high cysteine containing albumin storage proteins in oilseeds of diverse species', *Am. J. Bot.*, vol. 68, no. 1, pp. 44–48, 1981, https://doi.org/10.1002/j.1537-2197.1981.tb06354.x.

69 L. Radomir, 'The Chemistry of Cereal Proteins', Routledge, 2017.

70 C. Y. Ma and V. R. Harwalkar, 'Chemical characterization and functionality assessment of oat protein fractions', *J. Agric. Food Chem.*, vol. 32, no. 1, pp. 144–149, 1984, https://doi.org/10.1021/jf00121a035.

71 L. S. Robert, C. Nozzolillo, A. Cudjoe, and I. Altosaar, 'Total solubilization of groat proteins in high protein oat (*Avena sativa* L. cv. Hinoat): evidence that glutelins are a minor component', *Can. Inst. Food Sci. Technol. J.*, vol. 16, no. 3, pp. 196–200, 1983, https://doi.org/10.1016/S0315-5463(83)72207-8.

72 K. Kitamura and K. Shibasaki, 'Isolation and some physico-chemical properties of the acidic subunits of soybean 11S globulin', *Agric. Biol. Chem.*, vol. 39, no. 5, pp. 945–951, 1975, https://doi.org/10.1080/00021369.1975.10861718.

73 G. Walburg and B. A. Larkins, 'Oat seed globulin', *Plant Physiol.*, vol. 72, no. 1, pp. 161–165, 1983, https://doi.org/10.1104/pp.72.1.161.

74 D. M. Peterson, 'Subunit structure and composition of oat seed globulin', *Plant Physiol.*, vol. 62, no. 4, pp. 506–509, 1978, https://doi.org/10.1104/pp.62.4.506.

75 M. A. Shotwell, 'Oat globulins', In: Seed Proteins (ed. P. R. Shewry and R. Casey), Dordrecht: Springer Netherlands, pp. 389–400, 1999.

76 T.-N. Wen and D. S. Luthe, 'Biochemical characterization of rice glutelin', *Plant Physiol.*, vol. 78, no. 1, pp. 172–177, 1985, https://doi.org/10.1104/pp.78.1.172.

77 N. Kamal et al., 'The mosaic oat genome gives insights into a uniquely healthy cereal crop', *Nature*, vol. 606, no. 7912, pp. 113–119, 2022, https://doi.org/10.1038/s41586-022-04732-y.

78 L. Amagliani, J. O'Regan, A. L. Kelly, and J. A. O'Mahony, 'The composition, extraction, functionality and applications of rice proteins: a review', *Trends Food Sci. Technol.*, vol. 64, pp. 1–12, 2017, https://doi.org/10.1016/j.tifs.2017.01.008.

79 E. Derbyshire, D. J. Wright, and D. Boulter, 'Legumin and vicilin, storage proteins of legume seeds', *Phytochemistry*, vol. 15, no. 1, pp. 3–24, 1976, https://doi.org/10.1016/S0031-9422(00)89046-9.

80 D. Fukushima, 'Structures of plant storage proteins and their functions', *Food Rev. Int.*, vol. 7, no. 3, pp. 353–381, 1991, https://doi.org/10.1080/87559129109540916.

81 S. Moelbert, E. Emberly, and C. Tang, 'Correlation between sequence hydrophobicity and surface-exposure pattern of database proteins', *Protein Sci.*, vol. 13, no. 3, pp. 752–762, 2004, https://doi.org/10.1110/ps.03431704.

82 S. Simm, J. Einloft, O. Mirus, and E. Schleiff, '50 years of amino acid hydrophobicity scales: revisiting the capacity for peptide classification', *Biol. Res.*, vol. 49, no. 1, p. 31, 2016, https://doi.org/10.1186/s40659-016-0092-5.

83 J. Jumper et al., 'Highly accurate protein structure prediction with AlphaFold', *Nature*, vol. 596, no. 7873, pp. 583–589, 2021, https://doi.org/10.1038/s41586-021-03819-2.

84 R. Schubert, H. Bäumlein, A. Czihal, and U. Wobus, 'Genomic sequence of a 12S seed storage protein gene from oat (*Avena sativa* L. cv. 'Solidor')', *Nucleic Acids Res.*, vol. 18, no. 2, pp. 377–377, 1990, https://doi.org/10.1093/nar/18.2.377.

85 M. Adachi, Y. Takenaka, A. B. Gidamis, B. Mikami, and S. Utsumi, 'Crystal structure of soybean proglycinin A1aB1b homotrimer', *J. Mol. Biol.*, vol. 305, no. 2, pp. 291–305, 2001, https://doi.org/10.1006/jmbi.2000.4310.

86 M. R. G. Tandang-Silvas et al., 'Conservation and divergence on plant seed 11S globulins based on crystal structures', *Biochim. Biophys. Acta - Proteins Proteomics*, vol. 1804, no. 7, pp. 1432–1442, 2010, https://doi.org/10.1016/j.bbapap.2010.02.016.

87 J. M. Dunwell, J. G. Gibbings, T. Mahmood, and S. M. Saqlan Naqvi, 'Germin and germin-like proteins: evolution, structure, and function', *CRC. Crit. Rev. Plant Sci.*, vol. 27, no. 5, pp. 342–375, 2008, https://doi.org/10.1080/07352680802333938.

88 M. A. Moreira, M. A. Hermodson, B. A. Larkins, and N. C. Nielsen, 'Partial characterization of the acidic and basic polypeptides of glycinin', *J. Biol. Chem.*, vol. 254, no. 19, pp. 9921–9926, 1979, https://doi.org/10.1016/S0021-9258(19)83605-0.

89 D. Yusuf, A. M. Davis, G. J. Kleywegt, and S. Schmitt, 'An alternative method for the evaluation of docking performance: RSR vs RMSD', *J. Chem. Inf. Model.*, vol. 48, no. 7, pp. 1411–1422, 2008, https://doi.org/10.1021/ci800084x.

90 L. F. De la Cruz-Torres et al., 'Physicochemical and functional properties of 11S globulin from chan (*Hyptis suaveolens* L. poit) seeds', *J. Cereal Sci.*, vol. 77, pp. 66–72, 2017, https://doi.org/10.1016/j.jcs.2017.06.017.

91 R. Jung et al., 'The role of proteolysis in the processing and assembly of 11S seed globulins', *Plant Cell*, vol. 10, no. 3, pp. 343–357, 1998, https://doi.org/10.1105/tpc.10.3.343.

92 T. Kumamaru et al., 'Vacuolar processing enzyme plays an essential role in the crystalline structure of glutelin in rice seed', *Plant Cell Physiol.*, vol. 51, no. 1, pp. 38–46, 2010, https://doi.org/10.1093/pcp/pcp165.

93 M. P. Scott, R. Jung, K. Muntz, and N. C. Nielsen, 'A protease responsible for post-translational cleavage of a conserved Asn-Gly linkage in glycinin, the major seed storage protein of soybean', *Proc. Natl. Acad. Sci.*, vol. 89, no. 2, pp. 658–662, 1992, https://doi.org/10.1073/pnas.89.2.658.

94 Y. Wakasa, L. Yang, S. Hirose, and F. Takaiwa, 'Expression of unprocessed glutelin precursor alters polymerization without affecting trafficking and accumulation', *J. Exp. Bot.*, vol. 60, no. 12, pp. 3503–3511, 2009, https://doi.org/10.1093/jxb/erp187.

95 P. Plietz, B. Drescher, and G. Damaschun, 'Structure and evolution of the 11S globulins: conclusions from comparative evaluation of amino acid sequences and X-ray scattering datal', *Biochem. und Physiol. der Pflanz.*, vol. 183, no. 2–3, pp. 199–203, 1988, https://doi.org/10.1016/S0015-3796(88)80100-8.

96 Y. Zhao, Y. Mine, and C.-Y. Ma, 'Study of thermal aggregation of oat globulin by laser light scattering', *J. Agric. Food Chem.*, vol. 52, no. 10, pp. 3089–3096, 2004, https://doi.org/10.1021/jf030735y.

97 G. Liu et al., 'Composition, secondary structure, and self-assembly of oat protein isolate', *J. Agric. Food Chem.*, vol. 57, no. 11, pp. 4552–4558, 2009, https://doi.org/10.1021/jf900135e.

98 R. A. Badley, D. Atkinson, H. Hauser, D. Oldani, J. P. Green, and J. M. Stubbs, 'The structure, physical and chemical properties of the soy bean protein glycinin', *Biochim. Biophys. Acta - Protein Struct.*, vol. 412, no. 2, pp. 214–228, 1975, https://doi.org/10.1016/0005-2795(75)90036-7.

99 P. Plietz, G. Damaschun, J. J. Müller, and K. Schwenke, 'The structure of 11-S globulins from sunflower and rape seed', *Eur. J. Biochem.*, vol. 130, no. 2, pp. 315–320, 1983, https://doi.org/10.1111/j.1432-1033.1983.tb07154.x.

100 P. Plietz, D. Zirwer, B. Schlesier, K. Gast, and G. Damaschun, 'Shape, symmetry, hydration and secondary structure of the legumin from *Vicia faba* in solution', *Biochim. Biophys. Acta - Protein Struct. Mol. Enzymol.*, vol. 784, no. 2–3, pp. 140–146, 1984, https://doi.org/10.1016/0167-4838(84)90120-1.

4

Extraction and Purification Technologies of Oat Protein

4.1 Introduction

Conventional plant protein extraction often consists of four stages: (i) cell disruption, (ii) protein solubilization, (iii) protein precipitation at the isoelectric point (pI) and (iv) protein concentration or separation [1]. Physical activities, such as seed coat removal and size reduction, damage plant cells and release their constituents. Following the removal of moisture and fat, the protein is solubilized in chemical solvents, resulting in complete dissolution. Amphiphilic proteins are zwitterions at their isoelectric pH. Protein surfaces are negatively charged above the pI and positively charged below the pI. The equilibrium of negative and positive charges at the pI reduces electrostatic forces, resulting in attractive forces that collect and precipitate proteins [2]. This provides the framework for protein extraction at the pI. The extraction process of protein produces a variety of components, including concentrates, isolate and hydrolysate [3]. Protein concentrate is created by removing non-protein components, mostly carbohydrates, using hydroalcoholic solutions and acidic water to enhance protein concentration. Protein isolate, on the other hand, is produced by solubilizing the protein in salt water or a solution with a pH that deviates considerably from the pI. Protein hydrolysate is composed of peptides and amino acids resulting from protein degradation via enzymatic action, acid treatment, alkaline treatment or fermentation [4–6].

Extraction conditions significantly influence the yield, purity and overall quality of oat protein [7]. Based on protein content and accompanying constituents, extracted oat proteins are commonly classified into three product types: (i) oat protein isolate (OPI), a relatively pure fraction containing > 80% protein; (ii) oat protein concentrate (OPC), containing 50–80% protein and retaining higher levels of native lipids, carbohydrates and dietary fibre; and (iii) protein-rich oat flour (OF), typically < 50% protein with proportionally greater amounts of non-protein components [8]. Because of its high purity, OPI is frequently employed in structure–function studies where non-protein constituents might confound rheological and microstructural measurements. It is important to note, however, that although OPI is dominated by globulins, it remains a mixture rather than a single, homogeneous protein. This compositional complexity complicates the attribution of specific functional roles, as individual proteins within the mixture may contribute differently to observed behaviours. Moreover, even low-level impurities can modulate protein structure and functionality and should therefore be considered when interpreting experimental results. From a practical standpoint, OPI is generally restricted to research and pilot-scale contexts and is not typically available through retail channels. In contrast, most commercial oat protein ingredients are OPCs with protein contents typically in the 50–60% range. This divergence between research materials and market-available products underscores a key translational challenge, findings generated with OPI may not directly extrapolate to applications where OPC is the prevalent ingredient. This chapter covers the traditional and advanced extraction and purification strategies, as well as highlights existing challenges for oat protein extraction. Table 4.1 presents the advantage and disadvantages of different protein extraction methods.

4.2 Defatting of Oat Flour

Oats are distinctive among cereal grains due to their relatively high fat content, which significantly influences the functionality, oxidative stability and aromatic profile of extracted oat protein [17]. Consequently, defatting is an essential pretreatment step to enhance protein yield and purity by minimizing the interference of lipids during extraction. Defatting of oat flour is most commonly achieved through solvent extraction, with hexane being widely employed owing to its chemical inertness and high extraction efficiency. Typically, oat flour is mixed with the organic solvent at a solid-to-solvent ratio ranging from 1 : 2 to 1 : 5 (w/v), and stirred for 45 minutes to 1 hour. Following extraction, the lipid containing is removed by filtration or centrifugation, leaving a nominally 'fat-free' flour, although trace amounts of residual lipids may remain. Studies has demonstrated that protein extracted from hexane-defatted oat flour exhibit improved purity, solubility and thermal stability compared with those obtained from non-defatted flour [18]. In addition, key functional properties, particularly emulsifying activity and emulsion stability, are significantly enhanced. These findings highlight the importance of lipid removal not only for improving protein extraction efficiency but also for optimizing protein functionality.

Beyond hexane, alternative strategies have been explored to improve lipid removal from oat flour. Recent investigations have shown that ethanol and supercritical carbon dioxide (SC-CO_2) treatment are both highly effective in reducing lipid content. In ethanol-based defatting, crude protein concentrate (OPC) is mixed with ethanol at a ratio of 1 : 6 (w/v) and heated at 65 °C for 4 hours. The solvent is then removed, and the residual biomass is dried at 65 °C for 24 hours. This process reduces the oil content from 20.6 to 4.9%, a performance that exceeds that of hexane extraction, likely due to the polarity of ethanol, which facilitates the extraction of phospholipids—one of the major lipid fractions in oat groats. Moreover, SC-CO_2 extraction, conducted at a CO_2 flow rate of 5.5 kg/h and pressures of 285–300 bar for 4 hours, demonstrated even greater efficiency, reducing oil content from 20.6 to 3.5% [19]. This technique is particularly attractive because of its non-toxic, solvent free and environmentally benign nature, positioning SC-CO_2, as a promising alternative to conventional organic solvent-based defatting methods.

Overall, the defatting approaches discussed not only enhance the purity of extracted oat proteins but also substantially improve their functional properties, thereby supporting more efficient and sustainable protein extraction processes.

Table 4.1 Advantages and disadvantages of different extraction methods.

Extraction method	Advantages	Disadvantages	References
Aqueous extraction	High solubility and stability of extracted protein	Energy intensive and time-taking process. Isolate protein with lower inferior quality	[9]
Chemical extraction	Economical with Improved digestibility and bioavailability of extracted protein	Non-ecofriendly, low yield, energy extensive, amino acid loss and low protein quality due to denaturation	[9, 10]
Ultrasonic-assisted extraction	Green, energy-efficient and low maintenance technology that require minimal solvent use and offer improved protein yield. Enhanced intramolecular bonding, decreases Hydrophobicity and improves emulsification and gelation properties	Potentially change protein structure, might alter nutritional and functional properties	[9, 11]
Enzyme-assisted extraction	Increase protein yield and solubility. Smaller protein fractions and prevent complex formation between proteins and other components	Require specific range of pH to execute. May cause excess protein degradation which reduce affect the functionality	[10]
Pulsed electric field (PEF)	Water can be used and minimize organic solvent usage, provide non-toxic extraction. Reduced extraction time and temperature. Processing not negatively effects the protein quality	Low yield compared to other methods and expensive	[12, 13]
Microwave-assisted extraction	Shorter extraction time, improved yield with better efficiency. Less solvent consumption and non-toxic, can be used for larger volume extraction	Generate high amount of thermal energy, may cause degradation of heat sensitive bioactive compounds	[14, 15]
High-pressure processing	Fast extraction and high yield with less impurities. Heat sensitive components can be extracted without degradation at ambient temperature	This process cannot extract higher amount of protein, also decrease the protein solubility	[16]

4.3 Liquid-assisted Protein Extraction

In liquid-assisted extraction methods, oat proteins are typically extracted using aqueous solutions and fractionated through processes such as centrifugation or decantation [20]. Isoelectric precipitation and membrane filtration are two procedures that can be used to produce a higher level of concentration. The innovative alkali extraction technique for oat protein was proposed by Cluskey, Wall and Inglett [21], who suggested that an alkaline solution (0.015 M NaOH, pH 7.83, with a solid to solvent ratio of 1 : 10) could be used to extract 88% of the total nitrogen in oats, which resulted in the production of an oat protein concentration (OPC) that had a protein content of 72.1%. This resulted in a much reduced nitrogen recovery at 57 and 19% respectively, when the extraction was performed at lower pH values (7.00 and 6.25) subsequent studies have adopted and refined variation of this method [22–24]. Alkaline extraction followed by isoelectric precipitation can yield both OPCs and OPIs with protein contents ranging from 72.4 to 92.6%, and protein recovery rates between 60.4 and 72.1% [25]. The wide variation in purity observed can primarily be attributed to differences in the defatting process and centrifugation conditions employed. Defatting oat raw material prior to extraction generally results in a higher protein content in the final oat protein fraction, though it does not significantly influence the protein recovery. Most of the increase in protein content can be attributed to the lower lipid content in the defatted material. Other studies have also demonstrated that protein recovery is often poorer with acid extraction ($pH \leq 4$) compared to alkaline extraction ($pH \geq 8$) [21, 23].

Optimization of both alkaline and acid extraction processes conducted by adjusting parameters such as pH, extraction duration, temperature and solid-to-solvent ratio. Under optimal conditions (solid: solvent ratio of 1 : 10), alkaline extraction at pH 11.5 (using NaOH) resulted in a protein recovery of 75.5%, while acid extraction at pH 3.0 (using HCl) yielded a lower recovery of 54.6% [23]. In contrast, recovery rates were much lower for salt extraction, with 1 M NaCl yielding around 38% recovery, and 0.5 M $CaCl_2$ resulting in only 25% recovery [21, 26]. As a result of investigations that have been conducted, it is clear that alkaline extraction, in particular when combined with isoelectric precipitation, has the potential to provide oat protein components that are of highest yield and purity. Alkaline extraction methods have also been successfully applied to defatted oat bran [22, 27, 28]. Oat bran, which is derived from oat groats or flakes, has a higher protein content (18–32%) compared to oat flour [21]. However, extracting protein from oat bran presents unique challenges due to the close association between proteins and fibre, particularly β-glucans, which increase the viscosity of the slurry and make extraction more difficult [29]. OPC with 73.4% protein was successfully produced from oat bran using the alkaline extraction method [22]. In addition, it was discovered that the effectiveness of protein extraction from oat bran might be enhanced by pretreating the bran with the commercial enzyme Viscozyme® L, which is a combination of various carbohydrates. Under optimum alkaline extraction conditions (30 minutes, 50 °C, pH 9.5 and a solid to solvent ratio of 1 : 10), this pretreatment enhanced protein recovery from 14.8% (without pretreatment) to 56.2% (with pretreatment) [27]. Other carbohydrases, such as α-amylase and amyloglucosidase, also improved extraction efficiency, with amyloglucosidase achieving the highest protein purity (82%) [28].

Despite the numerous studies showing successful protein extraction using alkaline methods, it is essential to note that alkaline treatments can adversely affect the nutritional and techno-functional properties of the extracted proteins. For example, prolonged exposure to high alkaline conditions can lead to the formation of lysinoalanine, which reduces the availability of lysine and can be toxic. Alkaline circumstances at high temperature (65 °C) have been reported to results in the synthesis of lysinoalanine in wheat gluten, soy protein and lactalbumin [30]. In addition, Ma and his colleagues evaluated the effects of oat globulins being exposed to an alkaline environment for a longer period of time (24–26 hours) at temperature ranging from 25 to 55 °C. After 96 hours of alkaline incubation, their findings showed that the denaturation temperature increased nearly 107 °C (without any exposure to alkaline) to approximately 111 °C. This indicates that more stable protein aggregates were formed. However, the incubation temperature also influenced other properties: surface hydrophobicity increased at 25 °C but decreased at 37 °C [30]. These findings highlight the need for careful optimization of extraction conditions to avoid compromising the nutritional and functional qualities of the extracted oat protein.

In conclusion, while alkaline extraction remains the most effective method for extracting high-yield, high-purity oat protein, the conditions must be carefully controlled to preserve both the protein's nutritional value and functional properties. The choice of extraction method and the pretreatment processes, such as defatting and enzymatic treatment, can significantly influence the final protein quality and yield, which is critical for applications in food and nutrition.

4.4 Protein Extraction with Dry Fractionation Method

Currently, the most frequently employed methods for producing plant protein concentrates and isolates are the wet extraction techniques previously discussed. Nevertheless, the processing method necessitates a significant amount of energy because of the extensive dilutions and the subsequent removal of water by drying [31]. The energy required for dry fractionation techniques, including air classification and electrostatic separation, is considerably lower. In contrast to wet techniques, dry fractionation methods offer the advantage of retaining a higher quantity of nutrients within the protein component. This represents a further competitive advantage. Protein ingredients derived from dry methods generally exhibit lower purity, indicated by reduced protein content, compared to those obtained via wet methods. The separation process is hindered by the variations in particle characteristics, such as size and charge, of the various components present in the raw material. A study indicates the effectiveness of dry fractionation of oat flours is significantly constrained by the small granule size of oat starches [32]. The presence of anti-nutritional components in the final protein fraction resulting from dry fractionation techniques represents a further drawback of these methods. These compounds may adversely affect certain plant protein sources.

First time categorization process of oat flour was introduced by Wu and Stringfellow in 1973. A protein-rich fraction comprising 83–88% protein was obtained from defatted oat flour using pentane and hexane, with a protein recovery of 7–16%. This was achieved following two successive air classification processes [33]. Subsequent research introduced refinements to the air classification process, notably by incorporating SC–CO_2 extraction as a lipid removal step prior to fractionation [34]. Sibakov et al. (2011) successfully obtained a protein concentrate containing 73% oat protein through a series of cascade air classification procedures [34]. Prior to the air classification phases, both procedures incorporated a step for the removal of lipids from oats through CO_2-supercritical extraction. It is evident that the removal of lipids from lipid-rich materials is beneficial. This is as a result of the fact that, lipid rich particles have a poor dispersion in air [34]. A finer oat flour was produce as a consequence of the defatting step that used CO2 supercritical, which ultimately led to an improvement in the air classification process that ultimately followed [34]. A modification in the structure of oat flour [35] and a reduction in the aggregation of starch granules [36], are proposed explanations for these results. These modifications occur when a defatting procedure is performed before the air classification process. The Technical Research Centre of Finland (VTT) has issued a patent outlining a technique for defatting oat flour via of CO_2-supercritical extraction, succeeded by sieving or air classification to yield diverse fractions. A fraction is enriched in oat protein was acquired, comprising 50–80% protein. Cascade air classification stages seem to be an efficient dry extraction technique, according to existing literature, for generating high purity techno-functional OPCs from CO_2-supercritical defatted oat flour.

In addition to the protein-rich fraction, it is important to note that both wet and dry fractionation procedures yield multiple fractions beyond the protein-rich component. The fractions contain substantial quantities of lipids, starch and β-glucans [33, 34]. These components must be employed for food or feed applications to be effectively utilized. A second advantage of dry fractionation over wet extraction techniques is the absence of the requirement for chemicals or salts. This enables the use of the remaining fractions without requiring additional treatment.

4.5 Advanced Protein Extraction Methods

Green chemistry is recognized as a significant development in scientific research aimed at promoting environmental sustainability. The extraction of natural products through green chemistry enhances the production of safer food components, boosts extraction yields, improves nutritional and functional attributes and offers opportunities for clean labelling [8, 37]. Furthermore, the novel protein extraction method has the potential to offer enhanced purity, reduced solvent usage, minimized energy costs and lower waste generation compared to conventional extraction methods [38]. This thoroughly examines the mechanisms, benefits and constraints of advanced protein extraction technologies, including deep eutectic solvents (DES), ultrasonic-assisted extraction (UAE), enzyme-assisted extraction (EAE), pulsed electric field (PEF), reverse micelles extraction (RME) and subcritical water extraction (SWE). These methods are frequently classified as environmentally friendly approaches, particularly for plant-based proteins. Furthermore, the utilization of these extraction technologies surpasses traditional protein extraction method, regarding yield and functional characteristics.

4.5.1 Deep Eutectic Protein Extraction

Traditional protein extraction methods including alkaline extraction and acid precipitation, contribute to the environmental pollution and can potentially denature the protein. In response to these limitations, DESs have emerged as promising green alternatives for biomolecule extraction due to their tuneable physicochemical properties, low toxicity and biodegradability [39].

In this context, the application of DESs for oat protein extraction has been explored to improve efficiency and reduce environmental impact. In particular, choline chloride (ChCl) and 1-hexyl-3-methylimidazolium chloride ([HMIm][Cl]) were employed as hydrogen bond acceptors (HBAs), while ethylene glycol, glycerol and 1,4-butanediol served as hydrogen bond donors (HBDs). Various combinations of these HBAs and

HBDs were systematically evaluated to determine the influence of solvent composition, solid-to-liquid ratio, extraction temperature and time on the overall protein recovery. Two optimal DES-based systems were identified. The first, termed DES-1, utilized an HBA : HBD ratio of 1 : 2, a solid–liquid ratio of 1 : 10, and was operated at 80 °C for 120 minutes. The second, DES-4, was optimized with a 1 : 1 HBA : HBD ratio, a solid–liquid ratio of 1 : 12, and an extraction temperature of 60 °C for the same duration. Comparative analysis indicated that DES-4 yielded a higher protein recovery than DES-1 under their respective conditions [39].

To further enhance the extraction process, a deep eutectic system (DESys)-based method was developed. This approach was intended to minimize processing steps and energy consumption while maintaining or improving recovery efficiency. Interestingly, although DESys-4 demonstrated lower protein recovery compared to DESys-1, this outcome was attributed to the direct interaction of [HMIm][Cl] with oat proteins, potentially disrupting protein folding, aggregation behaviour, and structural stability. Both DES- and DESys-based methods exhibited superior protein yields compared to conventional alkali-solubilization/acid-precipitation (ASAP) techniques. Characterization of the extracted proteins revealed that the choice of extraction method significantly influenced the physicochemical properties of the proteins, indicating that DESs and DESys may also serve as tools for tailoring protein functionality [39].

Despite these advantages, it is important to consider the potential toxicity associated with ionic liquids (ILs), such as [HMIm][Cl]. Although hydroxyl-functionalized ILs may exhibit reduced toxicity, they generally remain less biocompatible than ChCl-based systems. Therefore, from both environmental and safety perspective, ChCl-based DESys approaches are more suitable for oat protein extraction [40, 41]. Overall, the development and optimization of DES- and DESys-based extraction strategies present a promising direction for sustainable and efficient oat protein recovery. These systems offer valuable insights into the design of future green solvents for biomolecular extraction and may help bridge the performance gap between traditional ILs and emerging DES technologies.

4.5.2 Ultrasonic-assisted Protein Extraction

Ultrasonic technology employs mechanical waves generated at frequencies above 20 kHz, which lie beyond the audible range for humans (20 Hz–20 kHz). In food processing applications, ultrasonic frequencies typically ranges from 20 to 100 kHz are widely utilized. The fundamental mechanism of ultrasound-assisted extraction (UAE) is cavitation, a phenomenon involving the formation, growth, subsequent implosion of microbubbles within a liquid medium [42]. Cavitation generates intense localised mechanical and thermal energy, thereby facilitating the release of biomolecules from solid matrices. As a result, the plant cell wall structure is disrupted, leading to cell rupture and the formation of microchannels that enhance solvent penetration (e.g. alkalis or acidic solutions) through the cellular pores, ultimately promoting protein dissolution (Figure 4.1) [43].

Ultrasound represents a significant advancement over conventional extraction technologies in food sector, offering advantages such as reduced processing time and energy consumption, lower installation and maintenance costs and operation at relatively low temperatures [44]. Consequently, numerous studies have focused on optimizing key parameters, including pH, temperature and extraction time UAE to maximise protein

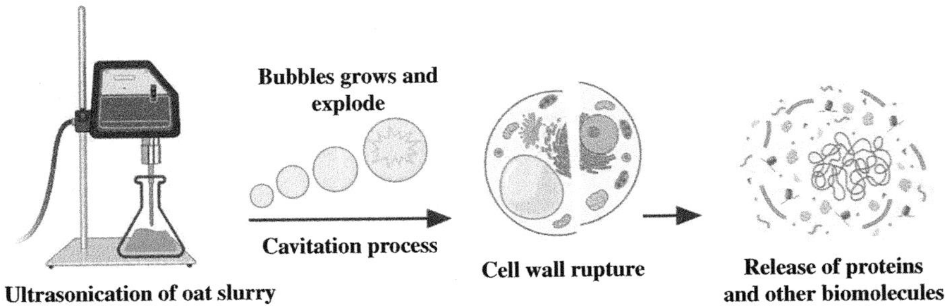

Figure 4.1 Ultrasound-assisted extraction of oat protein.

recovery during UAE. Orellana-Palacios [45] identified optimal extraction conditions at pH of 10.5, a temperature of 41.8 °C and an extraction time of 26.1 minutes, resulting in the highest extraction yield (17.3%) and protein content (65.6%). A distinct study indicated an 82.6% recovery of pea protein under particular extraction conditions: a solid-to-liquid ratio of 1 : 11.5 (g : mL), a pH of 9.6, an extraction duration of 13.5 minutes and an ultrasonic amplitude of 33.7% [46]. Protein yield increased significantly (76.83%) when ultrasonic conditions were applied at 80% amplitude for 30 minutes at 60% duty cycle when compared to the traditional extraction technique (32.48%) [47]. Ultrasound-assisted extraction has also been successfully employed to recover proteins from defatted mulberry seeds, with optimal conditions including a solid-to-liquid ratio of 1 : 40, a temperature of 60 °C, an extraction time of 9 minutes and an output power of 600 W [48].

Despite its potential, UAE has certain limitations. Optimal conditions vary depending on the type of plant protein source. Proteins are susceptible to degradation or denaturation if UAE temperatures are not properly controlled. Furthermore, free radicals generated during UAE can induce protein oxidation, potentially modifying the structure and functionality of the extracted proteins. The industrial application of UAE remains underexploited. Therefore, it is essential to optimise extraction parameters, maintain precise temperature control during sonication and expand pilot-scale studies to facilitate the industrial adoption of UAE.

4.5.3 Enzyme-assisted Extraction

The plant cell wall is composed primarily of a complex network of interconnected polysaccharides, including cellulose, hemicellulose, pectin and starch. This structural matrix acts as a physical barrier that restricts protein release during conventional extraction processes. Enzymes play a crucial role in enzyme-assisted extraction (EAE) by hydrolyzing cell wall components and disrupting the cellular matrix, thereby catalyzing the breakdown of structural barriers (Figure 4.2). This enzymatic action facilitates the release of intracellular proteins into the solvent, leading to accelerated extraction kinetics and improved extraction yields [49]. Commonly employed enzymes in EAE include pectinases, cellulases, hemicellulases, amylases and proteases, which may be applied individually or in combination depending on the substrate and extraction objectives [50].

EAE has demonstrated considerable potential in enhancing extraction efficiency, reducing processing time, minimizing damage to bioactive compounds and enabling the recovery

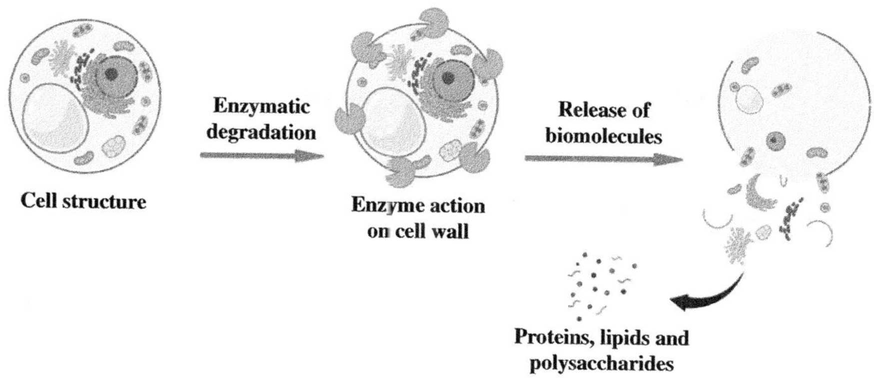

Figure 4.2 Enzyme-assisted extraction of oat protein.

of heat-sensitive and unstable components. Coniglio Díaz, Barua, Albertó and Zapata [51] conducted a comparative study between EAE, commercial EAE formulations and traditional extraction methods r, reporting that EAE yielded 557–827% higher protein content at 0 h compared with approaches. Furthermore, nanoparticles derived from enzymatically extracted proteins exhibited superior structural and functional features compared to those obtained via alkali-extraction [52]. Research comparing EAE with alkaline and salt extraction revealed that EAE exhibited the greatest protein content, excellent solubility and enhanced physiochemical qualities [53].

The efficiency of enzyme-assisted protein extraction is influenced by several key parameters, including temperature, pH, enzyme concentration, enzyme specificity and mode of action, extraction time, substrate accessibility and the solvent system employed. To optimize these variables, response surface methodology and orthogonal experimental designs are frequently applied. For instance, an earlier study reported optimal conditions for protein extraction from oilseed rape leaves at a temperature of 42.8 °C, an amylase activity of 18,446 U, and an extraction time of 4.44 h, resulting in an extraction yield of 9.56% and a protein purity of 89.41% [54]. In another study, a 70% extraction yield of green coffee proteins was achieved alongside an 80% reduction in enzyme usage by employing a solid–liquid ratio of 1 : 17.5 and an alkaline protease concentration of 0.1%.

Overall, enzyme-assisted extraction represents a highly effective approach for the recovery of plant proteins with enhanced techno-functional properties. However, large-scale commercial application remains limited by the cost, availability and efficiency of specific enzymes.

4.5.4 Pulsed Electric Field

PEF entails the use of short electrical pulses, lasting from 10^{-4} to 10^{-2} seconds, at high amplitudes of 0.1–80 kV/cm, operating as a non-thermal method. The method of using PEF to improve extraction is subjecting plant cell to an electric field, leading to mechanical disruption and the creation of temporary or permanent porous structure inside the tissues, a phenomenon termed electroporation [55]. This enhances the cell membrane's permeability to ions and macromolecules, therefore promoting the release the intercellular constituent like protein, lipid and carbohydrates (Figure 4.3).

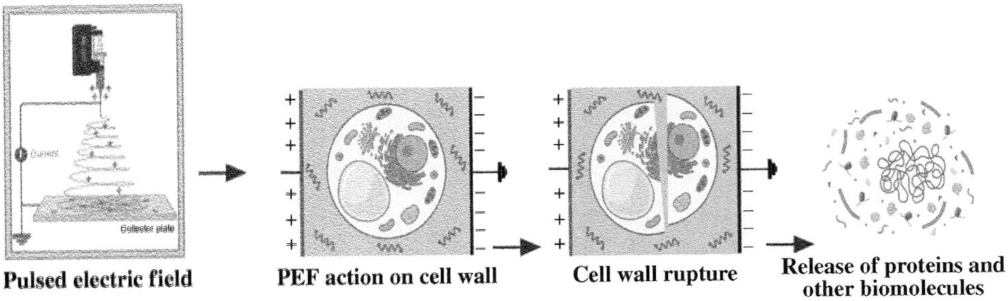

Figure 4.3 Pulsed electric field-assisted extraction of oat protein.

PEF-assisted protein extraction has emerged as an innovative approach, offering numerous advantages over traditional methods. These advantages include superior food quality, less water use, diminished emission, increased energy efficiency and the reclamation of by-products from food wastes [56]. Käferböck et al. [57] reported a about 90% improvement in C-phycocyanin extraction using PEF cell disruption relative to bead milling. The application of PEF at 2.3 kV for a period of 25 minutes resulted in a 20.71–22.8% boost in the efficiency of rice bran protein extraction compared to typical alkaline extraction techniques [58]. A separate study indicated that protein concentration obtained from samples pretreated with PEF rose by 28.1% in comparison to untreated samples, with an energy input of 6.41 kJ/kg [59]. The extraction effectiveness of PEF is often affected by variables like pH, temperature, length, operating time, electric field intensity, conductivity pulse frequency and processing energy. PEF being a relatively novel technology, has limited uses in the extraction of plant proteins. Consequently, additional research is necessary to determine appropriate extraction parameters and to identify the optimal integration of this approach with other extraction strategies.

4.5.5 Extraction with Combined Techniques

The previously mentioned novel extraction methods offer benefits compared to traditional techniques; nevertheless, they also present drawbacks, such as elevated costs and suboptimal equipment utilization. As a result, numerous studies have combined these extraction methods to tackle these challenges. Hildebrand et al. [60] combined UAE with a single solvent, sequential solvents and enzymes to enhance protein recovery. A study demonstrated that the recovery of mulberry leaf protein increased by 171.76% when employing multi-frequency ultrasound-assisted cellulase extraction in comparison to conventional extraction methods [61]. Sun et al. [62] employed an ultrasound-assisted salt method for the extraction of oleosin protein, resulting in a yield that exceeded conventional methods by 17.6% and a solubility that was 122.9% higher. Görgüç et al. [63] showed that vacuum-ultrasound-assisted extraction and vacuum-ultrasound-assisted enzymatic extraction improved protein yields by 31.0 and 41.6%, respectively, in comparison to traditional alkaline extraction methods. PEF can be employed in conjunction with other methods to achieve optimal extraction results. The integrated approaches resulted in a protein recovery of 19.6 ± 0.33%, surpassing the 10.8 ± 0.37% achieved by PEF alone and the 9.7 ± 0.42% obtained through EAE alone [64]. A distinct study utilized PEF alongside mechanical pressing to extract proteins from the green macroalgae *Ulva* spp., achieving a sevenfold increase in total protein extraction compared to osmotic shock extraction [65]. To attain selective and efficient recovery of water-soluble proteins from *Arthrospira platensis* suspensions during water extraction, PEF combined with high-shear homogenization was employed [66]. DES can be employed in conjunction with several techniques for extracting plant proteins, such as high voltage electrical discharges, microwaves and sequential ultrasound. The combination of DES and microwave technology has demonstrated improvements in protein extraction and functional characteristics, such as water/oil retention, emulsification, digestibility, solubility, gelling and foaming [67]. Naseri et al [68] successfully extracted up to 90% of protein content utilizing a combination of enzymes followed by alkaline extraction. Additional research is required to determine the ideal conditions for plant protein extraction, investigate the most effective combination of extraction methods, minimize economic costs, develop more environmentally sustainable extraction techniques and improve the utilization of plant materials.

4.6 Existing Challenges in Protein Extraction

The functionality of proteins plays a vital role in their applications within the food industry. The primary functional attributes include solubility, fat and water-binding capacity, foaming capacity and stability, emulsion capacity and stability, gelation, film-forming capability and viscosity [69]. The techno-functional characteristics of plant proteins are affected by various technical variables, including pH, ionic strength of the solvent, duration, temperature and particle size, which are parameters used in conventional protein extraction [70]. The extraction process conducted at high temperatures and pH has resulted in protein isolates exhibiting less-than-ideal nutritional and functional properties, primarily due to considerable protein denaturation induced by heat and increased protein aggregation at higher pH levels [71, 72]. Furthermore, alkaline extraction methods have been linked to the formation of nephrotoxic lysinoalanine compounds through the alteration of amino acid residues, such as cysteine and serine, leading to a reduction in protein bioactivity [73].

The dark colour of the extracted plant protein acquired through conventional methods presents a notable limitation. The dark or dismal colour may be associated with the co-extraction of various chemicals, primarily phenolic compounds. The application of a few plant proteins is limited because of their bitter taste, dark colour and astringent properties, which result from the co-extraction of polyphenols [74]. During alkaline extraction, these polyphenols undergo oxidation, leading to the formation of o-quinones or o-dihydroxy structures, which demonstrate considerable reactivity [75]. Additionally, these o-quinones/o-dihydroxy compounds can create covalent bonds with the thiol group (-SH) and amino group (-NH2) of proteins at higher pH levels or form non-covalent hydrogen bonds at lower pH levels, leading to a dark green to brown coloration of protein components [75]. Additionally, co-extracted phenolic compounds may negatively influence the functional properties of proteins. The polyphenols adversely influenced the foaming and interfacial properties of the isolate obtained from defatted sunflower cake.

Alongside the structural and functional challenges associated with traditional extraction processes, environmental safety remains a crucial concern. Organic solvents, particularly n-hexane utilized in the defatting of raw materials, are known to contribute to air pollution and are recognized as harmful [76]. Furthermore, sodium hydroxide and potassium hydroxide are utilized in the alkaline extraction process, and their neutralization generates considerable effluent that presents a notable risk to plant and animal life [77]. As a result, it is essential to develop innovative extraction methods that minimize environmental impact to ensure ecological safety.

4.7 Future Perspective for Industrial Scale Protein Extraction

Recent advancements in eco-friendly extraction technologies highlight improved safety, increased extraction yield and minimized negative impacts on the techno-functional properties of food proteins when compared to traditional methods. However, most of these methods have only been applied at the laboratory level, suggesting that commercial adaptation is still in its initial phases. It is crucial to conduct extensive research and development to understand, optimize and implement these intricate processes to improve their application in food industries. It is essential to assess the economic feasibility and cost efficiency of expanding processes for these innovative, environmentally sustainable technologies. The exploration of potential mechanisms or modifications of protein structures necessitates thorough investigation through innovative extraction methods, as these methods greatly impact the physicochemical and functional properties of proteins. Furthermore, it is crucial to prioritize energy efficiency, environmental impact and co-product generation in order to enhance technologies that elevate process efficiency, product quality and environmental sustainability.

References

1 L. Grossmann and J. Weiss, 'Alternative protein sources as technofunctional food ingredients', *Annu. Rev. Food Sci. Technol.*, vol. 12, no. 1, pp. 93–117, 2021, https://doi.org/10.1146/annurev-food-062520-093642.

2 P. Novák and V. Havlíček, 'Protein extraction and precipitation,' In: Proteomic Profiling and Analytical Chemistry: *The Crossroads* (ed. P. Ciborowski and J. Silberring), Elsevier, pp. 51–62, 2016.

3 M. Kumar et al., 'Advances in the plant protein extraction: mechanism and recommendations', *Food Hydrocoll.*, vol. 115, p. 106595, 2021, https://doi.org/10.1016/j.foodhyd.2021.106595.

4 N. Asaithambi, P. Singha, and S. K. Singh, 'Comparison of the effect of different desugarization techniques on the functionality of egg white protein hydrolysates', *Appl. Food Res.*, vol. 2, no. 2, p. 100152, 2022, https://doi.org/10.1016/j.afres.2022.100152.

5 N. Asaithambi, P. Singha, and S. K. Singh, 'Influence of hydrodynamic cavitation on functional, nutritional, and structural characteristics of egg-white protein hydrolysates', *Food Hydrocoll. Heal.*, vol. 4, p. 100153, 2023, https://doi.org/10.1016/j.fhfh.2023.100153.

6 E. Gençdağ, A. Görgüç, and F. M. Yılmaz, 'Recent advances in the recovery techniques of plant-based proteins from agro-industrial by-products', *Food Rev. Int.*, vol. 37, no. 4, pp. 447–468, 2021, https://doi.org/10.1080/87559129.2019.1709203.

7 J. Spaen and J. V. C. Silva, 'Oat proteins: review of extraction methods and techno-functionality for liquid and semi-solid applications', *LWT*, vol. 147, p. 111478, 2021, https://doi.org/10.1016/j.lwt.2021.111478.

8 M. Pojić, A. Mišan, and B. Tiwari, 'Eco-innovative technologies for extraction of proteins for human consumption from renewable protein sources of plant origin', *Trends Food Sci. Technol.*, vol. 75, pp. 93–104, 2018, https://doi.org/10.1016/j.tifs.2018.03.010.

9 J. Ampofo and M. Ngadi, 'Ultrasound-assisted processing: science, technology and challenges for the plant-based protein industry', *Ultrason. Sonochem.*, vol. 84, p. 105955, 2022, https://doi.org/10.1016/j.ultsonch.2022.105955.

10 S. Momen, F. Alavi, and M. Aider, 'Alkali-mediated treatments for extraction and functional modification of proteins: critical and application review', *Trends Food Sci. Technol.*, vol. 110, pp. 778–797, 2021, https://doi.org/10.1016/j.tifs.2021.02.052.

11 M. M. Rahman and B. P. Lamsal, 'Ultrasound-assisted extraction and modification of plant-based proteins: impact on physicochemical, functional, and nutritional properties', *Compr. Rev. Food Sci. Food Saf.*, vol. 20, no. 2, pp. 1457–1480, 2021, https://doi.org/10.1111/1541-4337.12709.

12 L.-G. Yan, L. He, and J. Xi, 'High intensity pulsed electric field as an innovative technique for extraction of bioactive compounds—a review', *Crit. Rev. Food Sci. Nutr.*, vol. 57, no. 13, pp. 2877–2888, 2017, https://doi.org/10.1080/10408398.2015.1077193.

13 S. Zhang, L. Sun, H. Ju, Z. Bao, X. Zeng, and S. Lin, 'Research advances and application of pulsed electric field on proteins and peptides in food', *Food Res. Int.*, vol. 139, p. 109914, 2021, https://doi.org/10.1016/j.foodres.2020.109914.

14 M. D. Luque de Castro and L. S. Castillo-Peinado, 'Microwave-assisted extraction of food components', In: Innovative Food Processing Technologies (ed. K. Knoerzer, P. Juliano, and G. Smithers), Elsevier, pp. 57–110, 2016.

15 L. Gomez, B. Tiwari, and M. Garcia-Vaquero, 'Emerging extraction techniques: microwave-assisted extraction', In: Sustainable Seaweed Technologies (ed. M. D. Torres, S. Kraan, and H. Dominguez), Elsevier, pp. 207–224, 2020.

16 J. Ahmed, N. Al-Ruwaih, M. Mulla, and M. H. Rahman, 'Effect of high pressure treatment on functional, rheological and structural properties of kidney bean protein isolate', *LWT*, vol. 91, pp. 191–197, 2018, https://doi.org/10.1016/j.lwt.2018.01.054.

17 J. A. Gerde, T. Wang, L. Yao, S. Jung, L. A. Johnson, and B. Lamsal, 'Optimizing protein isolation from defatted and non-defatted *Nannochloropsis* microalgae biomass', *Algal Res.*, vol. 2, no. 2, pp. 145–153, 2013, https://doi.org/10.1016/j.algal.2013.02.001.

18 J. Yue et al., 'Impact of defatting treatment and oat varieties on structural, functional properties, and aromatic profile of oat protein', *Food Hydrocoll.*, vol. 112, p. 106368, 2021, https://doi.org/10.1016/J.FOODHYD.2020.106368.

19 D. Sargautis, T. Kince, and I. Gramatina, 'Characterisation of the enzymatically extracted oat protein concentrate after defatting and its applicability for wet extrusion', *Foods*, vol. 12, no. 12, p. 2333, 2023, https://doi.org/10.3390/foods12122333.

20 O. E. Mäkinen, N. Sozer, D. Ercili-Cura, and K. Poutanen, 'Protein from oat: structure, processes, functionality, and nutrition', *Sustain. Protein Sources*, pp. 105–119, 2017, https://doi.org/10.1016/B978-0-12-802778-3.00006-8.

21 J. E. Cluskey, Y. V. Wu, G. E. Inglett, and J. S. Wall, 'Oat protein concentrates for beverage fortification', *J. Food Sci.*, vol. 41, no. 4, pp. 799–804, 1976, https://doi.org/10.1111/j.1365-2621.1976.tb00726_41_4.x.

22 X. Guan, H. Yao, Z. Chen, L. Shan, and M. Zhang, 'Some functional properties of oat bran protein concentrate modified by trypsin', *Food Chem.*, vol. 101, no. 1, pp. 163–170, 2007, https://doi.org/10.1016/j.foodchem.2006.01.011.

23 O. V Kriger, E. V Kashirskikh, O. O. Babich, and S. Y. Noskova, 'Oat protein concentrate production', *Foods Raw Mater.*, vol. 6, no. 1, p. 47, 2018.

24 C. Y. Ma, G. Khanzada, and V. R. Harwalkar, 'Thermal gelation of oat globulin', *J. Agric. Food Chem.*, vol. 36, no. 2, pp. 275–280, 1988, https://doi.org/10.1021/jf00080a009.

25 K. Liu, 'Fractionation of oats into products enriched with protein, beta-glucan, starch, or other carbohydrates', *J. Cereal Sci.*, vol. 60, no. 2, pp. 317–322, 2014, https://doi.org/10.1016/j.jcs.2014.06.002.

26 C. Yung Ma, 'Preparation, composition and functional properties of oat protein isolates', *Can. Inst. Food Sci. Technol. J.*, vol. 16, no. 3, pp. 201–205, 1983, https://doi.org/10.1016/S0315-5463(83)72208-X.

27 X. Guan and H. Yao, 'Optimization of Viscozyme L-assisted extraction of oat bran protein using response surface methodology', *Food Chem.*, vol. 106, no. 1, pp. 345–351, 2008, https://doi.org/10.1016/j.foodchem.2007.05.041.

28 S. Jodayree, J. C. Smith, and A. Tsopmo, 'Use of carbohydrase to enhance protein extraction efficiency and antioxidative properties of oat bran protein hydrolysates', *Food Res. Int.*, vol. 46, no. 1, pp. 69–75, 2012, https://doi.org/10.1016/j.foodres.2011.12.004.

29 H. Anttila, T. Sontag-Strohm, and H. Salovaara, 'Viscosity of beta-glucan in oat products', *Agric. Food Sci.*, vol. 13, no. 1–2, p. 80, 2008, https://doi.org/10.2137/1239099041838012.

30 C. Y. Ma, V. R. Harwalkar, and A. Paquet, 'Physicochemical properties of alkali-treated oat globulin', *J. Agric. Food Chem.*, vol. 38, no. 8, pp. 1707–1711, 1990, https://doi.org/10.1021/jf00098a017.

31 M. A. I. Schutyser and A. J. van der Goot, 'The potential of dry fractionation processes for sustainable plant protein production', *Trends Food Sci. Technol.*, vol. 22, no. 4, pp. 154–164, 2011, https://doi.org/10.1016/j.tifs.2010.11.006.

32 K. Autio and A.-C. Eliasson, 'Oat starch', In: Starch: Chemistry and Technology, 3rd ed., (ed. J. BeMiller and R. Whistler), Elsevier, pp. 589–599, 2009.

33 Y. V. Wu and D. C. Doehlert, 'Enrichment of β -glucan in oat bran by fine grinding and air classification', *LWT - Food Sci. Technol.*, vol. 35, no. 1, pp. 30–33, 2002, https://doi.org/10.1006/fstl.2001.0806.

34 J. Sibakov et al., 'Lipid removal enhances separation of oat grain cell wall material from starch and protein', *J. Cereal Sci.*, vol. 54, no. 1, pp. 104–109, 2011, https://doi.org/10.1016/j.jcs.2011.04.003.

35 D. G. Stevenson, F. J. Eller, M. Radosavljević, J. Jane, and G. E. Inglett, 'Characterisation of oat bran products with and without supercritical carbon dioxide extraction', *Int. J. Food Sci. Technol.*, vol. 42, no. 12, pp. 1489–1496, 2007, https://doi.org/10.1111/j.1365-2621.2006.01370.x.

36 D. G. Stevenson, F. J. Eller, J. Jane, and G. E. Inglett, 'Structure and physicochemical properties of defatted and pin-milled oat bran concentrate fractions separated by air-classification 4', *Int. J. Food Sci. Technol.*, vol. 43, no. 6, pp. 995–1003, 2008, https://doi.org/10.1111/j.1365-2621.2007.01547.x.

37 C. Wen et al., 'Advances in renewable plant-derived protein source: the structure, physicochemical properties affected by ultrasonication', *Ultrason. Sonochem.*, vol. 53, pp. 83–98, 2019, https://doi.org/10.1016/j.ultsonch.2018.12.036.

38 F. Chemat et al., 'Review of alternative solvents for green extraction of food and natural products: panorama, principles, applications and prospects', *Molecules*, vol. 24, no. 16, p. 3007, 2019, https://doi.org/10.3390/molecules24163007.

39 W. Ge, Z. Xiao, X. Ding, W. Bi, and D. D. Y. Chen, 'Deep eutectic system enhanced oat protein extraction', *J. Food Sci.*, vol. 90, no. 1, 2025, https://doi.org/10.1111/1750-3841.17645.

40 K. Kuroda, 'A simple overview of toxicity of ionic liquids and designs of biocompatible ionic liquids', *New J. Chem.*, vol. 46, no. 42, pp. 20047–20052, 2022, https://doi.org/10.1039/D2NJ02634A.

41 J. Zhang et al., 'Responsive switchable deep eutectic solvents: a review', *Chinese Chem. Lett.*, vol. 34, no. 5, p. 107750, 2023, https://doi.org/10.1016/j.cclet.2022.107750.

42 S. Bernardi et al., 'Ultrasound: a suitable technology to improve the extraction and techno-functional properties of vegetable food proteins', *Plant Foods Hum. Nutr.*, vol. 76, no. 1, pp. 1–11, 2021, https://doi.org/10.1007/s11130-021-00884-w.

43 C. R. Eze, E. M. Kwofie, P. Adewale, E. Lam, and M. Ngadi, 'Advances in legume protein extraction technologies: a review', *Innov. Food Sci. Emerg. Technol.*, vol. 82, p. 103199, 2022, https://doi.org/10.1016/j.ifset.2022.103199.

44 N. T. Flores-Jiménez, J. A. Ulloa, R. I. Ortiz-Basurto, and J. E. Urías-Silvas, 'Application of high-intensity ultrasound to modify the rheological properties of a guamuchil Pithecellobium dulce (Roxb.) seed protein isolate', *Int. J. Food Prop.*, vol. 26, no. 1, pp. 739–751, 2023, https://doi.org/10.1080/10942912.2023.2183171.

45 J. C. Orellana-Palacios et al., 'Extraction optimization, functional and thermal properties of protein from cherimoya seed as an unexploited by-product', *Foods*, vol. 11, no. 22, p. 3694, 2022, https://doi.org/10.3390/foods11223694.

46 F. Wang, Y. Zhang, L. Xu, and H. Ma, 'An efficient ultrasound-assisted extraction method of pea protein and its effect on protein functional properties and biological activities', *LWT*, vol. 127, p. 109348, 2020, https://doi.org/10.1016/j.lwt.2020.109348.

47 T. S. Purdi, A. D. Setiowati, and A. Ningrum, 'Ultrasound-assisted extraction of *Spirulina platensis* protein: physicochemical characteristic and techno-functional properties', *J. Food Meas. Charact.*, vol. 17, no. 5, pp. 5474–5486, 2023, https://doi.org/10.1007/s11694-023-02051-y.

48 W.-J. Li et al., 'Ultrasound-assisted extraction ameliorates the physicochemical properties of defatted mulberry seed protein to promote lipid production in *Schizochytrium* sp. SR21', *Biomass Conv. Bioref.*, vol. 11, no. 2, pp. 489–502, 2021, https://doi.org/10.1007/s13399-020-00626-z.

49 X. Lu, W. Li, Q. Wang, J. Wang, and S. Qin, 'Progress on the extraction, separation, biological activity, and delivery of natural plant pigments', *Molecules*, vol. 28, no. 14, p. 5364, 2023, https://doi.org/10.3390/molecules28145364.

50 A. Łubek-Nguyen, W. Ziemichód, and M. Olech, 'Application of enzyme-assisted extraction for the recovery of natural bioactive compounds for nutraceutical and pharmaceutical applications', *Appl. Sci.*, vol. 12, no. 7, p. 3232, 2022, https://doi.org/10.3390/app12073232.

51 R. O. Coniglio, G. V. Díaz, R. C. Barua, E. Albertó, and P. D. Zapata, 'Enzyme-assisted extraction of phenolic compounds and proteins from sugarcane bagasse using a low-cost cocktail from *Auricularia fuscosuccinea*', *Int. J. Food Sci. Technol.*, vol. 57, no. 2, pp. 1114–1121, 2022, https://doi.org/10.1111/ijfs.15477.

52 M. N. Perović and M. G. Antov, 'The influence of enzymatic pretreatment of chickpea on properties of protein nanoparticles prepared by heat treatment', *LWT*, vol. 163, p. 113545, 2022, https://doi.org/10.1016/j.lwt.2022.113545.

53 B. Koysuren, M. H. Oztop, and B. G. Mazi, 'Sesame seed as an alternative plant protein source: A comprehensive physicochemical characterisation study for alkaline, salt and enzyme-assisted extracted samples', *Int. J. Food Sci. Technol.*, vol. 56, no. 11, pp. 5471–5484, 2021, https://doi.org/10.1111/ijfs.15229.

54 G. Kaur and S. Bhatia, 'Alpha-amylase-assisted extraction of protein concentrates from *Raphanus sativus* L. leaves', *Biomass Conv. Bioref.*, vol. 13, no. 16, pp. 15051–15065, 2023, https://doi.org/10.1007/s13399-022-03611-w.

55 R. N. Arshad et al., 'Pulsed electric field: a potential alternative towards a sustainable food processing', *Trends Food Sci. Technol.*, vol. 111, pp. 43–54, 2021, https://doi.org/10.1016/j.tifs.2021.02.041.

56 W. Zhang, M. A. Sani, Z. Zhang, D. J. McClements, and S. M. Jafari, 'High performance biopolymeric packaging films containing zinc oxide nanoparticles for fresh food preservation: a review', *Int. J. Biol. Macromol.*, vol. 230, p. 123188, 2023, https://doi.org/10.1016/j.ijbiomac.2023.123188.

57 A. Käferböck, S. Smetana, R. de Vos, C. Schwarz, S. Toepfl, and O. Parniakov, 'Sustainable extraction of valuable components from *Spirulina* assisted by pulsed electric fields technology', *Algal Res.*, vol. 48, p. 101914, 2020, https://doi.org/10.1016/j.algal.2020.101914.

58 S. Thongkong et al., 'Impacts of electroextraction using the pulsed electric field on properties of rice bran protein', *Foods*, vol. 12, no. 4, p. 835, 2023, https://doi.org/10.3390/foods12040835.

59 V. Andreou, M. Psarianos, G. Dimopoulos, D. Tsimogiannis, and P. Taoukis, 'Effect of pulsed electric fields and high pressure on improved recovery of high-added-value compounds from olive pomace', *J. Food Sci.*, vol. 85, no. 5, pp. 1500–1512, 2020, https://doi.org/10.1111/1750-3841.15122.

60 G. Hildebrand, M. M. Poojary, C. O'Donnell, M. N. Lund, M. Garcia-Vaquero, and B. K. Tiwari, 'Ultrasound-assisted processing of *Chlorella vulgaris* for enhanced protein extraction', *J. Appl. Phycol.*, vol. 32, no. 3, pp. 1709–1718, 2020, https://doi.org/10.1007/s10811-020-02105-4.

61 J. Zhao, Y. Liu, C. Shen, O.-M. Lai, C.-P. Tan, and L.-Z. Cheong, 'Enhanced storage stability and in-vitro digestibility of powdered-solid lipid nanoparticles with high-algae oil-load', *Food Biosci.*, vol. 55, p. 102810, 2023, https://doi.org/10.1016/j.fbio.2023.102810.

62 Y. Sun, M. Zhong, L. Wu, Y. Huang, Y. Li, and B. Qi, 'Effects of ultrasound-assisted salt (NaCl) extraction method on the structural and functional properties of Oleosin', *Food Chem.*, vol. 372, p. 131238, 2022, https://doi.org/10.1016/j.foodchem.2021.131238.

63 A. Görgüç, P. Özer, and F. M. Yılmaz, 'Simultaneous effect of vacuum and ultrasound assisted enzymatic extraction on the recovery of plant protein and bioactive compounds from sesame bran', *J. Food Compos. Anal.*, vol. 87, p. 103424, 2020, https://doi.org/10.1016/j.jfca.2020.103424.

64 E. Steinbruch et al., 'Enzymatic cell wall degradation combined with pulsed electric fields increases yields of water-soluble-protein extraction from the green marine macroalga *Ulva* sp.', *Innov. Food Sci. Emerg. Technol.*, vol. 84, p. 103231, 2023, https://doi.org/10.1016/j.ifset.2022.103231.

65 A. Robin et al., 'Functional protein concentrates extracted from the green marine macroalga *Ulva* sp., by high voltage pulsed electric fields and mechanical press', *ACS Sustain. Chem. Eng.*, vol. 6, no. 11, pp. 13696–13705, 2018, https://doi.org/10.1021/acssuschemeng.8b01089.

66 D. Carullo, F. Donsì, G. Ferrari, and G. Pataro, 'Extraction improvement of water-soluble compounds from *Arthrospira platensis* through the combination of high-shear homogenization and pulsed electric fields', *Algal Res.*, vol. 57, p. 102341, 2021, https://doi.org/10.1016/j.algal.2021.102341.

67 O. A. Olalere and C.-Y. Gan, 'Extractability of defatted wheat germ protein and their functionalities in a deep eutectic solvent (DES)-microwave extraction approach compared to conventional processing', *Sustain. Chem. Pharm.*, vol. 32, p. 101002, 2023, https://doi.org/10.1016/j.scp.2023.101002.

68 A. Naseri, G. S. Marinho, S. L. Holdt, J. M. Bartela, and C. Jacobsen, 'Enzyme-assisted extraction and characterization of protein from red seaweed *Palmaria palmata*', *Algal Res.*, vol. 47, p. 101849, 2020, https://doi.org/10.1016/j.algal.2020.101849.

69 J. Boye, F. Zare, and A. Pletch, 'Pulse proteins: processing, characterization, functional properties and applications in food and feed', *Food Res. Int.*, vol. 43, no. 2, pp. 414–431, 2010, https://doi.org/10.1016/j.foodres.2009.09.003.

70 V. V. Kolpakova, N. D. Lukin, and I. S. Gaivoronskaya, 'Interrelation of functional properties of protein products from wheat with the composition and physicochemical characteristics of their proteins', In: Global Wheat Production (ed. S. Fahad, A. Basir, and M. Adnan), InTech, 2018.

71 Z. Gao et al., 'Effect of alkaline extraction pH on structure properties, solubility, and beany flavor of yellow pea protein isolate', *Food Res. Int.*, vol. 131, p. 109045, 2020, https://doi.org/10.1016/j.foodres.2020.109045.

72 C. Valenzuela, L. Abugoch, C. Tapia, and A. Gamboa, 'Effect of alkaline extraction on the structure of the protein of quinoa (*Chenopodium quinoa* Willd.) and its influence on film formation', *Int. J. Food Sci. Technol.*, vol. 48, no. 4, pp. 843–849, 2013, https://doi.org/10.1111/ijfs.12035.

73 J. Zhang et al., 'Structure of the zein protein as treated with subcritical water', *Int. J. Food Prop.*, vol. 21, no. 1, pp. 128–138, 2018, https://doi.org/10.1080/10942912.2017.1414839.

74 S. González-Pérez and J. M. Vereijken, 'Sunflower proteins: overview of their physicochemical, structural and functional properties', *J. Sci. Food Agric.*, vol. 87, no. 12, pp. 2173–2191, 2007, https://doi.org/10.1002/jsfa.2971.

75 M. A. Malik and C. S. Saini, 'Polyphenol removal from sunflower seed and kernel: effect on functional and rheological properties of protein isolates', *Food Hydrocoll.*, vol. 63, pp. 705–715, 2017, https://doi.org/10.1016/j.foodhyd.2016.10.026.

76 S. P. J. Kumar, S. R. Prasad, R. Banerjee, D. K. Agarwal, K. S. Kulkarni, and K. V. Ramesh, 'Green solvents and technologies for oil extraction from oilseeds', *Chem. Cent. J.*, vol. 11, no. 1, p. 9, 2017, https://doi.org/10.1186/s13065-017-0238-8.

77 C. Zhang, J. P. M. Sanders, T. T. Xiao, and M. E. Bruins, 'How does alkali aid protein extraction in green tea leaf residue: a basis for integrated biorefinery of leaves', *PLoS One*, vol. 10, no. 7, p. e0133046, 2015, https://doi.org/10.1371/journal.pone.0133046.

5

Physical and Chemical Processing of Oat Protein

5.1 Introduction

In recent years, plant-based proteins have attracted considerable attention due to their sustainability, cost-effectiveness and health-promoting functions compared with animal-derived counterparts [1, 2]. However, the broader utilization of many plant proteins remains limited because of their intrinsic functional shortcomings. These limitations are primarily associated with poor water absorption capacity, high sensitivity and structural instability under environmental stresses such as extreme pH, high salt concentration and temperature fluctuations [3]. Furthermore, plant proteins are often embedded within complex biomaterials, including lignin, hemicellulose and other poorly digestible polysaccharides, which restrict their bioavailability. To overcome these barriers, protein modification has emerged as a crucial strategy for enhancing the physicochemical properties of plant proteins. Protein modification generally refers to alterations in the structure of a protein or in its chemical groups with the aim of improving its techno-functional, nutritional, physicochemical and biological properties. Such modifications provide opportunities to expand the applications of proteins as multifunctional components in food systems and to overcome their inherent limitations. Common protein modification methods include physical, chemical, biological and novel approaches. Such modifications not only improve functional attributes but also expand their techno-functional and biological applications, making them more suitable for industrial use [3]. A careful selection of modification techniques is therefore essential, as these directly influence the functional, nutritional and organoleptic properties of proteins. This section of the book focuses on oat protein, highlighting various modification approaches aimed at improving its nutritional profile, flavour and techno-functional properties. These advancements offer promising opportunities to broaden the application of oat protein in food product development.

5.2 Physical Processing of Protein

Physical techniques for enhancing protein functionality are relatively straightforward processes that do not involve the use of chemicals or enzymes. Owing to the absence of chemical agents, these modification strategies have attracted significant attention, as they eliminate the risk of chemical contaminants. In this section, the physical modification methods applied to oat and another plant-based protein are discussed, with particular emphasis on the advantages and limitations associated with each technology.

5.2.1 Thermal Processing

The introduction of heat provides the activation energy to disrupt various protein interactions, including peptide bonds, electrostatic interactions, hydrogen bonds and disulphide bonds. Increased thermal mobility causes proteins to shift from their native conformation to a semi-molten globule state, thereby destroying the tertiary structure. This process also exposes hydrophobic, hydrophilic and sulfhydryl groups that were previously buried within the protein core [4]. Consequently, controlled thermal application can be used to modify the structure of dietary protein components and improve certain functional properties. Heat treatment of plant proteins has been shown to enhance gelation [5], foaming properties [6] and water absorption capacity [7], although its effect on protein solubility may be negligible [8–10]. The structure and function of plant-based proteins are significantly altered at high temperatures. For example, high-temperature treatment (HTT) of oat protein isolates (OPI) at 230 °C for different time durations has been shown to reduce the total amino acid content; however, the essential amino acid composition remains relatively stable, likely because some amino acids are involved in the Maillard reaction [11]. Heating duration also affects the secondary structure of the protein, particularly by converting β-turns into β-sheets. This denaturation of the protein contributes to the redistribution of chemical bonds, ultimately leading to an increase in disulphide bond content within OPI. Consequently, large particle sizes, aggregation and reduced digestibility are observed. Meanwhile, improvements in foaming properties, water-holding capacity and emulsification properties of OPI have been reported [11]. These findings provide valuable insights for the controlled processing of oat protein and highlight the potential of OPI as a functional component in the food industry. Similarly, pea proteins form aggregates of approximately 200 kDa when heated between 80 and 100 °C [8]. Heat treatment reduces emulsion stability at pH 3.0, resulting in large droplets and cooked pea protein samples display poor foaming characteristics across all pH levels. In hemp seed protein, heating above 80 °C decreases solubility and induces aggregation due to the exposure of hydrophobic residues [9]. Heating at 95 °C for 10 minutes improves emulsion activity and foam stability, while reducing oil absorption capacity. Similarly, a 30-minute heat treatment at 90 °C enhances protein surface hydrophobicity by releasing hydrophobic side chains from the native structure into the solvent [10].

Preheating at low concentration results in heat-stable proteins with large particles due to disulphide bond formation and hydrophobic interactions. Conversely, heating at low concentrations and elevated pH produces smaller particles [12]. It is reported that boiling rice glutelin at pH 12 for 60 minutes increased its solubility and foaming capacity. Heat treatment of albumin at 100 °C for 30 minutes improved in vitro digestibility up to 87.55%. This improvement was attributed to the disruption of disulphide bonds and conformational changes in glutelin, which reduced aggregate size beyond 100 nm and increased structural flexibility [6]. Heat treatment at 80, 90 and 100 °C for 15–30 minutes further induced structural modifications in albumin proteins, increased surface hydrophobicity and enhanced fluorescence intensity. In addition, heating albumin improved gelling properties, amino acid availability and in vitro protein digestibility [5]. The dry-heating of faba-bean protein concentrate at 75–175 °C increased water-holding capacity while reducing solubility, making its properties more comparable to those of soy protein concentrate [7]. Partial denaturation exposed hydrophobic regions, leading to protein aggregation through non-covalent interactions.

Thermal treatment is an effective method for reducing or eliminating the adverse effects of anti-nutritional compounds in plant proteins [13]. Its benefits for the inactivation of trypsin inhibitors in chickpeas and soyabeans have been extensively studied. The combination of heating and metabisulfite as a reducing agent achieved an inactivation rate of up to 99.4% for the trypsin inhibitors [13]. Trypsin inhibitors are recognized as anti-nutritional factors that restrict cereal and legume consumption by inhibiting the activity of pancreatic trypsin and chymotrypsin in the gastrointestinal tract. This inhibition can lead to various disorders, including impaired digestion, inadequate protein digestion and absorption, pancreatic enlargement, growth retardation and muscle wasting [13]. Thermal treatment enhances the digestibility and nutritional properties of plant-based proteins. For instance, heating of albumin protein at 100 °C for 30 minutes has been shown to improve the protein digestibility up to 87.55% and also increase the availability of essential amino acids [5]. Thermal treatment serves as a standalone modification method; however, heating can also facilitate additional changes by accelerating chemical or enzymatic reactions. Overall, controlled heat treatment can be used to modify the activity of plant-based proteins, thereby enhancing their applications in both culinary and industrial contexts.

5.2.2 High-pressure Processing

5.2.2.1 High Hydrostatic Pressure

High hydrostatic pressure (HHP) is a non-thermal food processing technology, widely used for milk preservation, that employs pressures ranging from 100 to 800 MPa for a duration of several minutes [14]. HHP fulfils multiple objectives, such as the inactivation of microorganisms, modification in texture and emulsification. This technology enables the modification of food proteins through the disruption of hydrophobic and electrostatic interactions, facilitating the formation of new bonds that result in aggregation and gelation [15, 16].

The HPP treatment modified the denaturation, aggregation and interactions of plant-based proteins. Following unfolding and denaturation, HHP treatment reveals concealed sulfhydryl groups, resulting in enhanced protein hydrophobicity and reduced solubility [17]. HPP treatment improved the heat stability and emulsifying properties of seed protein through increased surface hydrophobicity, elevated sulfhydryl group content and modifications in secondary structure [18]. Some studies indicate that HHP may reduce the solubility of plant-based proteins, especially at elevated pressures exceeding 400 MPa, due to aggregation [19, 20]. Conversely, other research suggests a beneficial effect, demonstrating that HHP at 200 and 400 MPa enhanced the solubility, water-holding capacity and oil holding capacity of pine nut protein [21, 22]. Similarly, increased pressure and treatment time significantly affect the conformational structure of oat protein, improving texture, flavour and structural attributes during industrial processing [23]. High pressure exceeding 600 MPa markedly enhanced the secondary structure of kidney bean protein, leading to improved water-holding capacity, foaming and emulsifying properties [24]. HPP processing of calcium-fortified soy protein improved solubility and colloidal stability, compared with conventional thermal treatment [25].

HPP is also considered an effective method for improving the nutritional quality of plant proteins. For instance, the allergenicity of soy protein used in infant formula was reduced more effectively by HHP processing than by high-intensity ultrasound, microwave processing and high-pressure homogenization (HPH) [18]. The most effective allergenicity reduction has been observed at pressures between 300 and 700 MPa [18]. Furthermore, HHP serves as a pretreatment for enzymatic hydrolysis of plant proteins, enhancing their susceptibility to enzyme action and improving hydrolysis efficiency. For example, HHP treatment increased the extent of trypsin hydrolysis of flaxseed protein, producing smaller peptides with enhanced antioxidant activity [26]. Similarly, HHP treatment (300 MPa for 15 minutes) facilitated the enzymatic proteolysis of kidney bean protein isolates using alcalase, ultimately improving their functionality and antioxidant activity [27].

5.2.2.2 Dynamic High-pressure Fluidization

Dynamic high pressure (DHP) is a technology that operates at pressures ranging from 250 to 300 MPa, facilitating the passage of fluids through a small aperture. Rapid velocity changes and sudden pressure drops induce significant shear, turbulence and cavitation. Colloidal dispersion, such as nanoemulsions, are frequently produced through DHP fluidization, commonly referred to as HPH [28]. This method has been employed to inactivate microbiological cells in milk, beverages and juices without the application of heat. Additionally, it can alter proteins and carbohydrates [29, 30]. Recent research has investigated DHP as a method and pretreatment for enhancing the flexibility of plant-based proteins. The mechanical forces generated by DHP fragment macromolecules, decreasing the particle size of plant-derived proteins and facilitating greater interactions between particles and solvent compared to interactions among particles.

For instance, DHP-treated OPI was shown to improve the functional properties, thereby enhancing its industrial application. Specifically, the particle size of OPI was reduced by 70.96% and zeta potential was recorded to increase at a pressure of 120 MPa [31]. Meanwhile, the secondary structure of OPI was altered with increasing α-helix, β-sheets and β-turn and decrease in random coils after DHP treatment, which affected the functional performance of OPI. Moreover, hydrophobicity and sulfhydryl content were significantly increased; also, DHP treatment at control pressure of 120 MPa notably improved the solubility as well as oil and water-holding properties, foaming and emulsifying properties of OPI. Therefore, DHP offers a promising approach for expanding the utilization of OPI in food processing industry [31]. Similarly, lentil protein isolate nanoparticles, which stabilized oil-in-water nanoemulsions, exhibited reduced size following DHP treatment [32]. Modified lentil protein isolate using HPH, resulting in reduced nanoparticle size and enhanced solubility, emulsifying and foaming properties at pressures up to 100 MPa. However, elevated pressures exceeding 100 MPa markedly diminished these functional characteristics. These findings indicate that DHP significantly reduced particle size only up to 100 MPa, with a slight decrease observed at 150 MPa [33]. A previous investigation demonstrated that HPH altered hazelnut protein, leading to a notable size reduction of up to 50 MPa; nonetheless, nanoparticle size exhibited no significant variation beyond 150 MPa [34].

Depending on the protein and solvent system, DHP can generate the smallest nanoparticles at maximum pressure; beyond this point, protein denaturation may lead to an increase in particle size. Mechanical stresses resulting from pressure drop and elevated temperatures in homogenized valves lead to denaturation [30]. DHP may induce more substantial structural alterations at pressures exceeding 150 MPa or when combined with heat treatment. Furthermore, DHP treatment enhances the digestibility of plant-based protein in HPH-stabilized lentil protein isolate emulsions [32]. This method also decreases the allergenic potential of animal proteins [30]. It can also alter the immunogenicity of plant-based proteins or facilitate further modifications. A study demonstrated that employing it as a pretreatment for soy protein isolate at 120 MPa enhanced pancreatin efficiency by improving subunit accessibility and augmenting the emulsifying capacity of the hydrolysate [35].

5.2.3 Extrusion Processing

Extrusion involves the application of mechanical shear, heat and pressure, during which mixed ingredients undergo continuous mixing and are subjected to significant mechanical stresses generated by a rotating screw operating under high pressures (1.5–30.0 MPa) and temperatures (90–200 °C). This process is classified as a high-temperature short time (HTST) cooking method, widely utilized for multiple purposes, including the inactivation of microorganisms, enzymes and naturally occurring toxic substances, as well as the gelatinization of starch and the shaping of food materials [29]. During extrusion, the unfolding, denaturation and realignment of vegetable protein molecules occur, improving their technofunctional properties and contributing to the formation of a meat-like texture. Textured vegetable proteins produced through extrusion serve as effective meat substitutes in various food applications [36]. The extrusion process alters the interactions that determine the native conformation of proteins, peptide bonds, the fundamental chemical linkages, remain intact [37]. Elevated temperatures during extrusion can lead to protein denaturation through the disruption of hydrogen bonds. As temperature increases, intramolecular disulphide bonds may cleave, followed by the formation of new intermolecular bonds, resulting in protein aggregation and an increase in overall molecular weight [38, 39].

For instance, oat protein concentrates (OPC) have been successfully used as a single ingredient in the production of meat analogues via both low-moisture and high-moisture extrusion processes [40]. It has been observed that OPC with low protein-to-starch ratio (P:S) forms a more porous structure at lower moisture contents during low-moisture extrusion compared to OPC with a higher P:S ratio. In contrast, under high-moisture extrusion, OPC with lower P:S ratio exhibits increased textural strength, whereas a higher P:S ratio enhances the apparent fibrousness of the final product [40]. These findings demonstrate the potential of oat protein as single-ingredient source for meat analogues and emphasize the influence of fractionation type and powder composition on the techno-functional characteristics of protein concentrates, ultimately affecting the structural formation of extruded products. Similarly, pea protein undergoes notable structural changes following low-moisture extrusion, as evidenced by modifications in its secondary structure, including alterations in α-helices, β-sheets, non-covalently bonded β-turns and anti-parallel β-sheet confirmations [39]. Elevated temperature and pressure during extrusion significantly reduce anti-nutrients and enhance the digestibility of plant-based proteins by improving amino acid availability. Furthermore, extrusion serves as an effective pretreatment for subsequent protein modification techniques, such as enzymatic hydrolysis [38, 41] and glycation [29], by exposing amino acid residues that are typically concealed within the native protein structure.

5.2.4 Cold Plasma Processing

Cold atmospheric plasma processing (CAPP) is fundamentally based on the utilization of cold plasma, which is often referred to as the fourth state of matter. This plasma can be generated through a combination of thermal, mechanical, nuclear and electrical energy sources under diverse temperature and pressure conditions. CAPP offers a consistent and uniform treatment without the risk of heat-induced damage while eliminating the need for hazardous chemical reagents. Due to its limited penetration capability, CAPP application has been primarily focused on the inactivation of viruses, spores and microorganisms present on food surfaces. The substantial energy of CAPP can disrupt covalent bonds or the initiate a variety of chemical processes [42, 43]. Previous studies have demonstrated its potential in surface treatment, biopolymer modification and more recently, in the structural and functional improvement of plant-derived proteins. Emerging research suggests that CAPP effectively reduces the size of protein aggregates and particles in plant-based proteins. For instance, higher voltage and extended plasma exposure have been shown to generate smaller protein nanoparticles in grass pea protein, with minimum particle size observed under conditions of 18.6 kVpp for 600 seconds. Furthermore, plasma treatment has been reported to enhance the disulphide bond composition of plant-based proteins, thereby modifying their secondary structure and rheological properties [44].

Recent studies on oat protein have revealed that plasma-treated samples exhibit markedly improved texture, firmness and juiciness when incorporated into plant-based patties [45]. The enhanced gelation and water-retention properties led to improved structural integrity, reducing cooking loss and maintaining an appealing mouthfeel. These improvements are critical for replicating the texture of conventional meat, positioning plasma-treated oat protein as a promising ingredient for plant-based meat formulations. In particular, oat proteins processed under 230-15 conditions demonstrated favourable rheological and textural properties, effectively serving as both a protein gel and a texturizing agent in plant-based patty applications [45]. Similarly, another investigation demonstrated that cold plasma treatment (Figure 5.1) reduced the pH of oat protein dispersion and promoted hydrophobic agglomeration [46]. Moderate plasma treatment conditions (170-15; 230-15) resulted in the formation of larger protein aggregates, whereas extended treatment durations (170-30; 230-30) caused their destruction. Oxidative cleavage of peptides resulted in increased carbonyl content, indicating notable structural alterations. Plasma exposure also increased α-helix content while reducing β-sheets and random coils, thereby improving the overall structural order of the protein. Furthermore, UV absorbance and fluorescence spectra confirmed significant changes in tertiary structure, while variations in sulfhydryl and disulphide contents reflected thiol oxidation processes. Importantly, plasma-treated oat proteins exhibited superior foaming properties owing to improved solubility and surface tension [46]. Hence, cold plasma is an environmentally sustainable method for altering oat protein, facilitating the preparation of solid powdered goods. Addressing scaling, commercialization and capital expenditures is essential in conjunction with studies on the toxicity of plasma-exposed products.

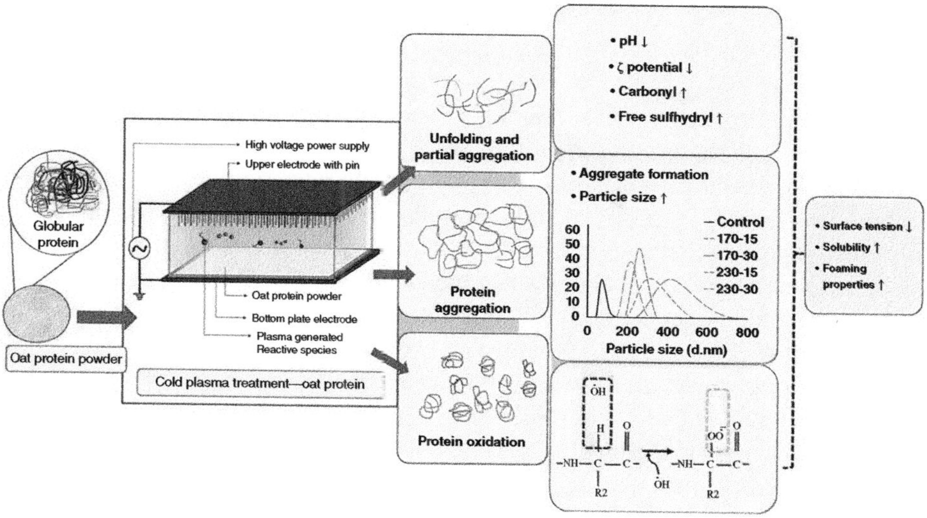

Figure 5.1 Effect of plasma-treatment on oat protein structural, chemical and foaming characteristics. *Source:* Ref. [46] with permission of Elsevier.

5.3 Chemical Processing of Protein

The chemical processing of dietary proteins is widely utilized due to its effectiveness, cost efficiency and simplicity of execution. To achieve chemical modification of proteins, one can either incorporate new functional moieties into the protein structure or eliminate existing components from it. Most chemical processing techniques have generated regulatory and clean label concerns because they utilize chemicals and often produce chemical by-products. Among these, several techniques are inappropriate for food applications. This section includes various methods of chemical modification, providing specific examples related to plant-derived proteins.

5.3.1 Glycation

Glycation and glycosylation are prevalent food-grade chemical reactions utilized to enhance protein functionalities due to their safety and the typical absence of exogenous chemicals [29]. Glycation is a process observed in nature, characterized by covalent bonds between proteins and polysaccharides in certain biopolymers, such as Arabic gum, which confer beneficial functional properties to this substance [47, 48]. Glycation can occur chemically via Maillard reactions or through the action of cross-linking enzymes, including transglutaminase and lactase. It involves the covalent conjugation of a free amino group from a protein, peptide or amino acid with the carbonyl group of a reducing sugar. This occurs through controlled heating in the presence of water, utilizing a chemical-reagent-free, safe and mild approach. Various methods, such as wet-heating, dry-heating and molecular crowding, can facilitate this process. The dry-heating method is the most prevalent among conventional approaches [49–51]. Recent developments in the preparation of protein–carbohydrate conjugates have garnered attention for enhancing the functionality of whey proteins [29]. Recent methodologies employed for the glycation of plant-proteins with saccharides include ultrasonication [52, 53], electrospinning [54, 55], microwave treatment [56, 57], spray drying [58], HHP [21] and cold plasma [59]. The characteristics and reactivity of saccharides significantly influenced the techno-functionality of plant-based proteins via the Maillard reaction [60]. A study demonstrated that xylose exhibits greater reactivity than fructose when conjugated with soy protein isolate under controlled wet-heating conditions, resulting in the formation of more complex and larger conjugates with a more relaxed structure [61]. A comparative analysis of black rice glutelin conjugates with various carbohydrates, including arabinose, sodium alginate, maltodextrin and lactose, indicated a higher degree of glycation associated with arabinose and maltodextrin [62]. The carbohydrate chain length is reported to depend on the structure and functionality of the conjugated protein [62].

Literature reports structural changes in various plant-proteins following glycation, leading to enhanced functionality. In recent study, oat protein conjugates resulting from glycation have been shown to enhance emulsifying properties, as characterized by zeta potential, droplet size and microstructure analysis. The extent of grafting and SDS-PAGE analysis confirm the covalent bonding of OPI with dextrin (Figure 5.2). The resultant OPI conjugates demonstrate enhanced emulsion stability, reduced particle size and improved storage stability [63]. Similarly, secondary structure modifications in sesame protein following dry heating-conjugation with maltodextrin, as evidenced by circular spectroscopy. This treatment resulted in increased protein solubility, leading to enhanced emulsifying capacity across a broad spectrum of pH levels, particularly at the isoelectric point. The wet heating glycosylation of black soybean protein isolate with chitosan enhanced its emulsifying capacity through induced secondary structural modifications [64]. Most studies

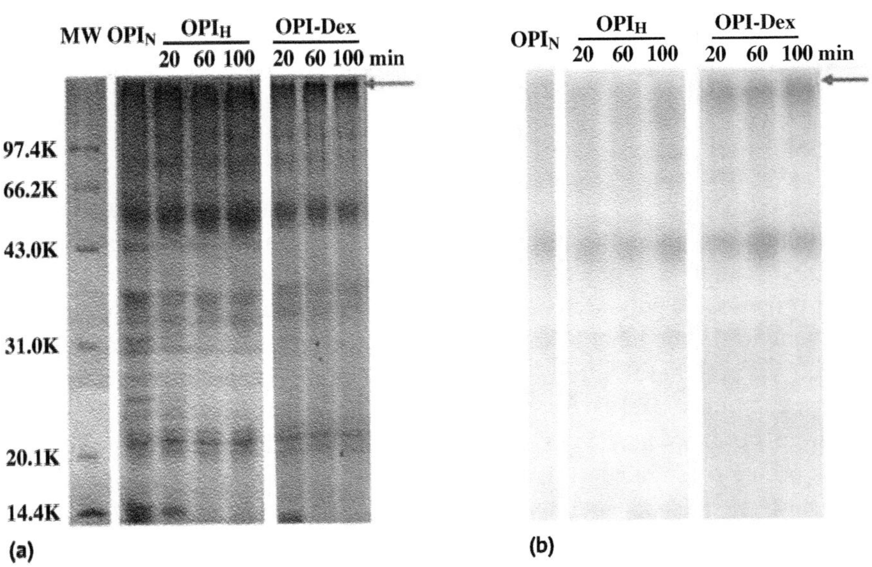

Figure 5.2 Confirmation of oat protein-dextrin (OPI-Dex) conjugates by SDS-PAGE. *Source:* Ref. [63] with permission of Elsevier.

indicate that the emulsifying performance of plant-based proteins improves after conjugation with various sugars, attributed to the formation of a thicker absorbed interfacial layer that provides steric and/or electrostatic hindrance [55, 65]. However, some researchers have reported a negative impact of this treatment on emulsifying functionality. For instance, wet-heating conjugation of soy protein isolate with xylose or fructose negatively impacts its emulsifying activity, even though it enhances solubility [66]. Improvements in other functional properties of plant-based proteins have been reported following glycation with various saccharides. The foaming and emulsifying properties of soy protein isolate were enhanced following wet-heating glycation with glucose [67]. Enhanced foaming ability was observed in soy protein isolate following its conjugation with lentinan through an ultrasonic-assisted Maillard reaction, alongside improvements in solubility, emulsifying capacity and thermal stability [68].

Furthermore, glycation has been employed to mitigate the beany flavour in certain plant-based proteins, such as pea protein conjugated with Arabic gum [69]. Glycation may also serve as a method for the immunomodulation of plant-based proteins, as demonstrated in a previous study, which identified significant immunomodulatory properties in rice protein–sodium alginate conjugates [56]. Although the glycation method of protein modification is efficient and safe, it has been reported to adversely affect the nutritional value of proteins by reducing the bioavailability of lysine [70]. Therefore, glycation is the most advantageous chemical modification of plant-proteins for food applications, as it does not require the use of chemicals and does not generate by-products. This method represents a favourable chemical modification approach for plant-based proteins, considering consumers preferences for clean labels and commercialization.

5.3.2 Acylation

Acylation refers to the process of adding an acyl group to a protein using anhydrides and halides. The process is termed as acetylation or succinylation, depending on the acylating agent utilized, namely acetic or succinic anhydride. All nucleophilic groups within the protein structure interact with reagents; however, the ε-amino group of lysine demonstrates the greatest affinity. Succinylation substitutes net positive charges on protein hydroxyl and lysine amino groups with net negative charges, whereas acetylation neutralizes basic groups [71]. Modifying the surface charge of plant-derived proteins via acylation influences their solubility and functionality. It has been demonstrated that acylation, particularly succinylation, reduced neutral pH zeta potential of oat protein [72]. Similarly, following succinylation, the neutral pH zeta potential of mung bean isolates decreased, resulting in enhanced emulsifying properties [73]. Acylation enhances the hydrophobicity of plant-proteins, thereby improving their functional properties while preserving their nutritional integrity. Furthermore, succinylation significantly affected the secondary structure and tertiary conformation of oat proteins, as shown FTIR and intrinsic fluorescence spectroscopy (Figure 5.3); it also led to an increase in the molecular weight of oat protein [72]. In parallel studies it has been found that the hydrophobicity and molecular weight of rapeseed protein increases, enhancing its thermal stability and gelling properties [66, 74]. Succinylation also brings modifications in the secondary structure of pea protein isolates, resulting in enhanced solubility, foaming ability, emulsion stability and water retention capacity [75].

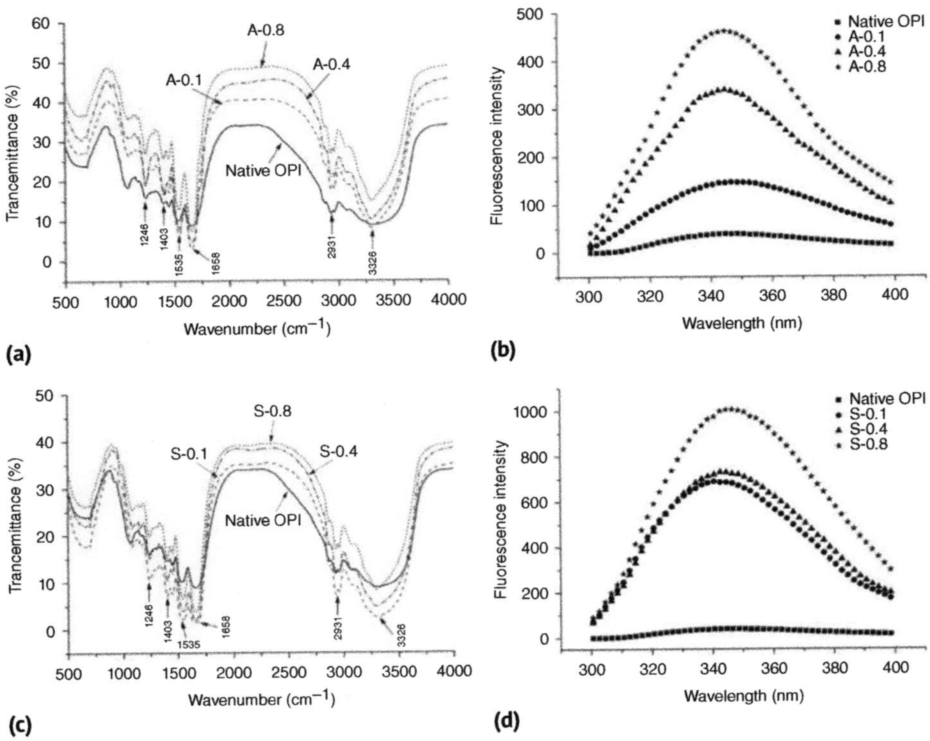

Figure 5.3 Post-acylated secondary structure and tertiary confirmation of oat protein. *Source:* Ref. [72] with permission of Elsevier.

5.3.3 Deamidation

Deamidation refers to the conversion of amide groups in glutamine and asparagine residues into carboxyl groups in a protein, thereby increasing the protein's negative charge. Deamidation can be performed under mild conditions and does not necessitate additional molecules, in contrast to acylation and alkylation, which require chemical agents. Consequently, this method is regarded as a source approach for modifying proteins in food systems. Due to high levels of glutamine and asparagine in cereals and legumes, deamidation serves as an appropriate modification method, particularly for their use in food products. Deamidation can be accomplished through various methods, including acid, alkali, enzyme and cation-exchange-resin treatments. Among these, acid treatment is the most common, while alkali treatment is the least common [76]. Glutaminase is the enzyme most extensively focused in literature regarding the deamidation of plant-based proteins. For instance, enzymatic deamidation of oat protein using glutaminase at 59 °C leads to a nearly twofold increase in protein solubility compared to native oat protein. Deamidated oat protein has demonstrated uniform oil droplet formation and enhanced stability over time. It also increases the flexibility of the secondary structure [77]. Another relevant study indicated that the deamidation of ultrafiltered oat protein concentrate decreases the zeta potential and enhances the repulsion in oat protein. Additionally, it eliminates non-polar lipids, thereby enhancing the foaming capacity and stability of oat protein [78].

A comparable study indicated that acid deamidation with citric acid, acetic acid and tartaric acid effectively reduce the bitterness of wheat gluten hydrolysates. Alkaline deamidation has been employed to enhance the solubility of rice bran protein. While acid deamidation is the predominant method, enzymatic deamidation is deemed more suitable for modifying plant-derived proteins due to substrate specificity, moderate reaction conditions and reduced side-chain reactions [79]. Improved solubility and enhanced techno-functionality of pea protein isolate have been observed, alongside a reduction in its beany flavour, grittiness and lumpiness [80]. Furthermore, deamidation has been identified as an effective method for reducing the allergenicity of plant-based proteins. For example, the gliadin protein, recognized as the primary allergen in wheat, exhibited reduced oral allergenicity in both in vitro and in vivo systems following deamidation [81, 82]. Another study reported a decrease in the transdermal allergenicity of wheat gliadin following deamidation [83]. These studies collectively demonstrate the effectiveness of deamidation in enhancing protein quality, thereby supporting the industrial application of oat protein.

5.3.4 pH Shifting

The pH of the liquid matrix in which proteins are dissolved significantly influences their structure and charge; consequently, acidic or alkaline treatments can induce changes in the structural and functional characteristics of proteins. At extreme pH levels, proteins experience denaturation and unfolding, exposing sulfhydryl and hydrophobic regions within their structure, thereby enabling new protein interactions. Alkaline conditions can be easily achieved through the application of chemical additives, including NaOH, NH4OH or urea [84, 85]. OPI undergo heating while the pH is shifted from 7 to 12 and then returned to 7, resulting in improved and maintained solubility (70–75%) at neutral pH. This discovery was supported by various physicochemical characteristics, such as particle size, the formation of short-chain peptides, thermal behaviour and a decrease in β-sheet content alongside an increase in random coil structures [86]. Another investigation revealed that the combined application of plasma treatment and pH adjustment to a mixture of OPI and casein resulted in an enhanced solubility of 82.63%. The combination treatment improved the surface hydrophobicity of the protein, promoting increased protein adsorption and redistribution at the water–oil interface. Furthermore, it enhances the emulsifying capacity of the combination of oat and casein protein isolates [87].

Numerous studies have employed pH shifting either prior to or alongside ultrasonic treatment for plant-based proteins. For instance, pH shifting at 12, followed by ultrasonication, to generate nano-sized soy protein aggregates with an average size of 22 nm. These aggregates demonstrated enhanced functionality, including increased solubility, surface hydrophobicity and emulsifying capacity [18]. Another similar study employed pH shifting at 12 and mano-thermo-sonication to generate soy protein isolate nano-aggregates with an average size of 27 nm. These aggregates demonstrated improved solubility, surface hydrophobicity, antioxidant activity, rheological characteristics and emulsifying properties [84]. The integration of alkali and ultrasonic treatment improved the solubility, emulsifying and foaming properties of rice protein [88]. The solubility, surface hydrophobicity and emulsifying properties of pea protein improved following pH-shifting at pH 12 combined with ultrasonic treatment [89]. The combined use of pH-shifting and sonication was utilized to improve the functionality of pea protein [90], and peanut protein for encapsulating bioactive compounds by addressing solubility challenges and enhancing their techno-functionality [59]. Proteins demonstrate optional solubility at higher levels; consequently, most studies in the literature have focused on adjusting the pH to alkaline conditions [89]. This highlights the important role of non-enzymatic processing method in improving plant protein solubility and its potential application in food products.

5.4 Biological Processing of Protein

Biological processing, primarily centred on enzymatic and fermentation procedures, is a renowned modification technique due to its lower energy consumption, environmental sustainability and the absence of non-toxic by-products. The costs of enzymes and culture must be considered for industrial-scale applications. In addition to enhancing the functional properties of target proteins, these processes also contribute to the nutritional quality of proteins, including protein digestibility, bioavailability and various bioactive properties, including antimicrobial, antioxidant and anti-diabetic effects. Consequently, the biological processing of proteins holds distinct advantages over other processing methods in various respects, rendering its distinctive and more advantageous.

5.4.1 Enzymatic Processing

Enzymatic processing is a common method for altering proteins, particularly for incorporation into food systems, owing to the non-toxic characteristics of the reactants and by-products involved. This alteration can be achieved under mild conditions with minimal by-products. In contrast to chemical modification, enzymatic modification preserves the chemical composition of the original proteins. The high specificity and efficiency of enzymes represent a significant advantage of enzymatic modification over chemical methods. This protein modification technique is classified into enzymatic hydrolysis and enzymatic cross-linking methods. The former occurs through the enzymatic formation of covalent bonds via transglutaminase and lactase, which catalyze the acyl transfer process between the γ-carboxamide group of protein-bound glutamine and lysine. In contrast, enzymatic hydrolysis involves the cleavage of peptide bonds by enzymes. Cross-linking can be performed using various enzymes to modify plant-derived proteins. Different enzymes, due to their unique mechanism of action, may display varying characteristics and functions in their end products. For instance, a study evaluated the effectiveness of two different crosslinking enzymes on oat protein and faba bean. The findings indicated that tyrosine displayed limited crosslinking capability on both proteins, whereas transglutaminase showed greater efficiency [91]. Transglutaminase, primarily sourced from bacteria such as *Streptoverticillium mobaraense*, serves as the main enzyme utilized for cross-linking of plant-derived proteins. In enzymatic cross-linking, time is one of the crucial factors, as incubation exceeding 60 minutes results in increased protein oxidation and a decline in its emulsifying properties. In addition to incubation duration, transglutaminase treatment may affect the content, structure and conformation of proteins, which is an important consideration for plant-derived proteins due to their composition of multiple fractions [92].

The albumin and globulin fractions of pea protein demonstrated differing responses during and after microbial transglutaminase treatment, with the albumin fraction proving ineffective for gelation through enzymatic treatment. Research suggests that changes in the conformation and structure of plant-based proteins contribute to the observed improvements in techno-functionality. Protein hydrolysis results in an increased number of ionizable groups and exposes hidden hydrophobic regions. The resulting hydrolysate demonstrates a lower molecular weight and improved functional characteristics and bioactivity compared to the original protein [71, 93]. The choice of enzyme, for example, (alcalase, chymotrypsin, chymosin, flavoenzyme, neutrase, papain, pepsin and trypsin) critically affects the properties of modified plant proteins, as their molecular differences relate to distinct cleavage sites [83, 94]. Trypsin specifically cleaves adjacent to the positively charged amino acids lysine and arginine, while maintaining the integrity of hydrophobic amino acid groups, thereby enhancing surface-active characteristics. The specific cleavage pattern of trypsin improved the solubility and interfacial properties of pea protein [95]. Tryptic hydrolysis resulted in oat protein peptides with improved foaming capacity [96]. Chymotrypsin, in contrast to trypsin, shows a preference for cleaving near hydrophobic amino acids like tryptophan or phenylalanine. It demonstrated the lowest degree of hydrolysis (DH) of pea protein among the evaluated enzymes [97]. Pepsin characterized by cleavage sites similar to those of chymotrypsin, it generates hydrophobic peptides that exhibit greater hydrophobicity than those produced by trypsin, likely due to the solubilization of hydrophobic amino acids following the action of pepsin. This could result in improved hydrophobicity and surface-active properties of the generated hydrolysates [93, 94].

The hydrolysis caused by papain was observed to enhance the bioactivity of plant-derived proteins. It shown the greatest capacity to enhance the in vitro antioxidant and metal chelating capabilities of oat bran proteins compared to a range of enzymes, including alcalase, flavourzyme and protamex. Alcalase, an endoenzyme, can liberate internal hydrophobic amino acids, whereas flavourzyme, an exopeptidase, can reveal those situated at the protein C and N terminals [98]. This resulted from the release of smaller peptides during alcalase action, which consequently exposed a greater number of antioxidant amino acids. The primary constraint in utilizing plant-based hydrolysates as an ingredient in the food business is their bitter flavour, attributed to low-molecular-weight peptides rich in hydrophobic amino acids. The bitterness of hydrolysates is associated with the DH, which can be mitigated by optimizing the hydrolyzing conditions to regulate the DH [97, 99]. Alcalase produces hydrolysates with increased bitterness owing to its elevated DH. Nonetheless, irrespective of its DH, the nature of the proteolytic enzyme is also a significant determinant in the bitterness of the hydrolysates. For instance, flavourzyme produces peptides with minimal bitterness, despite its capacity for extensive hydrolysis. The presence of hydrophobic amino acids and peptides near the N or C terminus of the protein may result in reduced bitterness compared to those situated within the peptide chain. Flavourzyme cleaves at the N or C terminus of proteins and peptides, producing hydrolysates with reduced bitterness compared to endopeptidases like alcalase [98].

5.4.2 Fermentation Processing

Fermentation serves as a traditional and cost-effective biological method for altering plant-based proteins. Multiple starter cultures, such as lactic acid bacteria, yeast, mould and

Bacillus strains, have been utilized for the fermentation of plant proteins, with lactic acid bacteria being the most common [100]. The fermentation of oats with *Lactiplantibacillus plantarum* B-16 demonstrated an increase in fermented oat soluble protein content from 7.05 to 14.43 mg/g. Electrophoresis and reversed-phase high-performance liquid chromatography indicated that the hydrolysis of fermented oat protein led to the formation of additional short peptides. Additionally, oat fermented by *L. plantarum* demonstrated enhanced angiotensin-converting enzyme (ACE) inhibitory activity relative to unfermented oats. Whole-grain oat products may serve as carriers for probiotics and represent potential therapeutic agents in the management of hypertension [101, 102]. Fermentation enhanced the solubility of soy protein, as well as its ability to retain water and oil, and its foaming capability [103]. Following solid-state fermentation using *Pediococcus pentosaceus*, lupin protein exhibited enhanced solubility and functional properties [104]. Fermented plant-based proteins have enhanced biological activity, as found that peanut protein had improved antioxidant capabilities post-fermentation [105]. Furthermore, the fermentation of plant proteins reduces their allergenic potential by degrading allergens and anti-nutritional compounds or altering their primary and tertiary structures. It has been discovered that fermentation is an effective method for reducing the bitter and beany off-flavours that are present in variety of plant-based proteins [100, 102, 103]. Collectively, fermentation processing is an effective technique to improve the functional and nutritional characteristics of oat proteins; however, the specific starters, their dose and duration must be controlled according to specifications and desired results.

5.5 Effect of Processing on Functional and Physicochemical Characteristics of Oat Proteins

5.5.1 Texturization Characteristics

Protein texturization refers to the inherent property of proteins to form organized tissue patterns through specific structural and functional arrangements within cells or in vitro. Plant protein texturization is a process wherein plant-derived proteins serve as the primary raw material and undergo structural modification, with or without exogenous additives. Through methods such as extrusion, protein molecular chains are functionally reorganized and cross-linked, ultimately yielding plant-based protein products featuring muscle-like anisotropic fibrous frameworks. Theoretically, all plant-derived proteins qualify as raw materials for textured plant protein production. Considering factors such as sourcing accessibility, cost-effectiveness and processing performance, wheat protein, soy protein and pea protein are extensively utilized in industrial texturization. Additionally, rice protein, peanut protein and others are increasingly utilized in extrusion-based protein texturization [106].

Plant proteins primarily consist of structurally substantial and compact storage proteins. Albumins and globulins predominantly occur in legumes and pseudocereals (e.g., soybean, oat and quinoa), while prolamins and glutenins are chiefly found in cereals (e.g., wheat, barley and millet). These proteins comprise polypeptide chains whose structural integrity is maintained through hydrophobic interactions, hydrogen bonding, electrostatic forces, van der Waals forces and disulphide bonds. During thermal processing, exposure of non-polar groups and sulfhydryl groups induces protein aggregation via hydrophobic interactions and disulphide crosslinking. This disrupts the equilibrium between protein–protein and protein–solvent interactions, ultimately forming orderly arranged matrix structures [107, 108].

As protein source, animal muscle tissue comprises three primary protein classes: sarcoplasmic proteins, stromal proteins and myofibrillar proteins (Table 5.1). Myofibrillar proteins constitute the dominant structural component of myofibrils in meat, primarily composed of myosin and actin. Myosin—a fibrous protein formed by ~4500 amino acids—contrasts with actin's globular conformation. Bundles of elongated myofibrils establish the foundation of muscle fibres, creating interstitial spaces where endogenous water is immobilized through capillary forces, hydrogen bonding and ion–dipole interactions. This hierarchical organization confers unique textural and masticatory properties to meat, an architectural complexity currently irreplaceable by alternative protein systems [109].

Comparative analysis of plant and animal protein structures (Table 5.1) reveals fundamental divergences: plant proteins predominantly adopt globular conformations with high molecular symmetry and enhanced solubility, whereas animal proteins typically exhibit fibrous, asymmetric architectures with limited aqueous solubility [110]. Thermally, plant proteins require significantly higher denaturation thresholds (e.g., soy glycinin ≈90 °C) compared to animal counterparts like myosin (initiating at 40 °C, peaking at 50 °C) and actin (66–73 °C), necessitating extended heating for structural reorganization and functional modification. Compositionally, plant proteins associate with carbohydrates and contain elevated

Table 5.1 Comparative characteristics of plant vs. animal proteins.

Feature	Plant proteins	Animal proteins
Protein types	Primarily compact storage proteins: albumins, globulins, prolamins and glutenins (composition varies by species)	Sarcoplasmic, stromal and myofibrillar proteins; myofibrillar proteins form irreplaceable fibrous architectures
Structure	Predominantly globular, high symmetry, generally soluble	Primarily fibrous, asymmetric, mostly water-insoluble
Denaturation temp	Higher thresholds (e.g., β-conglycinin ≈90 °C)	Lower thresholds (myosin: initiates at 40 °C, peaks at 50 °C; actin: 66–73 °C)
Secondary structure	β-sheet dominant (enhances thermal stability)	α-helix dominant (facilitates conformational changes)
Associated components	Complexed with carbohydrates (non-starch polysaccharides and dietary fibre)	Coexist with lipids (e.g., 25–30% fat in pork muscle)
Digestibility	Reduced bioavailability (PDCAAS 0.70–0.85) due to: cellulose encapsulation, antinutritional factors: phytates, protease inhibitors, lectins and tannins	Superior digestibility (PDCAAS 0.95–1.00): casein-dominated systems, efficient enzymatic hydrolysis

vitamins, minerals and dietary fibre, while animal proteins coexist with lipids (e.g., 25–30% fat in pork), leading to concomitant saturated fat and cholesterol intake. Digestibility favours animal proteins (≈95% PDCAAS bioavailability) due to efficient enzymatic hydrolysis of casein-dominated systems; plant proteins suffer reduced proteolysis (70–85% PDCAAS) from cellulose encapsulation and antinutritional factors (phytates, protease inhibitors, lectins and tannins) that impede enzyme accessibility [111].

High-moisture extrusion is a critical technology for texturizing plant proteins; it can simulate meat-like structures, effectively enhancing the textural deficiencies of current plant-based meats. Utilizing protein concentrates or isolates (>60% protein, <7% fat), this process generates macroscopically visible anisotropic fibres through hierarchical protein reorganization. During extrusion, proteins undergo sequential phase transitions: initial molecular unfolding (30–90 °C), where shear forces and hydration expose hydrophobic domains, transitioning into a fluidic state with partial denaturation; followed by molecular reorganization (90–120 °C, 2–5 MPa, 15–40 Nm torque), where polypeptide chains realign under thermo-mechanical stress, triggering dynamic bond exchange—disruption of non-covalent interactions (hydrogen/ionic bonds) and formation of disulphide crosslinks alongside hydrophobic associations [112, 113].

The alignment phase (120–160 °C) drives anisotropic structuring through flow-induced orientation in the die section (>100 s-1 shear rate) and cysteine oxidation-driven disulphide stabilization, yielding products with optimal elasticity (Young's modulus: 0.8–1.2 MPa) and chewiness (300–500 mJ). Exceeding 180 °C induces protein degradation via Maillard-driven lysine loss and pathological over-crosslinking, causing structural heterogeneity and toughness >700 mJ. Consequently, the 120–160 °C range represents the empirical thermal window for plant protein texturization, with source-specific optima: soy isolate (135–145 °C for glycinin dissociation), wheat gluten (125–135 °C for polymer reptation) and pea concentrate (140–155 °C for legumin denaturation). Successful texturization requires synchronizing thermal energy with protein-specific transition points, where only above critical temperatures (e.g., 115–125 °C for rice glutenin) can polypeptide chains fully unfold and reorganize into cohesive fibres. Process efficacy is quantified by a Fibre Formation Index >85% and PDCAAS >0.90, while avoiding lysinoalanine formation >150 ppm, a marker of thermal overprocessing that compromises nutritional and structural integrity in meat analogues.

Oat globulin exhibits a significantly higher denaturation temperature than other plant proteins, attributable to its elevated globulin content and stable hexameric quaternary structure [114]. Comparatively, soybean protein requires extrusion temperatures exceeding 120 °C to achieve well-defined fibrous textures in high-moisture textured products, while peanut protein necessitates temperatures above 130 °C to develop tightly packed fibrous matrices. Wheat protein demands even higher thermal inputs (>140 °C) due to its large molecular mass and extensive non-covalent interactions, which are essential for promoting crosslinking and generating complex fibrous networks. Although globulin-dominant plant proteins serve as primary raw materials for meat analogues, their inherent globular multimeric architecture may intrinsically limit the formation of densely packed fibrous structures during texturization. This structural constraint stems from the energy barrier involved in disrupting stable polymeric assemblies prior to polypeptide realignment, potentially compromising the ultimate tensile strength and anisotropic organization achievable compared to naturally fibrous proteins [114, 115].

5.5.2 Oat Dough Characteristics: High Hardness and Low Elasticity

The mixture formed during the kneading of flour and water, exhibiting both the elasticity of solids and the viscosity of liquids, is termed dough. Upon water addition, proteins and starch granules within flour particles hydrate and swell. During initial mixing, friction occurs between particles, where hydrophilic groups on protein surfaces hydrate without yet forming gluten [116]. Continued mixing allows water molecules to hydrate all polar groups along protein colloidal chains, with hydration proceeding from the surface inward. Soluble components within the protein colloids dissolve, generating internal osmotic pressure that drives water absorption into the colloidal interior until osmotic equilibrium is reached. Ultimately, gluten proteins develop hydrophobic regions externally and hydrophilic regions internally, retaining absorbed water. Throughout this process, the dough progressively softens, exhibits reduced stickiness and attains a smooth surface [116, 117].

Oat globulin exhibits a significantly higher denaturation temperature than other plant proteins, attributable to its elevated globulin content and stable hexameric quaternary structure. Comparatively, soybean protein requires extrusion temperatures exceeding 120 °C to achieve well-defined fibrous textures in high-moisture textured products, while peanut protein necessitates temperatures above 130 °C to develop tightly packed fibrous matrices. Wheat protein demands even higher thermal inputs (>140 °C) due to its large molecular mass and extensive non-covalent interactions, which are essential for promoting crosslinking and generating complex fibrous networks [114, 115].

Although globulin-dominant plant proteins serve as primary raw materials for meat analogues, their inherent globular multimeric architecture may intrinsically limit the formation of densely packed fibrous structures during texturization. This structural constraint stems from the energy barrier involved in disrupting stable polymeric assemblies prior to polypeptide realignment, potentially compromising the ultimate tensile strength and anisotropic organization achievable compared to naturally fibrous proteins [118]. At the protein structural level, glutenin subunits undergo sulfhydryl–disulphide interchange reactions, forming ordered fibrous polymeric assemblies through intermolecular disulphide bonding. Macroscopically, this manifests as progressive dough elasticity development—where larger polymer aggregates enhance elastic recovery via polymer chain reptation mechanisms. Gliadins adopt compact globular conformations stabilized by intramolecular disulphide bonds, hydrogen bonding and hydrophobic interactions. These become covalently integrated within the glutenin network framework, with their steric presence disrupting glutenin–glutenin interactions to impart dough viscosity.

The synergistic reorganization of disulphide linkages and secondary bonds among polypeptide chains generates an expansive, ordered gluten network architecture. This three-dimensional matrix confers simultaneous dough extensibility and elasticity. During dough formation, starch granules undergo minimal structural alteration, functioning as inert filler particles embedded within the continuous gluten phase to establish homogeneous dough microstructure [119]. Dough properties are modulated by multiple factors, including hydration level, protein characteristics, starch attributes, mixing methodology and duration. Starch granules and gluten proteins engage water molecules via hydrogen bonding with hydrophilic and polar groups, facilitating surface/internal hydration. As mechanical energy inputs (kneading, shearing, laminating) intensify, air incorporation accelerates thiol–disulphide interchange reactions. This drives orientation-specific protein deformation while dynamically reorganizing intermolecular forces, progressively establishing transitional regional gluten networks [120].

Dough hydration requirements vary significantly across flour types, with oat flour necessitating 90–120% water relative to flour weight-substantially exceeding wheat flour's typical ≈60% hydration level. Optimal dough cohesion in oat formulations is achieved specifically when using boiling water, attributable to three key factors: the inherent moisture disparity between raw flours, differential water absorption capacities of heat-treated oat flours and the enhanced solubility of oat β-glucan and protein denaturation at elevated temperatures. From Table 5.2, wheat dough exhibits significantly lower hardness (18.97 kg), while oat-based dough demonstrates substantially greater hardness, ranging from 41.37 to 58.03 kg under identical texture analyzer conditions—representing 2.5 to 3 times the hardness of wheat dough. Wheat dough demonstrates substantially greater springiness (0.91), while oat-based dough exhibits significantly lower springiness ranging from 0.60 to 0.84 under identical texture analyzer conditions. This primarily correlates with oat dough's hydration level of 85–95% flour weight. Notably, doughs from unroasted oats display the poorest springiness (0.60), whereas roasting improves springiness (0.63–0.95), though still inferior to wheat dough [121].

The heightened hardness and reduced springiness of oat dough stem from three interconnected mechanisms: oat proteins inherently fail to establish densely interconnected network structures; partial starch gelatinization induced by boiling water partially compensates by enhancing dough continuity; while β-glucan competitively sequesters water against starch and soluble polysaccharides. This multiphase hydration competition triggers water redistribution away from proteins, ultimately yielding elevated hardness and diminished elasticity [122].

5.5.3 Emulsifying Foaming Characteristics

Oat protein fractions demonstrate high solubility under alkaline conditions (pH 8–10), establishing alkaline extraction as the optimal method for comprehensive protein isolation. Albumin exhibits pH-independent solubility (>90% across all pH), while globulin displays a distinct bell-shaped solubility profile: minimal solubility at pH 6–7 (>90% solubility at pH 1.5–6 and 7–10) [123]. Prolamin similarly shows bell-shaped behaviour

Table 5.2 Dough hardness and springiness from wheat and oat flour.

Flour Type	Hydration (%)	Hardness (kg)	Springiness
Wheat flour	60	18.97 ± 0.90	0.91 ± 0.05
Yinshan oat flour	95	54.21 ± 0.95	0.77 ± 0.03
Sihai oat flour	90	44.19 ± 2.59	0.63 ± 0.19
Xibei oat flour	95	52.44 ± 1.45	0.69 ± 0.09
Wuchuan oat flour	90	41.37 ± 1.80	0.65 ± 0.07
Zhangjiakou oat flour	95	48.89 ± 0.94	0.84 ± 0.05
Raw oat flour	60	58.03 ± 1.53	0.60 ± 0.06

with minimum solubility at pH 5–6 and greater solubility in alkaline versus acidic environments. Glutelin maintains low solubility (≤20%) between pH 3 and 8, but exhibits dramatically higher solubility at pH 10.5 (≈90%) compared to pH 1.5 (≈30%). Critically, oat proteins surpass soy proteins in solubility across equivalent pH conditions. Beyond glutenin's poor foam stability, oat protein fractions generally exhibit favourable foaming properties and foam stability. Albumin demonstrates superior foamability (240% expansion) compared to globulin (100%), prolamin (50%) and glutenin (45%). After 50 minutes of quiescent standing, their respective foam stabilities measure 47, 60, 63 and 27%. Foam stability increases with rising pH for albumin, globulin and glutenin, while prolamin displays markedly lower stability under alkaline conditions relative to acidic and neutral pH environments [123].

Among oat protein fractions, prolamin demonstrates the highest emulsification stability (9.5 min), while albumin, globulin and glutenin exhibit significantly lower stability indices of 3.2, 3.0 and 2.0 minutes, respectively. Oat albumin and glutenin exhibit higher hydration capacities (2.4 mL/g and 1.9 mL/g, respectively) compared to globulin and prolamin (0.8 and 0.9 mg/L). Albumin demonstrates moderate fat-binding capacity (2.8 mg/L), while globulin, prolamin and glutenin show values of 1.6, 1.7 and 2.1 mg/L, respectively. Oil retention capacity is functionally critical for plant-based meat analogues, with oat albumin displaying significantly higher oil-holding properties than other protein components [123].

Oat proteins are characterized by globulin predominance (>50% composition), which inherently exhibits limited solubility; however, Osborne fractionation-derived oat globulin demonstrates optimal solubility at pH 9.0. Solubility minima (~10%) occur at the isoelectric point (pH 4.0–6.0), while significant solubility enhancement emerges under strongly acidic (<2.5) or alkaline (>8.0) conditions due to electrostatic repulsion effects. Roasted naked oat globulin undergoes structural reorganization where thermal processing exposes additional hydrophobic groups and enhances molecular ordering, thereby strengthening protein–water interactions and significantly elevating solubility. Controlled thermal denaturation facilitates protein unfolding to improve solubility, with both roasting and autoclaving substantially increasing protein content in oat beverages. Hydrothermal treatments—including autoclaving (high pressure) and atmospheric steaming—prove particularly effective for protein modification, promoting enzymatic proteolysis and solubility enhancement [123].

The inherently low solubility of oat proteins critically constrains functionalities such as foaming and emulsification, thereby limiting their industrial utilization. To address this, enzymatic hydrolysis and chemical modifications (e.g., deamidation and succinylation of OPI) have been successfully employed to markedly enhance solubility. Oat protein solutions exhibit characteristic non-Newtonian fluid behaviour, demonstrating pronounced shear-thinning where apparent viscosity decreases with increasing shear rate. Viscosity escalates progressively with rising protein concentration, while intensified shear-thinning effects emerge markedly at higher protein concentrations [123].

5.5.4 Protein Conversion Coefficient

The protein conversion factor is a fundamental concept in biology and nutrition, used to convert nitrogen content in food or biological samples into protein content. The Kjeldahl method—widely recognized for its accuracy—quantifies nitrogen to derive protein levels by applying a standard conversion factor. Typically, this factor remains constant: for meat and legumes, nitrogen constitutes approximately 16% of protein mass; thus, protein content is calculated as nitrogen value × 6.25 (i.e., 1/0.16). However, significant variations in nitrogen composition across materials result in conversion factors ranging from 5.50 to 6.38. Protein conversion coefficients vary across food categories (Table 5.3), with common coefficients including 6.25 and 5.70. For cereals, wheat, rye, barley, oats and millet share a coefficient of 5.83, while rice and rice flour use 5.95 and corn/sorghum employ 6.25. Soy products exhibit dual coefficients (5.71 or 6.25) due to processing-induced protein loss. Peanuts utilize 5.46, and oilseeds (cottonseed, sunflower, sesame and coconut) share 5.30. Among animal-derived foods, meat products and eggs apply 6.25, dairy products 6.38 and gelatin 5.50.

In summary, the Kjeldahl method and protein conversion factors enable precise quantification of protein content, with coefficient selection dictated by the intrinsic nitrogen-to-protein composition of each substance. Crucially, processing methods and cooking techniques significantly influence these factors, for instance, roasting meat induces protein concentration shifts through moisture evaporation and Maillard reactions, necessitating dynamic coefficient adjustments to maintain analytical accuracy.

5.5.5 High Lipase Activity

Lipase (EC 3.1.1.3), also termed triacylglycerol hydrolase, functions as a biocatalyst to hydrolyze triglycerides at oil–water interfaces and catalyzes ester synthesis, transesterification, acidolysis, alcoholysis and aminolysis in water-immiscible systems without coenzyme requirements, enabling broad applications in food processing, detergents, pharmaceuticals and bioenergy. Esterases preferentially hydrolyze short/medium-chain

Table 5.3 Protein conversion coefficient.

Source	Protein content (DW)	Coefficient
Cereals	Wheat/Rye/Barley/Oats/Millet	5.83
	Rice and Rice Flour	5.95
	Corn/Sorghum	6.25
Legumes and Nuts	Soy and Soy Products	5.71 or 6.25 (Based on varied procedure)
	Peanuts	5.46
	Cottonseed/Sunflower/Sesame/Coconut	5.30
Animal-Derived Foods	Dairy Products	6.38
	Eggs	6.25
	Meat and Meat Products	6.25
	Gelatin	5.50

DW: dry weight

esters in aqueous solutions but not long-chain esters; fatty acyl hydrolases target mono-dispersed or micellar fats while sparing water-soluble lipids; whereas lipases operate exclusively at oil–water interfaces, hydrolyzing long-chain esters but not solubilized fats [124].

Plant lipases, predominantly found in oilseed crops, catalyze the conversion of endogenous lipids into glycolytic energy substrates to support plant growth. Crucially, lipid hydroperoxides generated by lipase hydrolysis serve as substrates for peroxidase and catalase—enzymes pivotal to oat's stress resistance—thereby facilitating oat cultivation in alpine regions. These enzymes offer advantages including accessible sourcing, high substrate specificity and organic solvent tolerance, along with broader consumer acceptance. However, their low natural expression levels and significant activity loss during intricate purification processes have limited extensive research and utilization. Nevertheless, plant lipases represent promising candidates for industrial enzyme applications warranting in-depth investigation. Lipase activity is present in nearly all cereal grains, though with substantial variation across species. When quantified as released oleic acid (mg/g), oat lipase activity exceeds 20 mg/g—significantly higher than wheat (2–4.5 mg/g), brown rice (11–13 mg/g) and millet (6–10 mg/g). Remarkable intra-species differences exist: foreign hulled oat varieties exhibit up to eightfold activity divergence (67.7–523.1 μmol/g/h), while 31 domestic naked oat varieties show a coefficient of variation (CV) of 32.56% (30.92–120.44 μmol/g/h) [124].

Lipase in oats is predominantly localized in the grain pericarp, exhibiting uneven distribution throughout the kernel. Layer-by-layer abrasion analysis revealed that higher dehull rates (0–15.9%) corresponded with increased total lipid content (6.53–6.79%) and significantly reduced lipase activity (325.8~119.8 μmol/g/h), confirming enzyme concentration in the pericarp and aleurone layer. Post-harvest handling (cleaning, storage, processing) damages these layers, elevating lipase activity and compromising grain quality. Lipase activity further correlates with kernel size, large kernels (typically 2~4 per spikelet) show ≈80% activity of normal-sized grains, while small kernels exhibit ≈1.2-fold higher activity [124].

The lipase activity of oats is predominantly influenced by cultivation environment and varietal factors, with ANOVA indicating the effect hierarchy: environmental factors > genotype–environment interaction > varietal factors. Both cultivar selection and growing conditions significantly impact lipase activity, with environment being the dominant determinant. Reference indicators for selecting low-lipase activity varieties include: cool growing temperatures, low elevation, reduced precipitation, shorter growing season duration, low fat content and higher test weight. Oat lipase (36.5 kDa, 341 amino acids) functions as a serine hydrolase with a catalytic triad at Ser281-His315-Asp312, where Ser acts as the nucleophilic residue, His provides structural scaffolding, and Asp serves as the electrophilic component [125, 126]. Its activity is regulated by an α-helical lid that shields the active site in aqueous environments, hydrophobic groups facing inward block substrate access, while hydrophilic groups hydrogen-bond with water. Upon adsorption to oil–water interfaces, hydrophobic exposure triggers lid opening, initiating catalysis. The enzyme exhibits peak activity at 40 °C/pH 7.5 and maintains stability at 50 °C within pH 7.0–8.0. Divalent cations (Fe^{3+}, Cu^{2+}, Ba^{2+}, Mg^{2+}) and K^+ strongly inhibit activity, while Na+ shows no effect. Substrate specificity prioritizes oat oil and structurally similar triglycerides with analogous fatty acid profiles [125, 126].

Summary

With the growing global demand for plant-based proteins, there is an increasing emphasis on the industrialization and utilization of novel protein sources. Oat protein, known for its excellent nutritional and functional properties, still faces several constraints that limit its large-scale industrial application and incorporation into food products, including its use as an alternative protein source for meat analogues. To enhance its utilization and promote industrialization, modification of the structural and functional properties of oat protein is essential. Such improvements can increase its incorporation in food systems by enhancing water and oil-holding capacities, foaming ability and reducing the bitterness of bioactive oat protein hydrolysates. A range of physical, chemical and biological modification techniques may be required; however, achieving the desired structural and functional improvements necessitates careful selection and optimization of processing methods. Through these approaches, the industrial application of oat protein can be significantly expanded, making it a more valuable and sustainable cereal protein source for global use.

References

1 S. M. Jafari, A. Sedaghat Doost, M. Nikbakht Nasrabadi, S. Boostani, and P. Van der Meeren, 'Phytoparticles for the stabilization of Pickering emulsions in the formulation of novel food colloidal dispersions', *Trends Food Sci. Technol.*, vol. 98, pp. 117–128, 2020, https://doi.org/10.1016/j.tifs.2020.02.008.

2 M. Nikbakht Nasrabadi et al., 'Plant based Pickering stabilization of emulsions using soluble flaxseed protein and mucilage nano-assemblies', *Colloids Surf. A Physicochem. Eng. Asp.*, vol. 563, pp. 170–182, 2019, https://doi.org/10.1016/j.colsurfa.2018.12.004.

3 M. Nikbakht Nasrabadi, A. Sedaghat Doost, and R. Mezzenga, 'Modification approaches of plant-based proteins to improve their techno-functionality and use in food products', *Food Hydrocoll.*, vol. 118, p. 106789, 2021, https://doi.org/10.1016/j.foodhyd.2021.106789.

4 V. Raikos, G. Duthie, and V. Ranawana, 'Denaturation and oxidative stability of hemp seed (*Cannabis sativa* L.) protein isolate as affected by heat treatment', *Plant Foods Hum. Nutr.*, vol. 70, no. 3, pp. 304–309, 2015, https://doi.org/10.1007/s11130-015-0494-5.

5 N. A. Mir, C. S. Riar, and S. Singh, 'Structural modification in album (*Chenopodium album*) protein isolates due to controlled thermal modification and its relationship with protein digestibility and functionality', *Food Hydrocoll.*, vol. 103, p. 105708, 2020, https://doi.org/10.1016/j.foodhyd.2020.105708.

6 M. Zhao, W. Xiong, B. Chen, J. Zhu, and L. Wang, 'Enhancing the solubility and foam ability of rice glutelin by heat treatment at pH12: insight into protein structure', *Food Hydrocoll.*, vol. 103, p. 105626, 2020, https://doi.org/10.1016/j.foodhyd.2019.105626.

7 J. M. Bühler, B. L. Dekkers, M. E. Bruins, and A. J. van der Goot, 'Modifying faba bean protein concentrate using dry heat to increase water holding capacity', *Foods*, vol. 9, no. 8, p. 1077, 2020, https://doi.org/10.3390/foods9081077.

8 D. Chao and R. E. Aluko, 'Modification of the structural, emulsifying, and foaming properties of an isolated pea protein by thermal pretreatment', *CyTA - J. Food*, vol. 16, no. 1, pp. 357–366, 2018, https://doi.org/10.1080/19476337.2017.1406536.

9 S.-W. Yin, C.-H. Tang, J.-S. Cao, E.-K. Hu, Q.-B. Wen, and X.-Q. Yang, 'Effects of limited enzymatic hydrolysis with trypsin on the functional properties of hemp (*Cannabis sativa* L.) protein isolate', *Food Chem.*, vol. 106, no. 3, pp. 1004–1013, 2008, https://doi.org/10.1016/j.foodchem.2007.07.030.

10 Q. Wang, J. Jiang, and Y. L. Xiong, 'Genipin-aided protein cross-linking to modify structural and rheological properties of emulsion-filled hempseed protein hydrogels', *J. Agric. Food Chem.*, vol. 67, no. 46, pp. 12895–12903, 2019, https://doi.org/10.1021/acs.jafc.9b05665.

11 X. Wang, Y. Lei, H. Rafique, L. Zou, and X. Hu, 'Effect of stir-frying on physicochemical and functional properties of oat protein isolates', *Foods*, vol. 12, no. 14, p. 2670, 2023, https://doi.org/10.3390/foods12142670.

12 P. Choudhary, S. Dutta, J. A. Moses, and C. Anandharamakrishnan, 'Recent developments in encapsulation of α-lipoic acid for enhanced bioavailability and stability', *Qual. Assur. Saf. Crop. Foods*, vol. 15, no. 1, pp. 123–138, 2023, https://doi.org/10.15586/qas.v15i1.1081.

13 S. Avilés-Gaxiola, C. Chuck-Hernández, M. del R. Rocha-Pizaña, S. García-Lara, L. M. López-Castillo, and S. O. Serna-Saldívar, 'Effect of thermal processing and reducing agents on trypsin inhibitor activity and functional properties of soybean and chickpea protein concentrates', *LWT*, vol. 98, pp. 629–634, 2018, https://doi.org/10.1016/j.lwt.2018.09.023.

14 B. H. Hite, 'The Effect of Pressure in the Preservation of Milk: A Preliminary Report', Morgantown, WV, 1899. https://doi.org/10.33915/agnic.58.

15 P. Lv, D. Wang, L. Dai, X. Wu, Y. Gao, and F. Yuan, 'Pickering emulsion gels stabilized by high hydrostatic pressure-induced whey protein isolate gel particles: characterization and encapsulation of curcumin', *Food Res. Int.*, vol. 132, p. 109032, 2020, https://doi.org/10.1016/j.foodres.2020.109032.

16 A. Sedaghat Doost, F. Devlieghere, C. V. Stevens, M. Claeys, and P. Van der Meeren, 'Self-assembly of Tween 80 micelles as nanocargos for oregano and trans-cinnamaldehyde plant-derived compounds', *Food Chem.*, vol. 327, p. 126970, 2020, https://doi.org/10.1016/j.foodchem.2020.126970.

17 R. P. Queirós, J. A. Saraiva, and J. A. L. da Silva, 'Tailoring structure and technological properties of plant proteins using high hydrostatic pressure', *Crit. Rev. Food Sci. Nutr.*, vol. 58, no. 9, pp. 1538–1556, 2018, https://doi.org/10.1080/10408398.2016.1271770.

18 H. Lee et al., 'Soy protein nano-aggregates with improved functional properties prepared by sequential pH treatment and ultrasonication', *Food Hydrocoll.*, vol. 55, pp. 200–209, 2016, https://doi.org/10.1016/j.foodhyd.2015.11.022.

19 M. C. Condés, M. C. Añón, and A. N. Mauri, 'Amaranth protein films prepared with high-pressure treated proteins', *J. Food Eng.*, vol. 166, pp. 38–44, 2015, https://doi.org/10.1016/j.jfoodeng.2015.05.005.

20 J. Zhao, T. Zhou, Y. Zhang, Y. Ni, and Q. Li, 'Optimization of arachin extraction from defatted peanut (*Arachis hypogaea*) cakes and effects of ultra-high pressure (UHP) treatment on physiochemical properties of arachin', *Food Bioprod. Process.*, vol. 95, pp. 38–46, 2015, https://doi.org/10.1016/j.fbp.2015.03.009.

21 D. Liu, L. Zhang, Y. Wang, Z. Li, Z. Wang, and J. Han, 'Effect of high hydrostatic pressure on solubility and conformation changes of soybean protein isolate glycated with flaxseed gum', *Food Chem.*, vol. 333, p. 127530, 2020, https://doi.org/10.1016/j.foodchem.2020.127530.

22 B. Cao, L. Fang, C. Liu, W. Min, and J. Liu, 'Effects of high hydrostatic pressure on the functional and rheological properties of the protein fraction extracted from pine nuts', *Food Sci. Technol. Int.*, vol. 24, no. 1, pp. 53–66, 2018, https://doi.org/10.1177/1082013217726883.

23 S. Ma, M. Zhang, Y. Shi, H. Wang, and H. Chu, 'Effects of ultrahigh pressure treatment on eating quality of steamed oat and oat protein structure', *CyTA - J. Food*, vol. 19, no. 1, pp. 56–62, 2021, https://doi.org/10.1080/19476337.2020.1857847.

24 J. Ahmed, N. Al-Ruwaih, M. Mulla, and M. H. Rahman, 'Effect of high pressure treatment on functional, rheological and structural properties of kidney bean protein isolate', *LWT*, vol. 91, pp. 191–197, 2018, https://doi.org/10.1016/j.lwt.2018.01.054.

25 L. Piccini, A. Scilingo, and F. Speroni, 'Thermal versus high hydrostatic pressure treatments on calcium-added soybean proteins. Protein solubility, colloidal stability and cold-set gelation', *Food Biophys.*, vol. 14, no. 1, pp. 69–79, 2019, https://doi.org/10.1007/s11483-018-9558-z.

26 M. Franck, V. Perreault, S. Suwal, A. Marciniak, L. Bazinet, and A. Doyen, 'High hydrostatic pressure-assisted enzymatic hydrolysis improved protein digestion of flaxseed protein isolate and generation of peptides with antioxidant activity', *Food Res. Int.*, vol. 115, pp. 467–473, 2019, https://doi.org/10.1016/j.foodres.2018.10.034.

27 N. Al-Ruwaih, J. Ahmed, M. F. Mulla, and Y. A. Arfat, 'High-pressure assisted enzymatic proteolysis of kidney beans protein isolates and characterization of hydrolysates by functional, structural, rheological and antioxidant properties', *LWT*, vol. 100, pp. 231–236, 2019, https://doi.org/10.1016/j.lwt.2018.10.074.

28 A. Sedaghat Doost, K. Dewettinck, F. Devlieghere, and P. Van der Meeren, 'Influence of non-ionic emulsifier type on the stability of cinnamaldehyde nanoemulsions: a comparison of polysorbate 80 and hydrophobically modified inulin', *Food Chem.*, vol. 258, pp. 237–244, 2018, https://doi.org/10.1016/j.foodchem.2018.03.078.

29 A. Sedaghat Doost, M. Nikbakht Nasrabadi, V. Kassozi, K. Dewettinck, C. V. Stevens, and P. Van der Meeren, 'Pickering stabilization of thymol through green emulsification using soluble fraction of almond gum – whey protein isolate nano-complexes', *Food Hydrocoll.*, vol. 88, pp. 218–227, 2019, https://doi.org/10.1016/j.foodhyd.2018.10.009.

30 B. C. Porto, A. A. L. Tribst, and M. Cristianini, 'Dynamic high pressure effects on biopolymers: polysaccharides and proteins', In: Biopolymers for Food Design (ed. A. M. Grumezescu and A. M. Holban), Elsevier, pp. 313–350, 2018, https://doi.org/10.1016/B978-0-12-811449-0.00010-4.

31 M. Cheng et al., 'Effect of dynamic high-pressure microfluidization on physicochemical, structural, and functional properties of oat protein isolate', *Innov. Food Sci. Emerg. Technol.*, vol. 82, p. 103204, 2022, https://doi.org/10.1016/j.ifset.2022.103204.

32 M. Primozic, A. Duchek, M. Nickerson, and S. Ghosh, 'Formation, stability and in vitro digestibility of nanoemulsions stabilized by high-pressure homogenized lentil proteins isolate', *Food Hydrocoll.*, vol. 77, pp. 126–141, 2018, https://doi.org/10.1016/j.foodhyd.2017.09.028.

33 F. T. Saricaoglu, 'Application of high-pressure homogenization (HPH) to modify functional, structural and rheological properties of lentil (*Lens culinaris*) proteins', *Int. J. Biol. Macromol.*, vol. 144, pp. 760–769, 2020, https://doi.org/10.1016/j.ijbiomac.2019.11.034.

34 F. T. Saricaoglu, O. Gul, A. Besir, and I. Atalar, 'Effect of high pressure homogenization (HPH) on functional and rheological properties of hazelnut meal proteins obtained from hazelnut oil industry by-products', *J. Food Eng.*, vol. 233, pp. 98–108, 2018, https://doi.org/10.1016/j.jfoodeng.2018.04.003.

35 H. Li, K. Zhu, H. Zhou, W. Peng, and X. Guo, 'Comparative study of four physical approaches about allergenicity of soybean protein isolate for infant formula', *Food Agric. Immunol.*, vol. 27, no. 5, pp. 604–623, 2016, https://doi.org/10.1080/09540105.2015.1129602.

36 I. Zahari et al., 'Development of high-moisture meat analogues with hemp and soy protein using extrusion cooking', *Foods*, vol. 9, no. 6, p. 772, 2020, https://doi.org/10.3390/foods9060772.

37 R. Osen, S. Toelstede, P. Eisner, and U. Schweiggert-Weisz, 'Effect of high moisture extrusion cooking on protein–protein interactions of pea (*Pisum sativum* L.) protein isolates', *Int. J. Food Sci. Technol.*, vol. 50, no. 6, pp. 1390–1396, 2015, https://doi.org/10.1111/ijfs.12783.

38 W. Ma, B. Qi, R. Sami, L. Jiang, Y. Li, and H. Wang, 'Conformational and functional properties of soybean proteins produced by extrusion-hydrolysis approach', *Int. J. Anal. Chem.*, vol. 2018, pp. 1–11, 2018, https://doi.org/10.1155/2018/9182508.

39 S. M. Beck, K. Knoerzer, and J. Arcot, 'Effect of low moisture extrusion on a pea protein isolate's expansion, solubility, molecular weight distribution and secondary structure as determined by Fourier transform infrared spectroscopy (FTIR)', *J. Food Eng.*, vol. 214, pp. 166–174, 2017, https://doi.org/10.1016/j.jfoodeng.2017.06.037.

40 S. M. Gaber, T. Dessev, D. Knezevic, G. Haustveit, and S. H. Knutsen, 'A feasibility study on Oat concentrates as a single source of protein for production of meat analogues', *LWT*, vol. 222, p. 117626, 2025, https://doi.org/10.1016/j.lwt.2025.117626.

41 L. Chen, J. Chen, L. Yu, K. Wu, and M. Zhao, 'Emulsification performance and interfacial properties of enzymically hydrolyzed peanut protein isolate pretreated by extrusion cooking', *Food Hydrocoll.*, vol. 77, pp. 607–616, 2018, https://doi.org/10.1016/j.foodhyd.2017.11.002.

42 C. Sarangapani, A. Patange, P. Bourke, K. Keener, and P. J. Cullen, 'Recent advances in the application of cold plasma technology in foods', *Annu. Rev. Food Sci. Technol.*, vol. 9, no. 1, pp. 609–629, 2018, https://doi.org/10.1146/annurev-food-030117-012517.

43 H. Tolouie, M. A. Mohammadifar, H. Ghomi, and M. Hashemi, 'Cold atmospheric plasma manipulation of proteins in food systems', *Crit. Rev. Food Sci. Nutr.*, vol. 58, no. 15, pp. 2583–2597, 2018, https://doi.org/10.1080/10408398.2017.1335689.

44 H. Mahdavian Mehr and A. Koocheki, 'Physicochemical properties of grass pea (*Lathyrus sativus* L.) protein nanoparticles fabricated by cold atmospheric-pressure plasma', *Food Hydrocoll.*, vol. 112, p. 106328, 2021, https://doi.org/10.1016/j.foodhyd.2020.106328.

45 G. Eazhumalai, R. G. T. Kalaivendan, and U. S. Annapure, 'Cold plasma enhanced gelation and thermal properties of oat protein and its application in a selected model food system', *Sustain. Food Technol.*, vol. 3, no. 4, pp. 1203–1217, 2025, https://doi.org/10.1039/D5FB00129C.

46 G. Eazhumalai, R. G. T. Kalaivendan, and U. S. Annapure, 'Effect of atmospheric pin-to-plate cold plasma on oat protein: structural, chemical, and foaming characteristics', *Int. J. Biol. Macromol.*, vol. 242, p. 125103, 2023, https://doi.org/10.1016/j.ijbiomac.2023.125103.

47 M. N. Nasrabadi, S. A. H. Goli, and A. Nasirpour, 'Evaluation of biopolymer-based emulsion for delivering conjugated linoleic acid (CLA) as a functional ingredient in beverages', *J. Dispers Sci. Technol.*, vol. 36, no. 6, pp. 778–788, 2015, https://doi.org/10.1080/01932691.2014.921858.

48 M. Nikbakht Nasrabadi, S. A. H. Goli, and A. Nasirpour, 'Stability assessment of conjugated linoleic acid (CLA) oil-in-water beverage emulsion formulated with acacia and xanthan gums', *Food Chem.*, vol. 199, pp. 258–264, 2016, https://doi.org/10.1016/j.foodchem.2015.12.001.

49 M. Nikbakht Nasrabadi, S. A. H. Goli, A. Sedaghat Doost, K. Dewettinck, and P. Van der Meeren, 'Bioparticles of flaxseed protein and mucilage enhance the physical and oxidative stability of flaxseed oil emulsions as a potential natural alternative for synthetic surfactants', *Colloids Surf. B Biointerfaces*, vol. 184, p. 110489, 2019, https://doi.org/10.1016/j.colsurfb.2019.110489.

50 A. Sedaghat Doost et al., 'Maillard conjugation of whey protein isolate with water-soluble fraction of almond gum or flaxseed mucilage by dry heat treatment', *Food Res. Int.*, vol. 128, p. 108779, 2020, https://doi.org/10.1016/j.foodres.2019.108779.

51 Q. Zhang et al., 'Protein glycosylation: a promising way to modify the functional properties and extend the application in food system', *Crit. Rev. Food Sci. Nutr.*, vol. 59, no. 15, pp. 2506–2533, 2019, https://doi.org/10.1080/10408398.2018.1507995.

52 L. Chen, J. Chen, K. Wu, and L. Yu, 'Improved low pH emulsification properties of glycated peanut protein isolate by ultrasound Maillard reaction', *J. Agric. Food Chem.*, vol. 64, no. 27, pp. 5531–5538, 2016, https://doi.org/10.1021/acs.jafc.6b00989.

53 W. Qu, X. Zhang, W. Chen, Z. Wang, R. He, and H. Ma, 'Effects of ultrasonic and graft treatments on grafting degree, structure, functionality, and digestibility of rapeseed protein isolate-dextran conjugates', *Ultrason. Sonochem.*, vol. 42, pp. 250–259, 2018, https://doi.org/10.1016/j.ultsonch.2017.11.021.

54 I. Kutzli, D. Griener, M. Gibis, L. Grossmann, S. K. Baier, and J. Weiss, 'Improvement of emulsifying behavior of pea proteins as plant-based emulsifiers via Maillard-induced glycation in electrospun pea protein–maltodextrin fibers', *Food Funct.*, vol. 11, no. 5, pp. 4049–4056, 2020, https://doi.org/10.1039/D0FO00292E.

55 I. Kutzli et al., 'Influence of Maillard reaction conditions on the formation and solubility of pea protein isolate-maltodextrin conjugates in electrospun fibers', *Food Hydrocoll.*, vol. 101, p. 105535, 2020, https://doi.org/10.1016/j.foodhyd.2019.105535.

56 X. Meng et al., 'Solubility, structural properties, and immunomodulatory activities of rice dreg protein modified with sodium alginate under microwave heating', *Food Sci. Nutr.*, vol. 7, no. 8, pp. 2556–2564, 2019, https://doi.org/10.1002/fsn3.1105.

57 Q. Xing, S. Dekker, K. Kyriakopoulou, R. M. Boom, E. J. Smid, and M. A. I. Schutyser, 'Enhanced nutritional value of chickpea protein concentrate by dry separation and solid state fermentation', *Innov. Food Sci. Emerg. Technol.*, vol. 59, p. 102269, 2020, https://doi.org/10.1016/j.ifset.2019.102269.

58 L. Mao, Q. Pan, Z. Hou, F. Yuan, and Y. Gao, 'Development of soy protein isolate-carrageenan conjugates through Maillard reaction for the microencapsulation of *Bifidobacterium longum*', *Food Hydrocoll.*, vol. 84, pp. 489–497, 2018, https://doi.org/10.1016/j.foodhyd.2018.06.037.

59 J. Yu et al., 'Analysis of the glycosylation products of peanut protein and lactose by cold plasma treatment: solubility and structural characteristics', *Int. J. Biol. Macromol.*, vol. 158, pp. 1194–1203, 2020, https://doi.org/10.1016/j.ijbiomac.2020.04.255.

60 W. Li, H. Zhao, Z. He, M. Zeng, F. Qin, and J. Chen, 'Modification of soy protein hydrolysates by Maillard reaction: effects of carbohydrate chain length on structural and interfacial properties', *Colloids Surf. B Biointerfaces*, vol. 138, pp. 70–77, 2016, https://doi.org/10.1016/j.colsurfb.2015.11.038.

61 L.-H. Wang, X. Sun, G.-Q. Huang, and J.-X. Xiao, 'Conjugation of soybean protein isolate with xylose/fructose through wet-heating Maillard reaction', *J. Food Meas. Charact.*, vol. 12, no. 4, pp. 2718–2724, 2018, https://doi.org/10.1007/s11694-018-9889-y.

62 P. Liu, Y. Li, L. Gao, X. Zhou, P. Ma, and Q. Wang, 'Effect of different carbohydrates on the functional properties of black rice glutelin (BRG) modified by the Maillard reaction', *J. Cereal Sci.*, vol. 93, p. 102979, 2020, https://doi.org/10.1016/j.jcs.2020.102979.

63 B. Zhang, X. Guo, K. Zhu, W. Peng, and H. Zhou, 'Improvement of emulsifying properties of oat protein isolate–dextran conjugates by glycation', *Carbohydr. Polym.*, vol. 127, pp. 168–175, 2015, https://doi.org/10.1016/j.carbpol.2015.03.072.

64 A. Saatchi, H. Kiani, and M. Labbafi, 'A new functional protein-polysaccharide conjugate based on protein concentrate from sesame processing by-products: functional and physico-chemical properties', *Int. J. Biol. Macromol.*, vol. 122, pp. 659–666, 2019, https://doi.org/10.1016/j.ijbiomac.2018.10.122.

65 B. Hiller and P. C. Lorenzen, 'Functional properties of milk proteins as affected by Maillard reaction induced oligomerisation', *Food Res. Int.*, vol. 43, no. 4, pp. 1155–1166, 2010, https://doi.org/10.1016/j.foodres.2010.02.006.

66 Z. Wang, C. Zhang, T. Zhang, X. Ju, and R. He, 'Effects of acylation and glycation treatments on physicochemical and gelation properties of rapeseed protein isolate', *RSC Adv.*, vol. 8, no. 70, pp. 40395–40406, 2018, https://doi.org/10.1039/C8RA07912A.

67 R. Li et al., 'Relationship between surface functional properties and flexibility of soy protein isolate-glucose conjugates', *Food Hydrocoll.*, vol. 95, pp. 349–357, 2019, https://doi.org/10.1016/j.foodhyd.2019.04.030.

68 C. Wen et al., 'Structure and functional properties of soy protein isolate-lentinan conjugates obtained in Maillard reaction by slit divergent ultrasonic assisted wet heating and the stability of oil-in-water emulsions', *Food Chem.*, vol. 331, p. 127374, 2020, https://doi.org/10.1016/j.foodchem.2020.127374.

69 Q. Zhang et al., 'Selective and efficient removal of fluoride from water: in situ engineered amyloid fibril/ZrO 2 hybrid membranes', *Angew. Chem. Int. Ed.*, vol. 58, no. 18, pp. 6012–6016, 2019, https://doi.org/10.1002/anie.201901596.

70 C. M. Oliver, L. D. Melton, and R. A. Stanley, 'Creating Proteins with Novel Functionality via the Maillard Reaction: a Review', *Crit. Rev. Food Sci. Nutr.*, vol. 46, no. 4, pp. 337–350, 2006, https://doi.org/10.1080/10408690590957250.

71 A. N. A. Aryee, D. Agyei, and C. C. Udenigwe, 'Impact of processing on the chemistry and functionality of food proteins', In: Proteins in Food Processing (ed. R. Y. Yada), Elsevier, pp. 27–45, 2018, https://doi.org/10.1016/B978-0-08-100722-8.00003-6.

72 C.-B. Zhao et al., 'Effect of acetylation and succinylation on physicochemical properties and structural characteristics of oat protein isolate', *Process Biochem.*, vol. 57, pp. 117–123, 2017, https://doi.org/10.1016/j.procbio.2017.03.022.

73 D. Charoensuk, R. G. Brannan, W. Chanasattru, and W. Chaiyasit, 'Physicochemical and emulsifying properties of mung bean protein isolate as influenced by succinylation', *Int. J. Food Prop.*, vol. 21, no. 1, pp. 1633–1645, 2018, https://doi.org/10.1080/10942912.2018.1502200.

74 C. Chen, C. Zhang, R. Zhang, X. Ju, R. He, and Z. Wang, 'Enzyme-catalyzed acylation improves gel properties of rapeseed protein isolate', *J. Sci. Food Agric.*, vol. 100, no. 11, pp. 4182–4189, 2020, https://doi.org/10.1002/jsfa.10457.

75 N. N. Shah, U. K.V., and R. S. Singhal, 'Hydrophobically modified pea proteins: synthesis, characterization and evaluation as emulsifiers in eggless cake', *J. Food Eng.*, vol. 255, pp. 15–23, 2019, https://doi.org/10.1016/j.jfoodeng.2019.03.005.

76 H. Kumagai and R. Urade, 'Deamidation of gluten proteins as a tool for improving the properties of bread', In: Flour and Breads and their Fortification in Health and Disease Prevention (ed. V. R. Preedy and R. R. Watson), Elsevier, pp. 3–11, 2019, https://doi.org/10.1016/B978-0-12-814639-2.00001-0.

77 Z. Jiang, T. Sontag-Strohm, H. Salovaara, J. Sibakov, P. Kanerva, and J. Loponen, 'Oat protein solubility and emulsion properties improved by enzymatic deamidation', *J. Cereal Sci.*, vol. 64, pp. 126–132, 2015, https://doi.org/10.1016/j.jcs.2015.04.010.

78 M. Immonen, A. Chandrakusuma, S. Hokkanen, R. Partanen, N. Mäkelä-Salmi, and P. Myllärinen, 'The effect of deamidation and lipids on the interfacial and foaming properties of ultrafiltered oat protein concentrates', *LWT*, vol. 169, p. 114016, 2022, https://doi.org/10.1016/j.lwt.2022.114016.

79 M. Hadidi, A. Ibarz, and S. Pouramin, 'Optimization of extraction and deamidation of edible protein from evening primrose (*Oenothera biennis* L.) oil processing by-products and its effect on structural and techno-functional properties', *Food Chem.*, vol. 334, p. 127613, 2021, https://doi.org/10.1016/j.foodchem.2020.127613.

80 L. Fang, H. Xiang, D. Sun-Waterhouse, C. Cui, and J. Lin, 'Enhancing the usability of pea protein isolate in food applications through modifying its structural and sensory properties via deamidation by glutaminase', *J. Agric. Food Chem.*, vol. 68, no. 6, pp. 1691–1697, 2020, https://doi.org/10.1021/acs.jafc.9b06046.

81 R. Abe et al., 'Evaluation of reduced allergenicity of deamidated gliadin in a mouse model of wheat-gliadin allergy using an antibody prepared by a peptide containing three epitopes', *J. Agric. Food Chem.*, vol. 62, no. 13, pp. 2845–2852, 2014, https://doi.org/10.1021/jf4034078.

82 R. Abe, N. Matsukaze, Y. Yamaguchi, M. Akao, H. Kumagai, and H. Kumagai, 'Wheat gliadin deamidated by cation-exchange resins induces oral tolerance in a mouse model of wheat allergy', *J. Food Bioact.*, vol. 2, pp. 119–128, 2018, https://doi.org/10.31665/JFB.2018.2147.

83 R. Abe et al., 'Allergenicity of deamidated and/or peptide-bond-hydrolyzed wheat gliadin by transdermal administration', *Foods*, vol. 9, no. 5, p. 635, 2020, https://doi.org/10.3390/foods9050635.

84 G. Yildiz, J. Andrade, N. E. Engeseth, and H. Feng, 'Functionalizing soy protein nano-aggregates with pH-shifting and mano-thermo-sonication', *J. Colloid Interface Sci.*, vol. 505, pp. 836–846, 2017, https://doi.org/10.1016/j.jcis.2017.06.088.

85 G. Yildiz, J. Ding, J. Andrade, N. J. Engeseth, and H. Feng, 'Effect of plant protein-polysaccharide complexes produced by mano-thermo-sonication and pH-shifting on the structure and stability of oil-in-water emulsions', *Innov. Food Sci. Emerg. Technol.*, vol. 47, pp. 317–325, 2018, https://doi.org/10.1016/j.ifset.2018.03.005.

86 A. Suryamiharja, X. Gong, and H. Zhou, 'Heating and neutralization significantly impact pH-shifting treatment: a case study on oat protein isolate', *Int. J. Biol. Macromol.*, vol. 320, p. 145789, 2025, https://doi.org/10.1016/j.ijbiomac.2025.145789.

87 Y. Teng et al., 'Emulsifying properties of oat protein/casein complex prepared using atmospheric cold plasma with pH shifting', *Foods*, vol. 14, no. 15, p. 2702, 2025, https://doi.org/10.3390/foods14152702.

88 Y. Zhang et al., 'Effects of modified processing methods on structural changes of black soybean protein isolate', *Molecules*, vol. 23, no. 9, p. 2127, 2018, https://doi.org/10.3390/molecules23092127.

89 S. Jiang et al., 'Modifying the physicochemical properties of pea protein by pH-shifting and ultrasound combined treatments', *Ultrason. Sonochem.*, vol. 38, pp. 835–842, 2017, https://doi.org/10.1016/j.ultsonch.2017.03.046.

90 S. Jiang et al., 'Pea protein nanoemulsion and nanocomplex as carriers for protection of cholecalciferol (vitamin D3)', *Food Bioproc. Tech.*, vol. 12, no. 6, pp. 1031–1040, 2019, https://doi.org/10.1007/s11947-019-02276-0.

91 O. Nivala, O. E. Mäkinen, K. Kruus, E. Nordlund, and D. Ercili-Cura, 'Structuring colloidal oat and faba bean protein particles via enzymatic modification', *Food Chem.*, vol. 231, pp. 87–95, 2017, https://doi.org/10.1016/j.foodchem.2017.03.114.

92 B. Zeeb, D. J. McClements, and J. Weiss, 'Enzyme-based strategies for structuring foods for improved functionality', *Annu. Rev. Food Sci. Technol.*, vol. 8, no. 1, pp. 21–34, 2017, https://doi.org/10.1146/annurev-food-030216-025753.

93 A. G. B. Wouters, I. Rombouts, E. Fierens, K. Brijs, and J. A. Delcour, 'Relevance of the functional properties of enzymatic plant protein hydrolysates in food systems', *Compr. Rev. Food Sci. Food Saf.*, vol. 15, no. 4, pp. 786–800, 2016, https://doi.org/10.1111/1541-4337.12209.

94 A. G. B. Wouters et al., 'Air–water interfacial properties of enzymatic wheat gluten hydrolyzates determine their foaming behavior', *Food Hydrocoll.*, vol. 55, pp. 155–162, 2016, https://doi.org/10.1016/j.foodhyd.2015.11.017.

95 M. Klost and S. Drusch, 'Functionalisation of pea protein by tryptic hydrolysis – characterisation of interfacial and functional properties', *Food Hydrocoll.*, vol. 86, pp. 134–140, 2019, https://doi.org/10.1016/j.foodhyd.2018.03.013.

96 M. Brückner-Gühmann, T. Heiden-Hecht, N. Sözer, and S. Drusch, 'Foaming characteristics of oat protein and modification by partial hydrolysis', *Eur. Food Res. Technol.*, vol. 244, no. 12, pp. 2095–2106, 2018, https://doi.org/10.1007/s00217-018-3118-0.

97 V. García Arteaga, M. Apéstegui Guardia, I. Muranyi, P. Eisner, and U. Schweiggert-Weisz, 'Effect of enzymatic hydrolysis on molecular weight distribution, techno-functional properties and sensory perception of pea protein isolates', *Innov. Food Sci. Emerg. Technol.*, vol. 65, p. 102449, 2020, https://doi.org/10.1016/j.ifset.2020.102449.

98 K. Schlegel, K. Sontheimer, P. Eisner, and U. Schweiggert-Weisz, 'Effect of enzyme-assisted hydrolysis on protein pattern, technofunctional, and sensory properties of lupin protein isolates using enzyme combinations', *Food Sci. Nutr.*, vol. 8, no. 7, pp. 3041–3051, 2020, https://doi.org/10.1002/fsn3.1286.

99 K. Schlegel, K. Sontheimer, A. Hickisch, A. A. Wani, P. Eisner, and U. Schweiggert-Weisz, 'Enzymatic hydrolysis of lupin protein isolates—changes in the molecular weight distribution, technofunctional characteristics, and sensory attributes', *Food Sci. Nutr.*, vol. 7, no. 8, pp. 2747–2759, 2019, https://doi.org/10.1002/fsn3.1139.

100 K. Schlegel, A. Leidigkeit, P. Eisner, and U. Schweiggert-Weisz, 'Technofunctional and sensory properties of fermented lupin protein isolates', *Foods*, vol. 8, no. 12, p. 678, 2019, https://doi.org/10.3390/foods8120678.

101 H. Wu, X. Rui, W. Li, Y. Xiao, J. Zhou, and M. Dong, 'Whole-grain oats (*Avena sativa* L.) as a carrier of lactic acid bacteria and a supplement rich in angiotensin I-converting enzyme inhibitory peptides through solid-state fermentation', *Food Funct.*, vol. 9, no. 4, pp. 2270–2281, 2018, https://doi.org/10.1039/C7FO01578J.

102 S. Schindler et al., 'Lactic fermentation to improve the aroma of protein extracts of sweet lupin (*Lupinus angustifolius*)', *Food Chem.*, vol. 128, no. 2, pp. 330–337, 2011, https://doi.org/10.1016/j.foodchem.2011.03.024.

103 P. Meinlschmidt, E. Ueberham, J. Lehmann, U. Schweiggert-Weisz, and P. Eisner, 'Immunoreactivity, sensory and physicochemical properties of fermented soy protein isolate', *Food Chem.*, vol. 205, pp. 229–238, 2016, https://doi.org/10.1016/j.foodchem.2016.03.016.

104 D. Klupsaite, G. Juodeikiene, D. Zadeike, E. Bartkiene, Z. Maknickiene, and G. Liutkute, 'The influence of lactic acid fermentation on functional properties of narrow-leaved lupine protein as functional additive for higher value wheat bread', *LWT*, vol. 75, pp. 180–186, 2017, https://doi.org/10.1016/j.lwt.2016.08.058.

105 X. Yang et al., 'Enhancement of nutritional and antioxidant properties of peanut meal by bio-modification with *Bacillus licheniformis*', *Appl. Biochem. Biotechnol.*, vol. 180, no. 6, pp. 1227–1242, 2016, https://doi.org/10.1007/s12010-016-2163-z.

106 T. Zhang, S. Yu, Y. Pan, H. Li, X. Liu, and J. Cao, 'Properties of texturized protein and performance of different protein sources in the extrusion process: a review', *Food Res. Int.*, vol. 174, p. 113588, 2023, https://doi.org/10.1016/j.foodres.2023.113588.

107 W. Zhang, I. D. Boateng, J. Xu, and Y. Zhang, 'Proteins from legumes, cereals, and pseudo-cereals: composition, modification, bioactivities, and applications', *Foods*, vol. 13, no. 13, p. 1974, 2024, https://doi.org/10.3390/foods13131974.

108 J. R. N. Taylor, J. Taylor, O. H. Campanella, and B. R. Hamaker, 'Functionality of the storage proteins in gluten-free cereals and pseudocereals in dough systems', *J. Cereal Sci.*, vol. 67, pp. 22–34, 2016, https://doi.org/10.1016/j.jcs.2015.09.003.

109 X. Li et al., 'The solubility and structures of porcine myofibrillar proteins under low-salt processing conditions as affected by the presence of L-lysine', *Foods*, vol. 11, no. 6, p. 855, 2022, https://doi.org/10.3390/foods11060855.

110 C. K. Richter, A. C. Skulas-Ray, C. M. Champagne, and P. M. Kris-Etherton, 'Plant protein and animal proteins: do they differentially affect cardiovascular disease risk?' *Adv. Nutr.*, vol. 6, no. 6, pp. 712–728, 2015, https://doi.org/10.3945/an.115.009654.

111 S.-J. Ye, H.-J. Park, and M.-Y. Baik, 'Modification of plant proteins as alternatives to animal proteins: a review', *Food Sci. Biotechnol.*, vol. 34, no. 2, pp. 349–363, 2025, https://doi.org/10.1007/s10068-024-01705-x.

112 O. K. Ozturk and B. R. Hamaker, 'Texturization of plant protein-based meat alternatives: Processing, base proteins, and other constructional ingredients', *Future Foods*, vol. 8, p. 100248, 2023, https://doi.org/10.1016/j.fufo.2023.100248.

113 R. Aghagholizadeh and A. A. Rigi, 'High-moisture extrusion in plant-based meat: challenges and emerging trends', *J. Food Process. Eng.*, vol. 48, no. 4, 2025, https://doi.org/10.1111/jfpe.70107.

114 C.-Y. Ma and V. R. Harwalkar, 'Studies of thermal denaturation of oat globulin by differential scanning calorimetry', *J. Food Sci.*, vol. 53, no. 2, pp. 531–534, 1988, https://doi.org/10.1111/j.1365-2621.1988.tb07749.x.

115 C. Ma and G. Khanzada, 'Functional properties of deamidated oat protein isolates', *J. Food Sci.*, vol. 52, no. 6, pp. 1583–1587, 1987, https://doi.org/10.1111/j.1365-2621.1987.tb05884.x.

116 L. Guo, H. Chen, Y. Zhang, S. Yan, X. Chen, and X. Gao, 'Starch granules and their size distribution in wheat: biosynthesis, physicochemical properties and their effect on flour-based food systems', *Comput. Struct. Biotechnol. J.*, vol. 21, pp. 4172–4186, 2023, https://doi.org/10.1016/j.csbj.2023.08.019.

117 A. Lomonaco, F. Galgano, N. Condelli, C. Paganoni, L. Carmela Mecca, and M. Di Cairano, 'Influence of processing on the technological and sensory quality of bread: an overview', *Ital. J. Food Sci.*, vol. 37, no. 3, pp. 53–79, 2025, https://doi.org/10.15586/ijfs.v37i3.2941.

118 V. Bulgaru et al., 'Characterization of plant-based raw materials used in meat analog manufacture', *Foods*, vol. 14, no. 3, p. 483, 2025, https://doi.org/10.3390/foods14030483.

119 P. Zang, Y. Gao, P. Chen, C. Lv, and G. Zhao, 'Recent advances in the study of wheat protein and other food components affecting the gluten network and the properties of noodles', *Foods*, vol. 11, no. 23, p. 3824, 2022, https://doi.org/10.3390/foods11233824.

120 R. Jia, M. Zhang, T. Yang, M. Ma, Q. Sun, and M. Li, 'Evolution of the morphological, structural, and molecular properties of gluten protein in dough with different hydration levels during mixing', *Food Chem. X*, vol. 15, p. 100448, 2022, https://doi.org/10.1016/j.fochx.2022.100448.

121 M. S. Rashed, E. Gallagher, J. M. Frias, M. Pojić, and S. Pathania, 'Dough rheology properties as affected by the inclusion of oat drink residue flour: a multivariate analysis approach', *Int. J. Food Sci. Technol.*, vol. 60, no. 1, 2025, https://doi.org/10.1093/ijfood/vvae101.

122 Y. Gu et al., 'Structural modification of starch and protein: from the perspective of gelatinization degree of oat flour', *Int. J. Biol. Macromol.*, vol. 260, p. 129406, 2024, https://doi.org/10.1016/j.ijbiomac.2024.129406.

123 A. Mohamed, G. Biresaw, J. Xu, M. P. Hojilla-Evangelista, and P. Rayas-Duarte, 'Oats protein isolate: thermal, rheological, surface and functional properties', *Food Res. Int.*, vol. 42, no. 1, pp. 107–114, 2009, https://doi.org/10.1016/j.foodres.2008.10.011.

124 Xinzhong Hu, 'Oat Enzyme Activity and Its Deactivation for Oat Food Processing', Northwest A&F University, 2007.

125 Y. Xiang, X. Wang, X. Hu, C. Ren, L. Guo, L. Li, 'Study on lipase activity differences among oat varieties and predictive modeling for high-quality varieties with low lipase activity', *Sci. Agric. Sin.*, vol. 21, no. 5, pp. 4104–4117, 2022.

126 Y. Xiang, L. Zou, R. Dong, X. Wang, and X. Hu, 'Enzymatic characteristics and potential natural inhibitors of oat lipase', *J. Cereal Sci.*, vol. 114, p. 103794, 2023, https://doi.org/10.1016/j.jcs.2023.103794.

6

Functional Properties of Oat Protein

This chapter delves into the core functional properties of oat protein, deconstructing the science behind each property and linking it directly to practical applications. It explores the fundamental mechanisms, the impact of processing parameters and strategies for optimization. The goal is to provide food scientists, product developers and researchers with the knowledge required to harness the full potential of oat protein, enabling the creation of the next generation of nutritious, sustainable and high-quality plant-based foods.

6.1 The Importance of Functionality in Food Applications

The global shift towards sustainable and plant-centric diets has propelled plant proteins from being mere nutritional supplements to important ingredients in food product development. However, their successful integration into diverse food matrices is not solely dictated by their nutritional adequacy (e.g., amino acid profile) but rather by their functional properties. These techno-functional characteristics determine a protein's behaviour during processing, its interactions with other food components, and ultimately, the sensory attributes, stability and overall quality of the final product. For oat protein to transition from a niche supplement to a mainstream ingredient, a comprehensive understanding of its functionality is paramount.

6.1.1 Defining Functional Properties

Functional properties in food science are defined as the physicochemical characteristics that govern a protein's performance in food systems during processing, storage, preparation and consumption [1]. They are the manifestation of a protein's molecular structure—its amino acid sequence, folding, charge distribution and hydrophobicity—in a macroscopic, observable outcome. These properties can be broadly categorized into three groups: hydration properties, surface properties and structure-forming property [2]. Hydration properties include solubility, water absorption and swelling, which are critical for viscosity, dough formation and moisture retention. Surface properties encompass emulsification (forming and stabilizing fat droplets in water) and foaming (forming and stabilizing air cells), which are essential for creating structured, creamy, or aerated products such as beverages, ice cream and whipped toppings. Structure-forming properties include gelation, cohesion, adhesion and elasticity, which are fundamental for developing texture in meat analogues, cheese alternatives and baked goods.

These functionalities are not intrinsic or fixed; in fact, they are highly dependent on external factors such as pH, temperature, ionic strength and the presence of other ingredients. Therefore, characterizing oat protein's functionality under various conditions is the first step towards its effective utilization.

6.1.2 Why Oat Protein's Functionality Matters

While numerous plant proteins are vying for market attention, oat protein presents a compelling, albeit challenging, profile that distinguishes it from competitors like soy, pea or wheat. Consumers increasingly seek products with minimal and recognizable ingredients. Oat protein, often derived from a familiar and well-perceived grain, aligns perfectly with this trend. Its ability to function effectively (e.g., as an emulsifier or texturizer) can reduce or even eliminate the need for synthetic additives, catering to the demand for clean-label products. In addition, unlike soy protein, oat protein is not a major allergen. Unlike wheat, its native form can be gluten-free (if processed to avoid cross-contamination). This makes it a safe and attractive option for a growing segment of health-conscious and allergy-sensitive consumers.

Oat protein is rarely isolated in its pure form. It often coexists with oat's signature soluble fibre, β-glucan. This polysaccharide is renowned for its health benefits (such as cholesterol-lowering effect) and its exceptional functional properties, such as high viscosity and water-binding capacity. The inherent interaction between oat protein and β-glucan can create synergistic effects, leading to enhanced stability, texture and mouthfeel that are unique to oat-based ingredients, thus offering a distinct advantage over other protein isolates.

Finally, oats are a hardy crop with a relatively low environmental footprint compared with some other protein sources [3]. This sustainability story, combined with its strong functionality, enhances the market appeal to ethically minded consumers and brands.

6.1.3 Benchmarking Against the Competition

To position oat protein accurately, it is instructive to briefly benchmark its functional potential against common plant proteins. Soy protein is the long-established gold standard for functionality, particularly in gelation and texturization (e.g., in meat analogues). In contrast, oat protein typically forms weaker gels but offers a cleaner, more neutral flavour profile, which makes it preferable in applications where flavour neutrality is critical. Pea protein shares similar challenges with oat protein, such as limited solubility and potential off-flavours. However, oat protein often exhibits superior emulsification properties and a less pronounced "beany" or "earthy" note, which can be a significant formulation advantage. Wheat protein (gluten) is unparalleled in its viscoelastic properties, which are essential for breadmaking and other applications requiring dough strength and gas retention. In contrast, oat protein cannot replicate these properties, as it lacks the specific protein composition that enables gluten functionality. Nevertheless, oat protein serves as a vital gluten-free alternative in structured products, offering binding and moisture retention without triggering gluten-related disorders.

This preliminary comparison highlights that oat protein is not a direct one-to-one substitute for any single existing protein. Rather, it is a unique ingredient whose value lies in its specific blend of nutritional, allergenic and functional properties. Its success hinges on formulating products that play to its strengths—such as emulsification and synergy with β-glucan—while using processing technologies to overcome its weaknesses, such as limited solubility.

6.2 Solubility and pH Stability

6.2.1 The Fundamental Role of Solubility in Oat Protein Functionality

Solubility in aqueous systems is one of the most critical functional properties of oat protein, as it directly determines its feasibility in many food applications. Protein solubility generally refers to the ability of a protein to disperse and form an apparently homogeneous system in an aqueous solution or specific solvent. For oat protein, this characteristic is particularly important because its inherently low solubility, especially in the neutral pH range, is a major technical bottleneck that limits its wide application. This solubility challenge primarily arises from its unique protein composition. Oat protein mainly consists of salt-soluble globulins and alcohol-soluble glutelins (avenins), which are prone to denaturation during extraction and drying processes [4]. These proteins often form large aggregates through hydrophobic interactions and disulphide bonds, reducing their ability to disperse in water.

The solubility characteristics of oat protein are fundamentally governed by its unique structural composition and interactions with non-protein components. The primary protein fractions consist of globulins (50–60%) and avenins (20–30%), which exhibit distinct structural properties that influence solubility [5]. Globulins, with molecular weights ranging from 150 to 300 kDa, exist as hexamers stabilized by disulphide bonds and hydrophobic interactions [6]. These large quaternary structures present significant challenges for aqueous dispersion. Avenins, while smaller (20–30 kDa), contain high proportions of hydrophobic amino acids and glutamine-rich domains that promote aggregation through hydrogen bonding and hydrophobic associations [7].

The formation of disulphide bonds represents a critical mechanism governing solubility behaviour. During extraction and processing, sulfhydryl groups exposed by thermal or alkaline treatment undergo oxidation, forming intermolecular disulphide bridges that create large, insoluble aggregates. This phenomenon is particularly pronounced in oat protein due to the relatively high cysteine content in globulin fractions. The aggregation process follows a two-stage mechanism: initial unfolding of native structures exposes hydrophobic regions, followed by covalent cross-linking that stabilizes large insoluble complexes. This process is largely irreversible under normal food processing conditions.

Non-protein components significantly impact solubility through both physical and chemical mechanisms. Starch granules (accounting for 5–15% of protein isolates) act as physical barriers that impede protein hydration and increase the viscosity of system, thereby reducing effective protein–solvent interactions. β-Glucan (3–8% of isolates) exhibits dual effects: at low concentrations, it may enhance solubility through electrostatic stabilization, while at higher concentrations it forms viscous networks that restrict protein mobility and promote aggregation [8]. Lipids (2–5% of isolates) pose particularly complex challenges due to their surface activity and chemical degradation. Polar lipids may form complexes with proteins that alter their surface properties, while non-polar lipids can create hydrophobic domains that sequester protein molecules. Most significantly, unsaturated lipids undergo oxidation during processing, generating reactive aldehydes that can cross-link with lysine residues via Maillard-type reactions, leading to the formation of insoluble protein aggregates.

The compositional complexity of oat protein isolates means that solubility must be understood as an emergent property resulting from protein–protein and protein–non-protein interactions. The presence of these non-protein components indicates that conventional strategies for enhancing solubility must address not only the native protein structure but also these additional interactions. This understanding explains why oat protein often shows different solubility behaviour compared with more purified plant protein isolates and why processing strategies must consider the whole system rather than focusing exclusively on the protein component.

The external factors influencing the solubility of oat protein are multifaceted. Among them, pH is one of the most critical external factors. The solubility–pH curve of oat protein exhibits a typical "U-shaped" characteristic (Figure 6.1) [4]. Under extreme pH conditions far from its isoelectric point (strongly acidic or alkaline), protein molecules carry a large net charge. The strong electrostatic repulsion keeps the protein molecules dispersed,

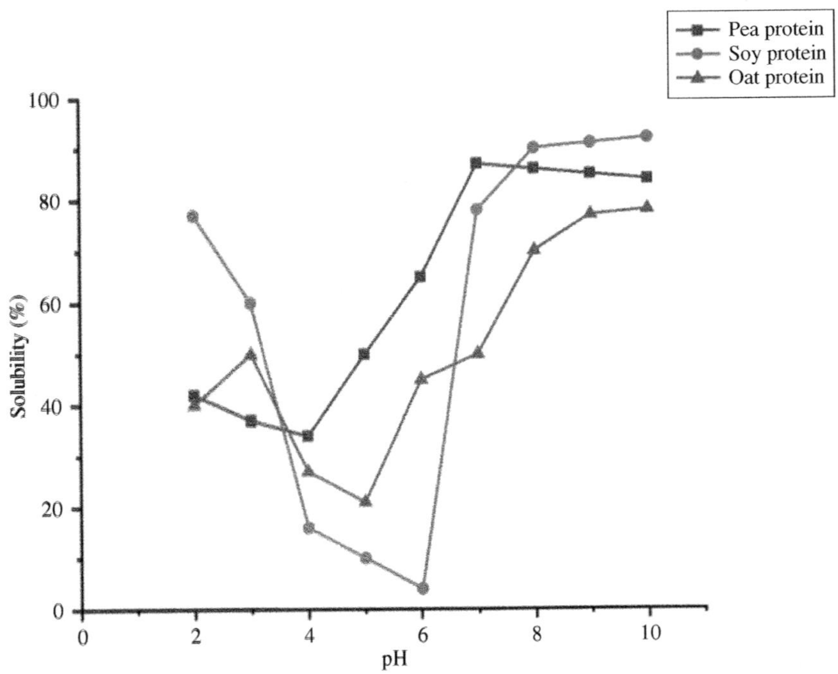

Figure 6.1 Graph comparing solubility vs. pH for oat, pea and soy proteins.
Source: Adapted from Ref. [4].

resulting in high solubility. When near its isoelectric point (typically around pH 4.0–5.5), the net charge on the protein molecules is zero and intermolecular electrostatic repulsion is minimized. Hydrophobic interactions then cause the proteins to rapidly aggregate and precipitate, at which point solubility reaches its lowest point. This property has direct implications for formulating acidic beverages (such as fruit juice drinks) and neutral foods (such as protein drinks). Besides pH, ionic strength is another important factor. Salt ions in the solution can shield the charges on the protein surface, weakening electrostatic repulsion. This generally reduces protein solubility when far from the isoelectric point, though under certain conditions, a "salting-in" effect can slightly enhance solubility.

6.2.2 Modification Strategies for Enhanced Solubility

To overcome the inherently low solubility of oat protein, a series of physical, chemical and biological modification technologies have been developed. Physical modification methods include high-intensity ultrasound treatment and high-pressure homogenization. The cavitation effect generated by high-intensity ultrasound creates extreme local conditions that effectively break down protein aggregates and partially unfold the protein structure, exposing more hydrophilic groups and significantly improving solubility [9]. High-pressure homogenization uses intense shear forces, cavitation and impact to disperse protein aggregates and reduce particle size, thus forming a more stable colloidal system [10]. Among chemical modifications, the alkaline pH-shifting treatment is the most commonly used. This technique involves dissolving the protein under extreme alkaline conditions to fully unfold it, then adjusting it back to neutral or the desired pH under controlled conditions. Partially denatured protein molecules undergo rearrangement during refolding, often exposing more polar groups and thereby achieving higher solubility than the native protein. Additionally, acylation reactions (such as acetylation) introduce negatively charged groups into the protein molecules, increasing their surface charge and hydrophilicity, which is also an effective chemical method to improve solubility.

In terms of biological modification, controlled enzymatic hydrolysis is particularly noteworthy. Using specific proteases (such as alkaline protease, neutral protease or complex protease) to perform limited hydrolysis on oat protein can cleave large, insoluble protein molecules into smaller, more hydrophilic peptide fragments [11]. These peptides, due to their low molecular weight and high surface charge density, usually exhibit excellent water solubility. However, this is a process that requires a fine balance, as excessive hydrolysis, while maximizing solubility, may sacrifice other functional properties such as emulsification and gelation, because small peptides have less ability to stabilize interfaces or form network structures. Therefore, controlling the degree of hydrolysis is key to enzymatic modification.

Solubility characteristics directly determine the oat protein's suitability for various applications. High solubility is essential for clear beverages, protein-fortified drinks and emulsion-based products in which sedimentation causes quality defects. In neutral pH systems like oat milk and nutritional beverages, solubility challenges manifest as undesirable sedimentation, gritty texture and phase separation. These practical considerations underscore the importance of solubility optimization through appropriate modification strategies and processing conditions to ensure successful product development and consumer acceptance.

6.2.3 Characterization Techniques

Accurate assessment of solubility employs several methodologies. The nitrogen solubility index (NSI) method quantifies soluble protein content after centrifugation. Turbidimetric analysis measures light scattering to assess dispersion quality. Chromatographic techniques such as size-exclusion HPLC characterize the molecular size distribution of soluble fractions. Electrophoretic methods, including SDS-PAGE, analyze protein composition in soluble vs. insoluble fractions. These analytical approaches provide comprehensive understanding of solubility behaviour and guide modification strategy selection for specific application requirements.

Emerging technologies offer promising avenues for solubility improvement. Cold plasma treatment modifies the surface properties without thermal degradation. Enzymatic cross-linking with transglutaminase can create soluble aggregates with improved functionality. Novel extraction methods using deep eutectic solvents preserve native protein structure better than conventional alkaline extraction [12]. Computational approaches, including molecular modelling, help predict modification effects on solubility, enabling more targeted development of oat protein ingredients with tailored functionality for specific food applications.

6.3 Emulsification and Foaming Capacity

6.3.1 Fundamental Principles of Interfacial Activity

The emulsification and foaming capacities of oat protein derive from its amphiphilic nature, enabling adsorption at oil–water and air–water interfaces. These functionalities depend on the protein's ability to rapidly adsorb to interfaces, undergo structural rearrangement, and form cohesive viscoelastic films that stabilize dispersed phases. Emulsification involves the formation and stabilization of oil droplets in aqueous media, while foaming encompasses the entrapment and stabilization of air cells. The effectiveness in these roles is quantified through the emulsifying activity index (EAI), the emulsifying stability index (ESI), the foam capacity (FC) and the foam stability (FS). Oat protein's particular molecular structure, containing both hydrophobic regions and hydrophilic segments, provides the necessary balance for these interfacial activities, though its performance is distinctly influenced by extraction methods and compositional factors [13].

6.3.2 Oat Protein as an Emulsifier

Oat protein stabilizes emulsions through a multistep process involving diffusion, adsorption, unfolding and film formation. Upon adsorption at the oil–water interface, protein molecules undergo structural reorientation with hydrophobic groups extending into the oil phase and hydrophilic regions remaining in the aqueous phase. This rearrangement reduces interfacial tension and creates a physical barrier against droplet coalescence. The performance is highly dependent on environmental conditions, with pH exerting a particularly strong influence. Maximum emulsification capacity typically occurs away from the isoelectric point, where enhanced solubility and increased electrostatic repulsion contribute to better droplet separation and stability [14]. Comparative studies show oat protein exhibits intermediate emulsification properties, outperforming rice protein but requiring higher concentrations than soy protein for equivalent stability (Table 6.1). Industrial applications leverage these properties in plant-based dairy alternatives, dressings and sauces where stable oil-in-water emulsions are essential.

6.3.3 Foaming Behaviour and Stabilization Mechanisms

Foaming properties involve air incorporation and bubble stabilization through protein adsorption at the air–water interfaces. Oat protein's ability to form and stabilize foams depends on its rate of adsorption, molecular flexibility and intermolecular interactions. During whipping or bubbling, proteins rapidly migrate to the air–water interfaces, lower surface tension and form protective membranes around air cells. The stability of these foams is determined by the viscoelasticity of the interfacial film and its resistance to drainage and disproportionation. Oat protein typically produces foams with moderate volume

Table 6.1 Comparative emulsification and foaming properties of plant proteins.

Protein source	Emulsifying property	Sparkling property
Soya bean isolate protein SPI (7S/11S)	EAI 43.4–44.2; ESI 25–86	FC 22–69; FS 67–100 [1]
Pea isolate protein PPI (vicilin/legumin)	EAI 31.1-42.9; ESI 10.9-12.4; some studies emulsified better than SPI at pH 7	FC 15-132; FS 27-96; foaming better than SPI at pH 3 and 7 (formulation/concentration dependent) [1, 15, 16]
Lentil protein (green/red lentil)	EAI 37.2–44.5; ESI 11–86.8	FC ~35 (flour-based); FS ~97 (flour-based) [1]
Potato protein/potato globulin (patatin dominant)	Native patatin has excellent emulsification with its peptides; EAI/stability is significantly enhanced by succinate/phosphorylation/glycosylation or complexation with polysaccharides	Excellent foaming: overrun of powder separates up to approx. 443–685% (>egg white); best foaming at low pH (~3) [17]
Wheat (alcohol soluble protein/gluten)	Emulsification can be enhanced by ultrasound/polyphenol combination	Alcohol soluble proteins foam well at neutral/alkaline pH; ultrasound increases gluten FC from ~70 to ~160% [18, 19]
Rice/rice bran protein	Emulsification capacity EC (mL/g): ~424 for pH4 (~262 for >SP), ~530 for pH7 (~845 for <SP)	Pure RBP has low FC (~43) but relatively high FS; combination with casein increases FC/FS to ~178/80 [20, 21]
Oat protein	Solubility limits emulsification/foaming; better at pH 7, worse at pH 4; significantly improved by limited enzymatic digestion (also forms viscoelastic interfacial films at low pH)	Most studies report limited foaminess in non-degreased or poorly soluble samples; increased albumin percentage/degreasing favourable [22–24]

Note: EAI = emulsifying activity index, m^2/g; ESI = emulsifying stability index, min; FC = foaming capacity, %; FS = foam stability, %.

but relatively poor stability compared to egg white or whey proteins, primarily due to its lower molecular flexibility and the presence of higher molecular weight aggregates [25]. The presence of non-protein components, particularly lipids, significantly impacts foaming by competing for the interfaces and destabilizing protein films through surface activity.

6.3.4 Oat Protein as a Foaming Agent

Oat protein demonstrates unique foaming characteristics that position it as a promising foaming agent in various food applications. Its foaming capacity stems from the ability to rapidly adsorb at the air–water interface, reduce surface tension and form viscoelastic films that stabilize air cells. The protein's moderate molecular flexibility allows for adequate unfolding and rearrangement at interfaces, while its amino acid composition provides the necessary balance of hydrophilic and hydrophobic domains required for effective foam formation and stabilization.

The foaming performance of oat protein is significantly influenced by several factors. pH conditions markedly affect FC, with optimal performance typically observed away from the isoelectric point, where enhanced solubility and electrostatic repulsion facilitate better air cell formation. Ionic strength modifies interfacial behaviour through charge screening effects, while temperature impacts protein flexibility and adsorption kinetics. The presence of non-protein components, particularly residual lipids, substantially impacts foaming properties. Even small amounts of lipids can severely destabilize foams through competitive adsorption at interfaces, where lipids typically displace proteins and weaken the interfacial film structure. This sensitivity to lipid content represents a major challenge in utilizing oat protein as a foaming agent and necessitates careful processing to minimize lipid co-extraction.

Compared to other plant proteins, oat protein exhibits intermediate foaming properties (Table 6.1). It generally produces foams with smaller bubble size distribution but lower overall stability than egg white or dairy proteins [25]. The FS, typically measured through drainage half-life, ranges from 20 to 40 minutes depending on protein concentration and environmental conditions [26]. This places oat protein ahead of rice and some pea protein isolates but behind soy protein in terms of FS. The moderate performance is attributed to the protein's molecular weight distribution and the presence of higher molecular weight aggregates that reduce molecular mobility at interfaces.

Practical applications leverage oat protein's foaming properties in several areas. In whipped toppings and desserts, it provides a plant-based alternative to traditional foaming agents while contributing a neutral flavour profile. In aerated beverages and protein shakes, it helps create and stabilize desired foam heads. Bakery applications utilize its foaming capacity in angel food cakes, soufflés and other aerated products where egg replacement is desired. The clean label appeal and allergen-free status make it particularly valuable in these applications, even when functional performance may not match conventional animal-based foaming agents.

Modification strategies can significantly enhance oat protein's foaming properties (Figure 6.2). Enzymatic hydrolysis enhances flexibility and interfacial activity by breaking rigid structures into more mobile peptides, though excessive hydrolysis reduces film strength [27]. Glycosylation through the Maillard reaction with carbohydrates increases

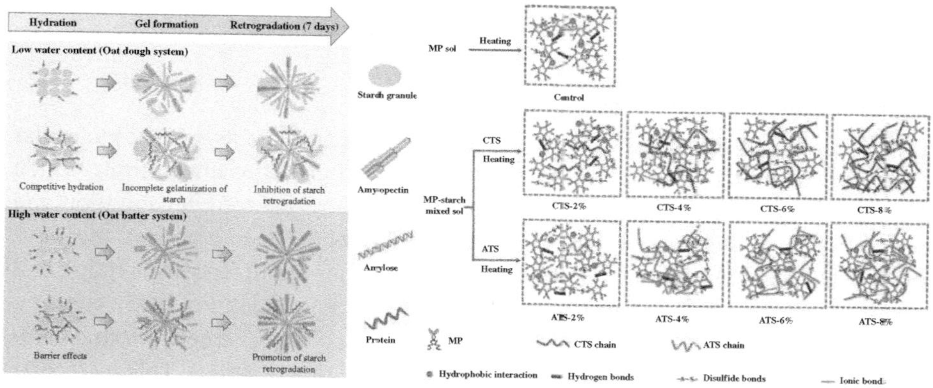

Figure 6.2 The interaction between oat protein and starch in the oat dough/batter system during heating, *Source:* Ref. [29] with permission of Elsevier; proposed mechanisms for the formation of network of mixed MP gels containing different levels (0, 2, 4, 6 and 8 %, w/w) of CTS or ATS, *Source:* Ref. [30] with permission of Elsevier.

hydrophilicity and steric stabilization [28]. Chemical acetylation modifies charge distribution and enhances electrostatic stabilization. Physical treatments, including thermal processing and high-pressure homogenization, improve functionality by altering protein structure and aggregation state. The combination with hydrocolloids such as guar gum or xanthan gum improves FS through enhanced viscosity and water-holding capacity. These approaches help overcome inherent limitations and make oat protein more competitive as a functional foaming ingredient in food applications.

6.3.5 Practical Applications

The emulsification properties make oat protein valuable in a wide range of applications. In plant-based milk alternatives, it prevents oil separation and improves mouthfeel [31]. Meat analogues utilize its emulsification capacity for fat binding and texture development. Bakery products benefit from its dual emulsification and foaming functions in aerated structures. Foaming properties find application in whipped toppings, desserts and aerated beverages where air cell stabilization is required. Industry adoption requires consideration of cost-effectiveness compared to alternative proteins, with oat protein's advantages lying in its clean label appeal, allergen-free status and sustainable perception rather than in outright functional superiority.

Standardized methods evaluate emulsification and foaming properties. Emulsification capacity is typically measured by creating model emulsions and determining the EAI through turbidimetric analysis and the ESI by monitoring stability over time. Foaming properties are assessed by measuring the volume increase upon whipping and the stability through liquid drainage and bubble size changes over time. Interfacial rheology characterizes the viscoelastic properties of protein films at interfaces. Microscopy techniques, including confocal laser scanning microscopy, visualize emulsion droplet size distribution and foam bubble structure. These analytical approaches provide a comprehensive understanding of performance under different conditions and guide product development and quality control.

6.4 Gelation and Texturization

6.4.1 Molecular Basis of Oat Protein Gelation

Oat protein possesses unique gelation properties that originate from its distinct molecular composition. The protein fraction consists primarily of 12S globulins and avenins, which exhibit different gelation behaviours. Globulins undergo heat-induced denaturation and aggregation through both disulphide bonding and hydrophobic interactions. Avenins, though less abundant, contribute to network formation through hydrogen bonding and Van der Waals interactions. The unique aspect of oat protein gelation lies in the cooperative interaction between these protein fractions, creating a composite network that demonstrates exceptional water-binding capacity and viscoelastic properties. This molecular synergy allows oat protein to form gels at concentrations as low as 8% (w/v), significantly lower than many other plant proteins, while maintaining structural integrity and moisture retention [31].

The gelation process of oat protein follows complex kinetics that distinguish it from other plant proteins. Differential scanning calorimetry reveals two major endothermic peaks at approximately 75 and 90 °C, corresponding to the denaturation of globulin and avenin fractions, respectively [32]. This two-stage denaturation process enables gradual network formation, resulting in more homogeneous gel structures. Rheological measurements during temperature sweeps show that the storage modulus (G') begins to increase significantly above 70 °C, reaching plateau values that are strongly dependent on protein concentration and pH conditions. The gel point, defined as the temperature where G' exceeds G', typically occurs between 75 and 80 °C for 10% protein solutions at neutral pH [32]. This relatively low gelation temperature provides energy-saving advantages in industrial processing compared to proteins requiring higher gelation temperatures.

The microstructure of oat protein gels reveals unique architectural features that explain their functional properties. Confocal laser scanning microscopy shows a continuous protein network with well-distributed pores ranging from 10–50 μm in diameter [33]. The network consists of both thick, primary strands (0.5–2.0 μm in diameter) and finer, secondary connections that create a hierarchical structure. This architecture contributes to the characteristic soft-yet-cohesive texture of oat protein gels. Cryo-scanning electron microscopy further reveals that the protein strands contain embedded starch granules and β-glucan fibres, which act as natural reinforcement elements within the protein matrix. This composite structure provides exceptional water-holding capacity (85–90%) and resistance to syneresis, even under prolonged storage or thermal stress [34].

6.4.2 Factors Influencing Gel Properties

Multiple factors significantly affect the gelation properties of oat protein, with heating rate and temperature playing particularly crucial roles in determining the final gel characteristics. The thermal processing parameters directly impact the denaturation kinetics, aggregation behaviour and ultimate network formation of oat protein gels.

Heating rate exerts a profound influence on gel microstructure and texture. Rapid heating typically leads to faster protein denaturation and aggregation, resulting in gels with finer network structures and more uniform pore size distribution. This accelerated heating promotes simultaneous unfolding of various protein fractions, creating a more homogeneous network. However, excessively rapid heating may cause localized over-aggregation and the formation of coarse, irregular structures with reduced water-holding capacity. In contrast, slow heating rates allow for gradual protein unfolding and more controlled aggregation, often producing stronger gels with better elastic properties due to more orderly network development. The optimal heating rate for oat protein gelation strikes a balance between sufficient denaturation time and practical processing constraints.

Heating temperature and temperature history critically determine the extent of denaturation and network cross-linking. Isothermal heating at different temperatures reveals distinct gelation mechanisms. At temperatures below 70 °C, limited protein unfolding occurs primarily through hydrophobic interactions, forming weak and thermo-reversible gels. Between 70 and 110 °C, both globulins and avenins undergo significant denaturation, with disulphide bond formation becoming increasingly important for network stabilization. Heating above this range promotes extensive aggregation and covalent cross-linking, creating strong, irreversible gels with enhanced mechanical properties. The maximum gel strength for oat protein is typically achieved through heating to 110–120 °C followed by holding at this temperature for 15–30 minutes, allowing complete network development [3, 22].

These thermal parameters interact with other factors previously discussed, including pH and ionic strength. At neutral pH, oat protein requires lower heating temperatures for gelation but may form weaker networks, while slightly acidic conditions necessitate higher temperatures but yield firmer gels. The presence of salts can modify thermal transitions by screening electrostatic repulsions, thereby lowering the required gelation temperature. Understanding these complex interactions enables precise control over oat protein gelation for specific application requirements, allowing manufacturers to tailor texture, moisture retention and stability through optimized thermal processing conditions.

The interaction between oat protein and β-glucan represents a particularly unique aspect of its functionality [35]. β-Glucan, a soluble fibre component naturally present in oat extracts, interacts with protein molecules through both physical entanglement and specific molecular interactions. This synergy creates a dual-network structure where the β-glucan phase provides enhanced water-binding and viscous properties, while the protein network contributes elasticity. The combination results in gels with improved texture, enhanced thermal stability and reduced syneresis compared to pure protein gels [34]. This natural synergy allows formulators to achieve desired textural properties with lower protein usage levels, providing both economic and nutritional benefits.

6.4.3 Comparative Analysis with Other Plant Proteins

Oat protein exhibits distinct advantages and differences compared to other plant proteins in gelation behaviour. While soy protein forms stronger, more elastic gels, oat protein provides superior moisture retention and smoother texture [36]. Pea protein gels often exhibit granular textures and weaker water-holding capacity, whereas oat protein gels show a homogeneous structure and excellent stability [37]. Wheat protein requires gluten for effective gelation and produces chewier textures, while oat protein creates softer, more versatile gels. Table 6.2 provides a detailed comparison of gel properties among major plant proteins.

Table 6.2 Comprehensive comparison of gel properties among plant proteins.

Parameter	Oat protein	Soy protein	Pea protein	Wheat gluten
Minimum gelation concentration (%)	6–8	4–6	8–10	10–12
Optimal gelation temperature (°C)	75–85	85–95	80–90	70–80
Gel strength (g, 10% solution)	120–150	200–250	100–130	180–220
Water-holding capacity (%)	85–90	75–80	70–75	60–65
Elasticity (G', Pa)	800–1200	1500–2000	600–900	1200–1600
Syneresis after 7 days (%)	5–8	10–15	15–20	20–25
Texture profile	Soft, cohesive	Firm, elastic	Granular, brittle	Chewy, rubbery

Source: [38] / MDPI / CC BY 4.0.

Several approaches can optimize the gelation properties of oat protein for specific applications. Enzymatic modification using transglutaminase significantly improves gel strength through covalent cross-linking, increasing storage modulus by 50–100% [39]. Limited enzymatic hydrolysis (1–10% degree of hydrolysis) using neutral proteases enhances protein flexibility and network formation, particularly beneficial for creating smoother textures [40]. Thermal pretreatment at sub-gelation temperatures (60–70 °C) followed by rapid cooling can induce partial unfolding that facilitates better network formation during subsequent gelation. Combination with specific hydrocolloids (0.1–0.3% xanthan gum or 0.5–1.0% carrageenan) can tailor rheological properties for specific applications, from spreadable textures to firm gels [41].

6.4.4 Industrial Applications

The unique gelation properties of oat protein enable diverse applications across food categories. In plant-based meat alternatives, it provides a juicy texture and fat-like mouthfeel that addresses common dryness issues. For dairy alternatives, it enables the creation of products with creamy textures and excellent melt characteristics in vegan cheeses. In bakery products, it improves moisture retention and softness while providing structure in gluten-free formulations. The pharmaceutical industry utilizes its gelling properties for controlled drug delivery systems, while cosmetic applications include its use as stabilizers for creams and lotions. Recent innovations include the development of thermo-reversible gels for specialized applications and the creation of textured protein ingredients through high-moisture extrusion processing.

Current research focuses on the enhancing understanding of structure–function relationships through advanced analytical techniques, including small-angle X-ray scattering and atomic force microscopy. Emerging processing technologies such as cold plasma treatment and high-pressure processing show promise for modifying gelation properties without thermal degradation [42]. Sustainable extraction methods that preserve native functionality are being developed, along with precision fermentation approaches to produce specific protein fractions with enhanced gelling properties [40]. The integration of computational modelling and machine learning techniques promises to accelerate the development of tailored oat protein ingredients for specific applications, potentially revolutionizing plant-based food formulation [43].

6.5 Interactions with Polysaccharides

6.5.1 Unique Synergistic Effects with Polysaccharides

Oat protein exhibits exceptional synergistic interactions with β-glucan that distinguish it from other plant protein–polysaccharide systems. This natural synergy stems from their coexistence in the oat kernel, leading to evolutionary compatibility that is rarely observed in blended systems. The interaction mechanism involves both thermodynamic compatibility and specific molecular recognition. β-Glucan chains form helical structures that specifically interact with hydrophobic patches on oat protein surfaces through van der Waals forces and CH-π interactions [44, 45]. Simultaneously, hydroxyl groups on β-glucan form hydrogen bonds with polar amino acid residues, creating a dual-mode interaction system [46]. This unique interaction results in complex coacervates with enhanced functional properties, including improved emulsion stability (up to a twofold increase in ESI), superior gel strength (12–25% enhancement) and exceptional thermal stability compared to pure protein systems [47, 48].

The interaction between oat protein and polysaccharides occurs through multiple mechanisms that vary with polysaccharide type and environmental conditions. With neutral polysaccharides like starch and β-glucan, the dominant interactions include hydrophobic associations and hydrogen bonding. The relatively high surface hydrophobicity of oat protein facilitates strong adsorption onto starch granules and β-glucan chains. With charged polysaccharides such as pectin or carrageenan, electrostatic interactions become predominant. At pH values above the protein's isoelectric point, oat protein carries a net negative charge but still contains localized positive patches that can interact with anionic polysaccharides through electrostatic attraction. This creates soluble complexes that enhance stability through both electrostatic and steric stabilization mechanisms. The unique amino acid profile of oat protein, particularly its balanced hydrophobic/hydrophilic residue distribution and specific sequence motifs, enables these diverse interaction modes.

The native association between oat protein and starch represents a unique structural feature that fundamentally differentiates oats from other cereals. In the native oat endosperm, protein bodies are physically embedded within the starch matrix in a highly organized architecture that has evolved for optimal nutrient storage and mobilization. This natural composite structure consists of three distinct interaction levels: molecular-level complexes between amylose/amylopectin and specific protein fractions; cellular-level organization where protein bodies are physically surrounded by starch granules; and tissue-level arrangement where the composite structure provides mechanical stability to the grain [49].

At the molecular level, oat protein forms specific complexes with starch through both non-covalent and covalent interactions. The prolamins (avenins) demonstrate particular affinity for amylose chains, forming helical inclusion complexes that modify both starch gelatinization and protein denaturation behaviour. These complexes increase starch gelatinization temperature by 5 °C while simultaneously raising protein denaturation temperature [50]. Additionally, natural Maillard reaction products formed during grain development create covalent bridges between lysine residues and reducing ends of starch molecules. These native conjugates exhibit enhanced emulsification properties and thermal stability compared to laboratory-prepared conjugates, demonstrating the sophistication of natural complex formation.

The cellular architecture reveals even more sophisticated interactions. Protein bodies are physically encapsulated within the starch matrix, creating natural microcapsules that protect proteins from degradation during processing. This structure also modifies water migration during hydration—water must first penetrate the starch phase before reaching protein bodies, creating sequential hydration kinetics that significantly impact functional properties. The encapsulation efficiency, measured by protein accessibility, varies among native oat varieties depending on variety and growing conditions.

During thermal processing, this native structure creates unique phase separation behaviour. Unlike blended systems where components separate randomly, native oat systems undergo directed phase separation where protein migrates to specific regions, creating controlled heterogeneity. This phenomenon is particularly valuable in extrusion processes where it enables the creation of anisotropic structures resembling muscle tissue without additional processing steps [51]. The natural structure also provides built-in stabilization against retrogradation—protein layers surrounding starch granules inhibit recrystallization.

Preservation of this native structure requires specialized processing approaches. Gentle dry fractionation using impact milling and air classification can separate oat fractions. Supercritical fluid extraction provides an alternative approach for lipid removal without disrupting protein–starch interactions. These processing strategies yield ingredients with functionality superior to conventional isolates, particularly in applications requiring water binding, texture modification and thermal stability.

6.5.2 Precision Modulation of Functional Properties

The interaction between oat protein and polysaccharides enables precise, multilevel modulation of functional properties that is unique in plant protein systems. This modulation occurs through three primary mechanisms: molecular-level complexation that modifies intrinsic protein properties; interface-level reorganization that enhances surface activity and bulk-phase structuring that determines macroscopic properties.

At the molecular level, complex formation with β-glucan creates molecular hybrids with fundamentally altered properties. The β-glucan chains wrap around protein molecules in helical configurations, increasing hydrodynamic volume and creating enhanced steric stabilization [34]. This wrapping also masks hydrophobic patches on the protein surface [52]. The complexes demonstrate unusual salt stability, unlike electrostatic complexes that dissociate at high ionic strength, oat protein-β-glucan complexes maintain integrity even at 200 mM salt concentration [53], making them particularly valuable in processed foods.

At the interface level, polysaccharides modify adsorption kinetics and interfacial architecture. In emulsion systems, oat protein rapidly adsorbs to interfaces, followed by subsequent polysaccharide attachment, creating multilayer interfaces with exceptional stability. The kinetics of this process are unique —oat protein's moderate surface activity allows controlled adsorption that leaves space for polysaccharide binding, unlike highly surface-active

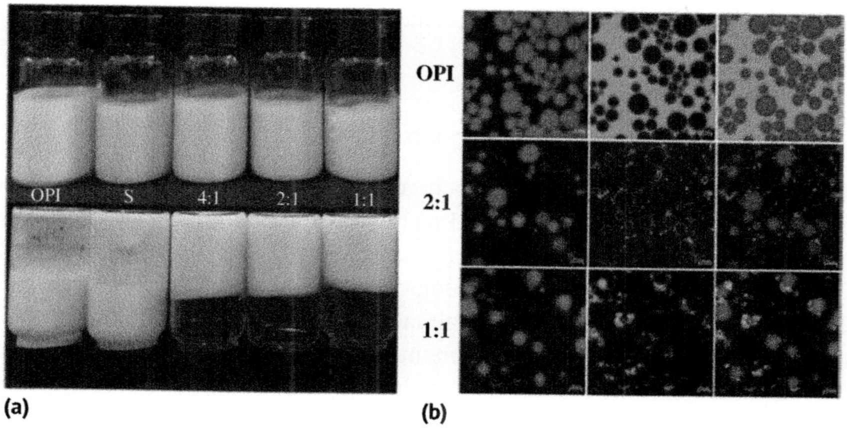

Figure 6.3 (a) Visual appearance, (b) CLSM images of the emulsion stabilized by OPI and OPI/S nanoparticles with different mass ratios. *Source*: Ref. [54] with permission of Elsevier.

proteins that dominate interfaces. In Figure 6.3, the particle size of the resulting emulsion is 22–25 μm (compared with 35 μm for protein alone) [54].

In gel systems, polysaccharides act as multifunctional modifiers through three distinct mechanisms: as active fillers that reinforce existing protein networks; as network co-formers that create interpenetrating dual networks or as phase separators that create controlled heterogeneity. The unique aspect of oat protein–polysaccharide gels is their ability to transition between these states based on processing conditions. For example, slow heating rates promote interpenetrating network formation with β-glucan, creating homogeneous gels with enhanced elasticity. Rapid heating induces phase separation, creating heterogeneous gels with superior water-holding capacity. This tunability enables the creation of tailored textures from single-ingredient systems.

The modulation effects show remarkable polysaccharide specificity. With neutral galactomannans (guar gum), the primary interaction is through hydrophobic association, increasing viscosity but providing limited stabilization. With anionic pectins, electrostatic interactions dominate, creating pH-responsive systems that can be designed to release functionality at specific pH values [55]. With xanthan gum, both electrostatic and entanglement interactions occur, providing exceptional stability across wide pH and temperature ranges. This specificity enables precision design of functionality for particular applications.

Practical applications leverage this precise modulation across diverse product categories. In bakery systems, controlled protein–β-glucan interactions simultaneously improve dough handling (through moisture management), crust colouration (through Maillard reaction modulation) and crumb softness (through starch retrogradation inhibition). In meat analogues, directed phase separation during extrusion creates anisotropic structures that mimic muscle tissue without additional processing steps. In dairy alternatives, the interactions enable texture customization from liquid beverages to spreadable cheeses through simple process parameter adjustment rather than ingredient changes.

The commercial implications are significant. These natural interactions allow formulators to achieve functionality that previously required multiple synthetic additives while maintaining clean labels. The ability to predictably modulate functionality through process control rather than ingredient addition represents a paradigm shift in food product development, particularly valuable for manufacturers seeking to create differentiated products in competitive markets.

6.5.3 Environmental Factors Governing Interaction Behaviour

The nature and strength of oat protein–polysaccharide interactions are highly dependent on environmental conditions. The pH significantly influences electrostatic interactions, with the strongest complex formation occurring near the protein's isoelectric point (pH 4.5–5.5) for charged polysaccharides. Ionic strength modulates electrostatic interactions through charge screening, with optimal stability typically observed at low to moderate salt concentrations. Temperature affects both interaction strength and mechanism— lower temperatures favour hydrogen bonding, while higher temperatures promote hydrophobic interactions. The unique thermal stability of oat protein-polysaccharide complexes allows them to maintain functionality across typical food processing temperatures, a distinct advantage over many other plant protein systems.

6.5.4 Applications in Food System

The unique interaction properties of oat protein with polysaccharides enable sophisticated food system design opportunities. In bakery products, controlled protein–polysaccharide interactions can simultaneously improve dough handling properties, crust colour and crumb softness. In meat analogues, they facilitate the creation of anisotropic structures through directed phase separation during extrusion or shear cell processing. For dairy alternatives, they enable precise texture modulation from liquid beverages to firm cheeses through manipulation of interaction parameters. The clean-label advantage of using native oat components (protein + β-glucan) rather than synthetic hydrocolloids provides significant market advantages while maintaining superior functionality.

Several approaches can optimize oat protein–polysaccharide interactions for specific applications. Enzymatic modification of the protein using transglutaminase enhances cross-linking with polysaccharide hydroxyl groups. The Maillard reaction under controlled conditions creates covalent conjugates with significantly improved functionality, particularly for emulsion stabilization. Physical processing, including high-pressure homogenization and ultrasound, can enhance interaction intensity through increased contact surface area. Genetic selection of oat varieties with specific protein polymorphisms and β-glucan structures offers future opportunities for enhancing natural synergy at the raw material level [47].

Current research gaps include a detailed understanding of molecular recognition mechanisms and predictive modelling of interaction outcomes. Advanced analytical techniques, including surface plasmon resonance and isothermal titration calorimetry, are needed to quantify interaction thermodynamics. Computational approaches combining molecular dynamics with machine learning could predict optimal combination ratios and processing conditions. Sustainable extraction methods that preserve native complexes represent another promising direction. The development of precision fermentation-produced oat protein fractions with tailored interaction properties offers exciting opportunities for creating next-generation food ingredients with unprecedented functionality. The unique interaction properties of oat protein with polysaccharides represent one of the most promising areas in food protein science, offering opportunities for creating sustainable, healthy and superior food products through natural design rather than synthetic addition.

6.6 Conclusion and Future Perspectives

Unique Advantages: Oat protein demonstrates a distinctive functional profile that differentiates it from other plant proteins while complementing existing options in the market. Through detailed examination of its solubility, emulsification, gelation and interaction properties, several key advantages emerge. The protein's moderate solubility at neutral pH, while initially challenging, can be effectively enhanced through various modification strategies, particularly enzymatic hydrolysis and conjugation with polysaccharides. Its exceptional emulsification capabilities, often surpassing those of pea and rice proteins, make it particularly valuable in beverage and emulsion-based applications. While oat protein forms softer gels compared to soy, its outstanding water-holding capacity and unique interaction with native β-glucan create textural properties that are ideal for many modern food applications.

The most significant differentiators for oat protein lie in its flavour profile and native compositional advantages. The clean, neutral taste requires less flavour masking compared to many plant proteins, addressing a major formulation challenge. Furthermore, the natural synergy with oat β-glucan provides functional benefits that cannot be easily replicated in blended protein–polysaccharide systems, offering both technical and clean-label advantages.

Structure–function relationships: The functional properties of oat protein are fundamentally governed by its unique structural characteristics. The balance between globulins and avenins creates a protein system that responds differently to processing conditions compared to other plant proteins. The presence of specific amino acid motifs, particularly the relatively high proportion of hydrophobic amino acids and glutamine, contributes to both its interfacial activity and its interaction with polysaccharides. The natural association with starch and β-glucan in the native oat system provides built-in functionality that is largely lost in isolation but can be preserved through appropriate processing methods.

Understanding these structure-function relationships is crucial for optimizing oat protein's performance in various applications. The protein's behaviour under different pH, temperature and ionic strength conditions follows predictable patterns that can be leveraged for specific functionality targets. This knowledge enables precision in application development and process optimization.

Plant protein market: When positioned against major plant proteins, oat protein occupies a unique niche that leverages its balanced functional properties rather than excelling in any single parameter. Table 6.3 summarizes its competitive positioning:

Several promising research directions emerge from this comprehensive analysis of oat protein functionality. First, developing methods that better preserve native protein–polysaccharide complexes during extraction could significantly enhance functionality. This includes low-temperature extraction techniques, supercritical fluid processing and enzymatic methods that maintain native structure. In addition, advanced modification strategies using targeted enzymatic treatments, controlled Maillard conjugation and physical processing methods could create specialized oat protein ingredients with tailored

Table 6.3 Strategic positioning of oat protein in applications.

Product name	Product type	Protein characteristics
PrOatein Havreprotein	Oat proteins concentrate powder	Has a mild taste of oat Suitable for cooking, baking and can be mixed with liquid or in smoothie. Contain no additive
Ideal oats®Oat protein	Oat protein concentrate	Naturally contains all essential amino acids, including desirable BCAAs. Helps to boost up metabolism, muscle growth, tissue repair and may help lower cholesterol
Critical oats	Advanced protein porridge	Breakfast snack food supplement contains protein isolates. Helps increase energy, improve digestion and nutrients absorption
Protein oat	Protein oat milk	Protein-rich, creamy oat milk with 8 g of plant-based protein, calcium and vitamin D. Can be directly used as drink, pour over cereals or add to smoothies
Muscle feast oats + isolates	Oats and whey protein powder	Natural, hormones and gluten free Oat and whey protein powder provide 31 g protein per serving. Protein isolates can be mixed with water or other beverages. Suitable for muscle growth and tissue repair
Protein oatmeal drink mix	Oat drink	Oatmeal drink mix can be used as a shake after workout to keep gut healthy, boost immunity and accelerate muscle recovery
Oats and whey	Powder product	Oats and whey powder can be mixed with milk or water. It contains 35% protein, contributes to muscle mass growth and helps reduce catabolic processes in muscle cells. Ideal for pre- or post-workout meals
Optimum nutrition oats and whey	Drinkable protein shake	Drinkable shake, easy to prepare, providing 24 g of protein per serving. Made with whole oat flour and whey, free from artificial flavours, colours and sweeteners. Contains essential nutrients for athletes

Source: [56] / Frontiers Media SA / CC BY 4.0.

functionality for specific applications. Furthermore, developing oat varieties with optimized protein composition through traditional breeding or modern biotechnological approaches could enhance functional properties at the source. Finally, future research should focus on developing oat protein ingredients optimized for specific application categories, recognizing that different applications require different functional property balances.

In conclusion, oat protein represents a valuable addition to the plant protein portfolio, offering unique functional advantages that complement rather than replace existing options. Its future success will depend on strategic applications in areas where its distinctive properties provide clear benefits, continued research to overcome current limitations and effective communication of its value proposition to both manufacturers and consumers. As the plant protein market continues to evolve and diversify, oat protein is well-positioned to capture specific market segments where its balanced functionality and clean-label advantages provide competitive differentiation.

References

1 K. K. Ma, M. Greis, J. Lu, A. A. Nolden, D. J. McClements, and A. J. Kinchla, 'Functional performance of plant proteins', *Foods*, vol. 11, no. 4, p. 594, 2022.

2 L. Kumar, R. Sehrawat, and Y. Kong, 'Oat proteins: a perspective on functional properties', *LWT*, vol. 152, p. 112307, 2021.

3 U. Holopainen-Mantila, S. Vanhatalo, P. Lehtinen, and N. Sozer, 'Oats as a source of nutritious alternative protein', *J. Cereal Sci.*, vol. 116, p. 103862, 2024.

4 R. Li, A. D. True, L. Sha, and Y. L. Xiong, 'Structure–functionality relationship and modification strategies of oat protein: challenges and opportunities', *Compr. Rev. Food Sci. Food Saf.*, vol. 24, no. 1, p. e70091, 2025.

5 R. M. Mel, 'Determining the Impact of Genotype × Environment on Oat Protein Isolate Structure, Function, and Composition', University of Manitoba, 2024.

6 A. Singh, M. Meena, D. Kumar, A. K. Dubey, and M. I. Hassan, 'Structural and functional analysis of various globulin proteins from soy seed', *Crit. Rev. Food Sci. Nutr.*, vol. 55, no. 11, pp. 1491–1502, 2015.

7 R. Mel and M. Malalgoda, 'Oat protein as a novel protein ingredient: structure, functionality, and factors impacting utilization', *Cereal Chem.*, vol. 99, no. 1, pp. 21–36, 2022.

8 P. Nanta et al., 'β-glucan fragmentation by microfluidization and TNF-α-immunostimulating activity of fragmented β-glucans', *Heliyon*, vol. 10, no. 8, p. e29444, 2024.

9 S. Shokri, F. Javanmardi, M. Mohammadi, and A. M. Khaneghah, 'Effects of ultrasound on the techno-functional properties of milk proteins: a systematic review', *Ultrason. Sonochem.*, vol. 83, p. 105938, 2022.

10 Y. Ma, J. Zhang, J. He, Y. Xu, and X. Guo, 'Effects of high-pressure homogenization on the physicochemical, foaming, and emulsifying properties of chickpea protein', *Food Res. Int.*, vol. 170, p. 112986, 2023.

11 O. O. Olatunde et al., 'Enzymatic modification of plant proteins for improved functional and bioactive properties', *Food Bioprocess Technol.*, vol. 16, no. 6, pp. 1216–1234, 2023.

12 F. F. Ajayi, P. Mudgil, and S. Maqsood, 'Delving into the green extraction of proteins from underutilized lima beans using deep eutectic solvent versus conventional methods: a comprehensive investigation of physicochemical, structural, and functional properties', *Food Chem.*, vol. 484, p. 144262, 2025.

13 M. Immonen, A. Chandrakusuma, S. Hokkanen, R. Partanen, N. Mäkelä-Salmi, and P. Myllärinen, 'The effect of deamidation and lipids on the interfacial and foaming properties of ultrafiltered oat protein concentrates', *LWT*, vol. 169, p. 114016, 2022.

14 J. Wang, C. Yang, and J. Jiang, 'Pickering emulsions with controllable rheological properties stabilized by oat globulin at different pH levels', *Colloids Surf. A Physicochem. Eng. Asp.*, vol. 716, p. 136694, 2025.

15 R. E. Aluko, O. A. Mofolasayo, and B. M. Watts, 'Emulsifying and foaming properties of commercial yellow pea (*Pisum sativum* L.) seed flours', *J. Agric. Food Chem.*, vol. 57, no. 20, pp. 9793–9800, 2009.

16 S. Sridharan, M. B. J. Meinders, J. H. Bitter, and C. V. Nikiforidis, 'On the emulsifying properties of self-assembled pea protein particles', *Langmuir*, vol. 36, no. 41, pp. 12221–12229, 2020.

17 M. Bashash, G. Wang-Pruski, Q. S. He, and X. Sun, 'The emulsifying capacity and stability of potato proteins and peptides: a comprehensive review', *Compr. Rev. Food Sci. Food Saf.*, vol. 23, no. 5, p. e70007, 2024.

18 H. Zhang, I. P. Claver, K. X. Zhu, and H. Zhou, 'The effect of ultrasound on the functional properties of wheat gluten', *Molecules*, vol. 16, no. 5, pp. 4231–4240, 2011.

19 B. G. Thewissen, I. Celus, K. Brijs, and J. A. Delcour, 'Foaming properties of wheat gliadin', *J. Agric. Food Chem.*, vol. 59, no. 4, pp. 1370–1375, 2011.

20 Y. Zhang et al., 'Effect of rice bran protein on the foaming properties and foaming characteristics of rice bran protein–sodium caseinate and rice bran protein nanoparticles–sodium caseinate', *Foods*, vol. 13, no. 15, p. 2328, 2024.

21 S. J. Cho, S. D. Lee, and S. W. Han, 'Functional properties of rice bran proteins extracted from low-heat-treated defatted rice bran', *Molecules*, vol. 27, no. 21, p. 7212, 2022.

22 R. Mel, K. M. Gough, K. T. Nilsen, and A. D. Beattie, 'Determining the impact of genotype × environment on oat protein isolate structural and functional characteristics', *Cereal Chem.*, vol. 100, no. 4, pp. 986–1000, 2023.

23 D. Sargautis, T. Kince, and I. Gramatina, 'Characterisation of the enzymatically extracted oat protein concentrate after defatting and its applicability for wet extrusion', *Foods*, vol. 12, no. 12, p. 2333, 2023.

24 M. Brückner-Gühmann, T. Heiden-Hecht, N. Sözer, and S. Drusch, 'Foaming characteristics of oat protein and modification by partial hydrolysis', *Eur. Food Res. Technol.*, vol. 244, no. 12, pp. 2095–2106, 2018.

25 F. Janssen, A. Breugelmans, D. Z. Gunes, and A. G. B. Wouters, 'Relating the foaming properties of oat proteins to their air-water interfacial characteristics and thin film drainage dynamics', *Food Hydrocoll.*, vol. 167, p. 111426, 2025.

26 F. Zhan, M. Youssef, B. R. Shah, J. Li, and B. Li, 'Overview of foam system: natural material-based foam, stabilization, characterization, and applications', *Food Hydrocoll.*, vol. 125, p. 107435, 2022.

27 Y. Hu et al., 'Improvement of physicochemical properties and stabilization of oat milk by composite enzymatic hydrolysis', *Food Res. Int.*, vol. 219, p. 117146, 2025.

28 C. Shi et al., 'Enhanced calcium and thermal stability of whey protein hydrolysate stabilized emulsions by ultrasound-assisted glycosylation: influence of the degree of glycosylation', *Ultrason. Sonochem.*, vol. 119, p. 107413, 2025.

29 B. Sun, X. Qian, M. Zhou, Y. Gu, S. Ma, and X. Wang, 'Changes of gelation behavior, water distribution and digestibility of protein-starch mixtures in the oat dough/batter model affected by water', *LWT*, vol. 182, p. 114860, 2023.

30 S. Wei et al., 'Effects of cross-linked/acetylated tapioca starches on the gelling properties, rheological behaviors and microstructure of myofibrillar protein gels: perspective on molecular interactions and phase transition', *Meat Sci.*, vol. 220, p. 109703, 2025.

31 J. McLauchlan, A. I. I. Tyler, B. Chakrabarti, C. Orfila, and A. Sarkar, 'Oat protein: review of structure-function synergies with other plant proteins', *Food Hydrocoll.*, vol. 154, p. 110139, 2024.

32 N. Siu, C. Ma, and Y. Mine, 'Physicochemical and structural properties of oat globulin polymers formed by a microbial transglutaminase', *J. Agric. Food Chem.*, vol. 50, no. 9, pp. 2660–2665, 2002.

33 C. Yang et al., 'Cold-set oat protein isolate--gellan gum binary gels with various microstructures: fabrication, characterization, formation mechanism, and controlled release properties', *Food Hydrocoll.*, vol. 131, p. 107818, 2022.

34 H. Cao, R. Li, M. Shi, H. Song, S. Li, and X. Guan, 'Promising effects of β-glucans on gelation in protein-based products: a review', *Int. J Biol. Macromol.*, vol. 256, p. 127574, 2024.

35 J. McLauchlan, A. I. I. Tyler, C. Orfila, and A. Sarkar, 'Characterisation of an oat protein-beta-glucan co-extract', *Food Hydrocoll.*, vol. 171, p. 111756, 2025.

36 T. V. Nieto-Nieto, Y. X. Wang, L. Ozimek, and L. Chen, 'Effects of partial hydrolysis on structure and gelling properties of oat globular proteins', *Food Res. Int.*, vol. 55, pp. 418–425, 2014.

37 Y. Wang, W. Kim, R. R. Naik, P. T. Spicer, and C. Selomulya, 'Tuning the pea protein gel network to mimic the heterogenous microstructure of animal protein', *Food Hydrocoll.*, vol. 140, p. 108611, 2023.

38 Y. Ma and F. Chen, 'Plant protein heat-induced gels: formation mechanisms and regulatory strategies', *Coatings*, vol. 13, no. 11, p. 1899, 2023.

39 P. Vijayan, Z. Song, J. Y. H. Toy, L. L. Yu, and D. Huang, 'Effect of transglutaminase on gelation and functional proteins of mung bean protein isolate', *Food Chem.*, vol. 454, p. 139590, 2024.

40 J. Tang, D. Yao, S. Xia, L. Cheong, and M. Tu, 'Recent progress in plant-based proteins: from extraction and modification methods to applications in the food industry', *Food Chem. X*, vol. 23, p. 101540, 2024.

41 S. Zhang, J. Han, E. Kwok, X. Kan, M. Iordache, and L. Chen, 'The impact of κ-carrageenan on the pea protein gelation by high pressure processing and the gelling mechanisms study', *Food Hydrocoll.*, vol. 158, p. 110577, 2025.

42 S. Zhang, J. Han, and L. Chen, 'Fabrication of pea protein gels with modulated rheological properties using high pressure processing', *Food Hydrocoll.*, vol. 144, p. 109002, 2023.

43 J. Jumper et al., 'Highly accurate protein structure prediction with AlphaFold', *Nature*, vol. 596, pp. 583–589, 2021.

44 N. Kishida, H. Sasafuchi, T. Sawada, and M. Yoshizawa, 'Helicity control of a polyaromatic coordination capsule through stereoselective CH–π interactions', *Chem. Sci.*, vol. 15, no. 33, pp. 13234–13239, 2024.

45 T. J. Gutiérrez and L. A. Bello-Pérez, 'Self-assembled and assembled starch V-type complexes for the development of functional foodstuffs: a review', *Food Hydrocoll.*, vol. 125, p. 107453, 2022.

46 Y. Peng et al., 'Multi-scale structure and digestible process of wheat starch as affected by distribution behavior of rice glutelin amyloid fibril aggregates during gelatinization and digestion', *Int. J. Biol. Macromol.*, vol. 284, p. 138197, 2025.

47 L. Zhong et al., 'Characterization and functional evaluation of oat protein isolate-Pleurotus ostreatus β-glucan conjugates formed via Maillard reaction', *Food Hydrocoll.*, 87, pp. 459–469, 2019.

48 X. He et al., 'Effect of oat β-glucan on gel properties and protein conformation of silver carp surimi', *J. Sci. Food Agric.*, vol. 103, no. 7, pp. 3367–3375, 2023.

49 E. T. Donhowe and D. M. Peterson, 'Isolation and characterization of oat aleurone and starchy endosperm protein bodies', *Plant Physiol.*, vol. 71, no. 3, pp. 519–523, 1983.

50 J. Kuang, W. Zhang, X. Yang, and P. Ma, 'Controlling pea starch gelatinization behavior and rheological properties by modulating granule structure change with pea protein isolate', *Food Chem. X*, vol. 25, p. 102218, 2025.

51 T. Moisio, P. Forssell, R. Partanen, A. Damerau, and S. E. Hill, 'Reorganisation of starch, proteins and lipids in extrusion of oats', *J. Cereal Sci.*, vol. 64, pp. 48–55, 2015.

52 A. Kumar, N. K. Singh, D. Ghosh, and M. Radhakrishna, 'Understanding the role of hydrophobic patches in protein disaggregation', *Phys. Chem. Chem. Phys.*, vol. 23, no. 22, pp. 12620–12629, 2021.

53 M. Nooshkam, M. Varidi, Z. Zareie, and F. Alkobeisi, 'Behavior of protein-polysaccharide conjugate-stabilized food emulsions under various destabilization conditions', *Food Chem. X*, vol. 18, p. 100725, 2023.

54 C. Yang et al., 'Ca2+ induced irregular spherical oat protein-shellac nanoparticles as Pickering emulsions stabilizer to improve emulsion storage stability', *Food Chem.*, vol. 480, p. 143975, 2025.

55 A. M. Stephen and G. O. Phillips, 'Food Polysaccharides and Their Applications', CRC Press, 2016.

56 H. Rafique et al., 'Dietary-nutraceutical properties of oat protein and peptides', *Front. nutr.*, vol. 9, p. 950400, 2022.

7

Applications, Product Development and Regulations

7.1 Food Industry Applications

7.1.1 Plant-based Dairy Alternatives

The application of oat protein in plant-based dairy alternatives represents one of its most significant and commercially successful domains. This success is built upon the ingredient's unique functional properties, particularly its emulsification capacity, heat stability and naturally mild flavour, which align well with the technical and sensory requirements of dairy analogue products.

Oat Milk and Cream Products: Oat protein plays a multifaceted and indispensable role in the formulation and stability of oat-based dairy alternatives, including oat milk and cream. Its functionality extends beyond mere nutritional contribution to being a critical structural and stabilizing agent. In these oil-in-water emulsions, oat protein acts as a natural emulsifier, adsorbing at the oil–water interface during homogenization. This adsorption reduces interfacial tension and facilitates the formation of fine lipid droplets. Subsequently, oat proteins form a protective viscoelastic membrane around the droplets, which is crucial for preventing coalescence and Ostwald ripening during storage [1].

The efficacy of oat protein is profoundly modulated by processing conditions, particularly roasting pretreatments. Thermal processing induces partial denaturation of oat proteins and promotes Maillard reaction-induced glycosylation. These structural modifications enhance the protein's amphiphilicity, surface activity and emulsifying capacity. Research demonstrates that oat milk produced from roasted oat flour exhibits significantly higher protein content in the aqueous phase, indicating improved solubility and a greater proportion of proteins available for interfacial stabilization [1]. This translates to emulsions with superior stability, as evidenced by higher absolute ζ-potential values, which enhance electrostatic repulsion between droplets, and increased apparent viscosity, which retards gravitational separation.

A key synergy exists between oat protein and the native soluble fibre β-glucan. While protein stabilizes the interface, β-glucan contributes to the continuous phase viscosity and forms a weak gel network in the aqueous phase. This network synergistically impedes droplet movement and sedimentation, thereby enhancing long-term emulsion stability and imparting a desirable, creamy mouthfeel to the final product.

The primary stability challenge in oat milk production is mitigating phase separation, primarily through sedimentation. This is addressed through a combination of homogenization and strategic thermal processing. Homogenization is critical for reducing lipid droplet size and ensuring a uniform distribution, thereby increasing the total interfacial area available for oat protein adsorption. While ultra-high temperature (UHT) processing ensures microbial safety, excessive heat can lead to protein aggregation and instability. The unique advantage of oat protein lies in its ability to form stable complexes with starch and lipids during moderate roasting (e.g., 200 °C with prior tempering). The formation of these protein–lipid complexes and the glycosylation of proteins impart enhanced thermal stability to the interfacial layer. This allows the system to withstand necessary thermal treatments without excessive denaturation that would trigger large-scale aggregation, a common issue with other plant proteins. Consequently, oat milk produced from optimally roasted flour demonstrates the highest stability kinetic index, minimal turbidity and the most homogeneous microstructure, underscoring the central role of processed oat protein in creating a robust and stable colloidal system.

Vegan Cheese: In vegan cheese applications, oat protein contributes to both texture development and melt characteristics. Unlike traditional dairy cheeses that rely on casein micelle networks, the formulation of plant-based cheese utilizes plant proteins in combination with other ingredients such as starches and vegetable oils to form a composite matrix. The protein content in such formulations typically ranges from 0.5 to 8% [2].

A critical functional requirement is achieving the appropriate melt and stretch properties, which are modulated by controlling the protein and polysaccharide ratio. The addition of texturizing agents like hydrocolloids or modified starches is a key strategy to create the desired texture in the final product.

The manufacturing process for plant-based cheese often involves a pathway based on fractionated ingredients, including proteins, starches and lipids. Thermal processing under shear is a common step, which facilitates the gelatinization of starch and the denaturation of proteins, leading to the formation of a viscoelastic gel upon cooling. This process creates a composite structure where a protein and polysaccharide network incorporates lipid droplets. The physicochemical properties of the final product, including its microstructure and meltability, are significantly influenced by processing parameters such as agitation speed, which affects lipid globule size and distribution.

Yogurt Alternatives: The incorporation of oat protein into yogurt systems reveals a complex interplay of functional properties, with performance being highly dependent on the specific protein fraction utilized. Comparative research indicates that oat protein concentrate (OPC) can serve as an effective alternative to skim milk powder (SMP), conferring both nutritional and technological advantages. Yogurt enriched with OPC demonstrates a more rapid onset of gel formation during fermentation and, critically, exhibits significantly reduced syneresis compared to SMP-based formulations [3]. This improvement in whey retention translates directly to enhanced sensory attributes, notably a superior mouthfeel and creaminess. In contrast, yogurt formulated with oat protein isolate (OPI) tends to develop a weakened gel structure and undergoes pronounced syneresis, a phenomenon attributed to inherent incompatibilities between oat and milk proteins.

A key processing adaptation to mitigate these compatibility issues involves leveraging the synergistic effects of protein aggregation and starch gelatinization. The native starch present within the oat matrix, when subjected to appropriate thermal processing, undergoes gelatinization and contributes to the formation of a composite gel structure. This starch-based network can effectively compensate for the suboptimal protein–protein interactions, thereby stabilizing the overall product matrix [3]. Consequently, a successful formulation strategy often employs a dual-structure approach, relying on both the acid-induced protein network and the supportive physical gel from gelatinized starch.

From a sensory perspective, the inclusion of OPC introduces a detectable bitter note and a distinct cereal-like flavour, which must be considered during product development. Despite these flavour implications, the overall textural performance of OPC-enriched yogurt is favourable. In summary, OPC presents itself as a viable and sustainable functional ingredient for yogurt manufacture, effectively improving gelation kinetics and syneresis control. However, potential bitterness may necessitate flavour modulation for broader consumer acceptance.

Technical Considerations: The commercial success of oat protein in dairy alternatives hinges on several technical considerations. Ingredient functionality varies significantly based on extraction method, with alkaline extraction followed by isoelectric precipitation generally providing superior emulsion stability compared to enzymatic extraction. The mineral composition of the protein ingredient also affects performance, particularly in fermented products where calcium and magnesium ions can influence gelation behaviour.

From a manufacturing perspective, the scalability of oat protein applications has been well demonstrated in commercial production. However, specific attention must be paid to the sequencing of ingredient incorporation, with optimal results achieved when proteins are fully hydrated before lipid addition, and starch components are incorporated after protein hydration. This sequencing ensures proper development of the composite structure that characterizes successful oat-based dairy alternatives.

The regulatory compliance of these applications varies by jurisdiction, with most markets accepting oat protein as a traditional food ingredient, though specific claims regarding protein content or nutritional benefits may require additional substantiation. The clean-label advantage of oat-based systems is particularly valuable in this category, as they typically require fewer additives than comparable soy or nut-based alternatives while delivering comparable or superior sensory properties.

7.1.2 Meat Analogues and Structured Products

Oat protein has emerged as a valuable functional ingredient in the development of meat analogues, offering unique advantages in texture modification, moisture management and flavour delivery. Its application spans various categories of meat alternative products, each requiring specific functional properties and processing approaches.

Burger Patties and Ground Meat Analogues: In ground beef patty applications, oat protein serves as a functional ingredient to enhance cooking yield and modify textural properties. Studies incorporating oat protein at low to moderate inclusion levels have demonstrated a significant improvement in cooking yield, which is attributed to the ingredient's capacity for moisture and fat retention during thermal processing [4, 5]. This characteristic is particularly valuable for improving the juiciness of leaner formulations.

The impact of oat protein on texture is concentration-dependent. While it contributes to a firmer texture, as evidenced by increased objective shear force measurements, this effect must be balanced against desired tenderness targets [6]. Furthermore, the inclusion of oat protein influences the visual characteristics of the product. At higher addition levels, it can lead to a lighter fresh colour and may accelerate the discolouration process during retail display, as indicated by a more rapid decline in redness and colour stability. A key functional advantage of oat protein in this context is its neutral flavour profile, which does not promote lipid oxidation, thereby helping to maintain oxidative stability comparable to that of a pure meat control during shelf life [7].

Whole-muscle Analogues: Oat protein is increasingly recognized as a critical functional ingredient in the formulation of whole-muscle plant-based analogues, such as those designed to mimic the fibrous texture of chicken breast or steak. Its incorporation into these products is driven by a combination of moderate gelation capacity, emulsifying stability and lipid-binding properties, which collectively contribute to the development of anisotropic structures and desirable mouthfeel. Unlike proteins that provide extreme firmness or elasticity, oat protein operates synergistically within multi-protein systems-complementing the cross-linking behaviour of soy protein and the cohesiveness of wheat gluten-to create a balanced and meat-like matrix. This cooperative interaction is essential during high-moisture extrusion, where conditions such as barrel temperatures of 130–150 °C, screw speeds of 200–400 rpm and moisture levels of 60–70% facilitate protein alignment and network formation [8]. Under these parameters, oat protein helps stabilize the emulsion of lipids within the protein matrix, preventing fat separation and ensuring uniform texture throughout the product. Its ability to bind water and fat also enhances juiciness and reduces undesired oil leakage during cooking, addressing common sensory shortcomings in plant-based meat alternatives.

Beyond its role in formulation design, the functional performance of oat protein can be further enhanced through targeted modification techniques. Physical methods such as ultrasound treatment improve protein solubility and surface activity, promoting better interaction with other ingredients during mixing and extrusion. Enzymatic approaches, including deamidation via glutaminase, have been shown to significantly increase oat protein's emulsifying capacity and solubility, leading to finer and more homogeneous gel structures. Additionally, cross-linking enzymes like transglutaminase introduce covalent bonds between oat protein molecules, reinforcing the network integrity and chewiness of the final analogue. These modifications allow oat protein to better mimic the structural and textural properties of animal muscle, positioning it as a versatile and valuable component in next-generation plant-based meats. As demand for clean-label and sustainable protein sources grows, oat protein offers a promising alternative that aligns with both technological and consumer-driven trends in the food industry.

Seafood Alternatives: In seafood analogue applications, oat protein typically contributes to the characteristic flaky texture and moist mouthfeel of products mimicking fish and other seafood. The technical challenge involves replicating the specific textural properties of seafood, which is addressed through a combination of oat protein with other functional ingredients, such as starch and hydrocolloids.

The manufacturing process for seafood analogues often utilizes thermo-mechanical treatment followed by cooling to develop the desired gel structure. Oat protein's ability to form soft, cohesive gels makes it particularly suitable for these applications, as it helps achieve the delicate texture characteristic of seafood products. The protein's light colour and neutral flavour profile are additional advantages, allowing for accurate flavour replication and colour matching without requiring extensive masking or adjustment.

Technical Considerations: The successful application of oat protein in meat analogues requires careful consideration of several technical factors. Protein purity and extraction method significantly influence functionality, with higher purity isolates generally providing better gelation and emulsification properties. Particle size distribution affects hydration kinetics and texture development, while the presence of native oat components like β-glucan can influence water mobility and texture modulation.

Processing parameters must be optimized for each specific application. In extrusion processes, temperature profiles, screw configuration and residence time all impact the final product characteristics. For bound products like burger patties, the sequence of ingredient incorporation and mixing intensity are critical for developing the proper protein matrix. Thermal processing conditions must be carefully controlled to achieve sufficient protein denaturation and gelation while avoiding excessive hardening or textural defects.

The compatibility of oat protein with other ingredients is another important consideration. While oat protein generally shows good synergy with most plant proteins, the specific ratios and combinations must be optimized for each application [9]. The interaction with starches, gums and other texture modifiers should be carefully evaluated to ensure optimal product performance.

7.1.3 Bakery and Confectionery Applications

Oat protein has established significant value in bakery and confectionery applications due to its multifunctional properties, including water binding, emulsification and structure formation. Its incorporation addresses several technical challenges while meeting consumer demands for clean-label and nutritionally enhanced products.

Gluten-free Bakery: In gluten-free formulations, the absence of a viscoelastic gluten network presents a major technological hurdle. While oat protein itself can contribute to structure, its functionality can be significantly enhanced through enzymatic cross-linking. The oxidative enzyme tyrosinase (TYR) has been demonstrated to specifically cross-link oat globulins, the major storage proteins in oats. This enzymatic treatment induces the formation of high molecular weight protein aggregates, which strengthens the protein network within the dough [10].

Microstructural analysis of oat dough confirms that TYR treatment leads to more intensive protein aggregation compared to untreated dough. This enzyme-induced protein cross-linking modifies the dough's rheological properties, resulting in increased firmness. When applied in baking, TYR alone, or in combination with xylanase (XYL), significantly increases the specific volume of gluten-free oat bread. Furthermore, the combination of TYR and XYL yields a bread that retains significantly greater softness after two days of storage compared to control breads, indicating an improvement in shelf life. This improvement is attributed to the TYR-strengthened protein network, which can better retain gas and maintain crumb structure, potentially working in synergy with the AX-modifying action of XYL [10].

In contrast, laccase (LAC), another oxidative enzyme, was found not to cross-link oat globulins under the tested conditions. While LAC alone did not affect bread volume, its combination with XYL did lead to a significant increase in the specific volume of gluten-free oat bread, though it did not impact crumb softness [10].

Protein-enriched Baked Products: For nutritionally enhanced bakery products, oat protein incorporation levels range from 10 to 15%, providing both amino acid supplementation and functional benefits. The protein's neutral flavour profile allows higher inclusion rates without compromising sensory qualities, though careful attention to particle size distribution is necessary to avoid textural defects [1].

Technical optimization focuses on balancing protein addition with other formula components. The high water-binding capacity requires adjustment of liquid additions, typically increasing by 5–8% for each 5% protein addition [11]. Emulsifier systems often need modification, with oat protein itself contributing to emulsion stability through its surface-active properties. Processing adaptations include extended mixing times and controlled fermentation conditions to accommodate the additional protein while maintaining desired volume and texture characteristics.

Confectionery Applications: In confectionery products, oat protein's functional properties are leveraged for aerated structures, emulsion stabilization and texture modification (Table 7.1). Proteins in aerated confections provide stable foam structures through the protein's ability to reduce surface tension and form viscoelastic interfacial films. The heat stability of oat protein proves particularly valuable in products requiring thermal processing, maintaining functionality across temperature ranges from 50 to 130 °C [12].

For chocolate and compound coatings, oat protein serves as an effective emulsifier at 1–2% concentration, preventing fat bloom and maintaining shelf stability [13]. The protein's compatibility with sugar systems and lipid phases enables smooth texture and clean flavour release. In fruit-based confections, oat protein's water-binding capacity controls water activity and prevents syrup separation while contributing to the desired chewiness [14].

Technical Considerations: Several critical factors influence oat protein's performance in bakery and confectionery applications. The extraction method significantly affects

Table 7.1 Oat protein applications in bakery and confectionery products.

Application type	Protein concentration (%)	Key functional role	Optimal processing conditions	Special considerations
Gluten-free bread	4–10 [15, 16]	Structure formation, Gas retention	Two-stage mixing, extended hydration	Hydration time critical
Protein-enriched products	8–18 [17, 18]	Nutritional enhancement, texture	Modified fermentation, adjusted baking	Particle size control important
Aerated confections	2–4	Foam stabilization, texture	Controlled aeration, temperature management	Heat stability advantageous
Chocolate products	1–2 [19, 20]	Emulsification, bloom prevention	Precise tempering, controlled cooling	Compatibility with lipid phases

functionality, with enzyme-assisted extraction generally providing better emulsion stability while alkaline extraction yields superior water-binding capacity. Native starch content in protein ingredients impacts gelatinization behaviour, requiring adjustment of thermal processing parameters.

The interaction between oat protein and other formula components necessitates careful formulation balance. In bakery systems, the protein–starch ratio directly influences crumb structure and softness, while in confectionery applications, the protein–sugar interaction affects crystallization behaviour and texture development.

Processing parameters require specific optimization for each application type. In bakery production, proofing time and temperature must accommodate the different hydration kinetics of oat protein compared to wheat gluten. For confectionery manufacturing, cooling rates and shearing conditions need adjustment to account for oat protein's influence on crystallization and aeration characteristics.

The successful integration of oat protein in bakery and confectionery products demonstrates its versatility and unique functional advantages. While each application presents specific technical challenges, proper formulation strategies and process adaptations enable manufacturers to leverage oat protein's beneficial properties while meeting consumer expectations for quality and clean-label products.

7.1.4 Beverages and Emulsions

Oat protein has gained traction in beverage and nutritional product applications due to its favourable solubility characteristics, emulsification properties and clean flavour profile. These functional attributes make it particularly suitable for various liquid-based formulations where stability and sensory qualities are paramount.

Ready-to-drink Protein Beverages: The application of oat protein in liquid beverages, particularly ready-to-drink formulations, is largely governed by its intricate solubility behaviour in response to pH and ionic strength. A fundamental understanding of these relationships is critical for successful product formulation, as they directly impact colloidal stability, mouthfeel and visual clarity.

The solubility of OPI exhibits a pronounced dependence on both pH and the concentration of dissolved salts. In the absence of salt, OPI displays a characteristic U-shaped solubility curve across the pH range of 2.0–8.0, with minimal solubility observed at the isoelectric point (pH ~4–5) and improved solubility under strongly acidic and neutral to alkaline conditions. However, this profile is profoundly altered by ionic strength. The presence of common salts like sodium chloride induces a well-defined 'salting-out' effect at intermediate ionic strengths, where protein solubility can plummet to below 1% due to charge screening that diminishes electrostatic repulsion and promotes hydrophobic aggregation. This is accompanied by a dramatic increase in particle size, exceeding 10,000 nm. Consequently, the formulation of oat protein beverages must meticulously control salt addition to avoid this insolubility zone [21].

For optimal solubility in beverage systems, two strategic approaches are indicated by the research. First, formulating at very low ionic strength combined with a pH away from the isoelectric point can achieve high solubility. Second, while very high salt concentrations can recover solubility at neutral pH through a 'salting-in' effect, this is generally impractical for sensory reasons. It is noteworthy that ion species also influence functionality; at comparable ionic strengths, sodium phosphate generally confers higher OPI solubility than NaCl.

To overcome the inherent solubility limitation at neutral pH without relying on extreme ionic conditions, physical modification techniques such as high-intensity ultrasound (HIU) present a viable solution. HIU treatment disrupts protein aggregates, significantly reduces particle size and increases surface charge. This mechanical intervention can elevate the solubility of OPI at pH 7.0 from approximately 41.5 to over 60%, while simultaneously imparting superior resistance to thermal aggregation—a critical attribute for beverages undergoing pasteurization [22].

The successful incorporation of oat protein into beverages requires a synergistic approach that carefully balances pH and ionic strength to navigate its complex solubility landscape. The strategic use of physical processing technologies like HIU can further expand its application window by fundamentally improving its dissolution and stability characteristics in aqueous systems, paving the way for the development of high-quality, shelf-stable oat protein beverages.

Salad Dressing Applications: OPI holds significant potential as a natural emulsifier in oil-in-water emulsions, such as salad dressings. However, its application is often constrained by its native compact globular structure, which limits its surface activity. To overcome this limitation, synergistic physical modification strategies, particularly the combination of thermosonication and high-pressure homogenization, have been demonstrated as effective means to enhance its functionality. The underlying principle involves the partial unfolding and dissociation of protein aggregates induced by thermosonication, a process significantly augmented by subsequent high-pressure treatment. This sequential intervention disrupts the quaternary and tertiary structures, leading to the exposure of previously buried functional groups.

This structural modification profoundly enhances the interfacial properties of oat protein. Specifically, treatments lead to a marked increase in surface hydrophobicity, promoting a stronger affinity for the oil–water interface. Concurrently, the absolute value of the ζ-potential increases, indicating enhanced electrostatic repulsion between adsorbed protein layers on adjacent oil droplets [23]. These combined effects contribute to improved interfacial stabilization.

The structural and interfacial improvements directly translate to superior macroscopic emulsion properties. Emulsions stabilized by the modified oat protein exhibit a finer and more homogeneous oil droplet distribution, attributable to more efficient protein adsorption and the formation of a cohesive, viscoelastic film at the interface. This robust interfacial membrane confers greater stability against coalescence and creaming during storage. In a model salad dressing system, the modified protein contributes to a homogeneous microstructure, improved viscosity and a smoother texture, demonstrating its efficacy in a complex food matrix.

The combination of thermosonication and high-pressure homogenization represents a viable physical strategy to fundamentally modify the structure of oat protein, thereby unlocking its emulsifying potential. This approach provides a theoretical foundation for the development of clean-label, plant-based emulsion-type products utilizing oat protein as a key functional ingredient.

Technical Specifications: The successful incorporation of oat protein into liquid food systems, such as beverages and dressings, is governed by a set of fundamental physicochemical properties. Understanding and controlling these parameters is essential for achieving desired product quality, stability and sensory attributes.

The performance of oat protein in beverage systems is primarily determined by its dissolution characteristics and colloidal stability. A high protein solubility across the target product pH range is a foundational requirement to prevent sedimentation and ensure a clear or uniformly turbid appearance. The particle size distribution of the protein ingredient and the resulting hydrated particles is critical; a predominance of submicron particles is necessary to minimize light scattering (for clarity) and to ensure a smooth mouthfeel without grittiness. Furthermore, stability against thermal aggregation is paramount for products undergoing pasteurization or UHT treatment. The native susceptibility of oat protein to aggregate upon heating can be significantly mitigated through structural modifications, such as high-intensity ultrasound, which enhances electrostatic repulsion and reduces particle size, thereby improving heat stability.

In emulsion systems like salad dressings, the functional specifications for oat protein shift towards its interfacial and structuring properties. The key parameter is its emulsifying capacity, which is intrinsically linked to its structural flexibility, surface hydrophobicity and charge characteristics. A high surface hydrophobicity promotes adsorption to the oil–water interface, while a substantial net charge enhances emulsion stability by increasing electrostatic repulsion between droplets. The protein's ability to form a viscoelastic film at the interface is crucial for preventing droplet coalescence during processing and storage. Additionally, the rheological contribution of the protein to the continuous phase and its interaction with other hydrocolloids directly influence the final product's viscosity, texture and resistance to phase separation. Physical processing can be employed to tailor these functional properties, making oat protein a viable structuring agent in oil-embedded food products.

7.1.5 Infant Formula and Clinical Nutrition

In infant nutrition, oat protein serves as a viable alternative to traditional protein sources, offering a hypoallergenic profile combined with excellent digestibility characteristics (Table 7.2). The protein's balanced amino acid composition, while requiring careful formulation to meet stringent regulatory standards for essential amino acids, provides a solid nutritional foundation for infant development. Manufacturing processes typically involve extensive enzymatic treatment to enhance protein digestibility and reduce potential allergenicity, resulting in protein hydrolysates with molecular weight profiles optimized for infant consumption.

The application of oat protein in clinical nutrition demonstrates its versatility in addressing specific medical needs. Enteral nutrition formulations utilize oat protein's favourable solubility and thermal stability to create products with excellent tube-passing characteristics and minimal risk of clogging. The protein's moderate viscosity profile allows for higher nutrient density formulations while maintaining appropriate flow properties. In oral nutritional supplements, oat protein contributes to improved product acceptability through its neutral flavour and smooth mouthfeel, particularly important for patients experiencing taste alterations or swallowing difficulties.

Technical considerations for these applications include rigorous quality control measures to ensure compliance with strict microbiological standards and heavy metal limits. Protein

Table 7.2 Oat protein applications in beverage and nutritional products.

Application type	Protein concentration (%)	Processing parameters	Stability considerations	Key functional attributes
Ready-to-drink beverages	1–5 [24–28]	Homogenization 100–150 bar, high-shear mixing	9–12 month shelf life, pH stability	Emulsification, solubility
Salad dressing	2–8 [29–32]	Spray drying 180–200 °C inlet	Vitamin compatibility, mixing stability	Neutral flavour, balanced nutrition
Infant formula	1.2–2 [33–35]	Spray drying 150–220 °C inlet	Calcium-to-phosphorus ratio, homogenization efficiency	Low allergenicity, digestibility
Clinical nutrition	3–10 [20, 27, 36–38]	Aseptic processing, pH control	Osmolality management, tube compatibility	Low allergenicity, digestibility

purification processes are optimized to remove anti-nutritional factors while preserving nutritional quality. Formulation strategies often incorporate oat protein in combination with other protein sources to achieve optimal amino acid profiles and meet specific nutritional requirements for different patient populations, from paediatric to geriatric applications.

7.1.6 Cosmetic and Pharmaceutical Uses

The functional properties of oat protein have enabled its successful application in cosmetic and pharmaceutical products, where its biological compatibility and multifunctional characteristics offer distinct advantages. In cosmetic formulations, oat protein serves as a natural alternative to synthetic polymers, providing film-forming, moisturizing and conditioning properties. The protein's ability to form elastic films on skin and hair surfaces contributes to improved barrier function and moisture retention, making it particularly valuable in products designed for sensitive or compromised skin conditions.

Pharmaceutical applications leverage oat protein's biocompatibility and biodegradability for drug delivery systems and topical formulations. The protein's molecular structure allows for the creation of controlled-release matrices that can be engineered to respond to specific physiological conditions [39]. In transdermal delivery systems, oat protein films facilitate gradual active ingredient release while maintaining skin hydration. The development of oat protein-based hydrogels and microcapsules demonstrates the material's versatility in addressing diverse pharmaceutical needs, from wound healing applications to targeted nutrient delivery.

The integration of oat protein in these advanced applications requires specialized processing approaches. Enzymatic modification techniques are employed to enhance specific functional properties, such as increasing water solubility for cosmetic serums or modifying gelation characteristics for pharmaceutical carriers. Quality parameters for these applications include precise molecular weight distribution control, standardized protein purity levels and consistent functional performance across production batches. The successful implementation in cosmetic and pharmaceutical products underscores oat protein's potential beyond traditional food applications, highlighting its value as a multifunctional biomaterial with diverse commercial possibilities.

These specialized applications demonstrate how oat protein's unique properties can be leveraged to create innovative products addressing specific needs in nutrition, healthcare and personal care markets. The continued development of processing technologies and formulation strategies will likely expand oat protein's utilization in these high-value applications, contributing to the growing recognition of plant proteins as versatile functional ingredients across multiple industries.

7.2 Product Development Strategies

7.2.1 Formulation Design Principles

The successful incorporation of oat protein into food products requires careful consideration of its unique chemical and physical properties. Formulation strategies must account for oat protein's specific hydration requirements, isoelectric point characteristics and interaction patterns with other food components. A fundamental principle involves the sequential hydration of oat protein, typically requiring 15–20 minutes for complete water absorption before introducing other ingredients. This ensures proper functionality development and prevents competitive hydration scenarios that could compromise final product texture.

The pH-dependent behaviour of oat protein necessitates careful buffer system design. Formulations typically target pH ranges either below 4.0 or above 6.5 to maintain optimal protein solubility and functionality [39]. In acidic systems, citrate buffers prove most effective, while in neutral to alkaline applications, phosphate-based systems provide superior stability. The ionic strength of the system must be carefully controlled, with optimal functionality observed at salt concentrations below 0.1 M to prevent charge screening effects that could impair protein solubility and interfacial activity.

Ingredient compatibility represents another critical consideration in formulation design. Oat protein demonstrates excellent synergy with select hydrocolloids, particularly high-acyl gellan gum and xanthan gum, which complement its emulsification properties without competing for hydration water [40]. The interaction with starch systems requires precise timing in thermal processing, as oat protein's gelation temperature range overlaps with typical starch gelatinization temperatures. This necessitates either staged heating protocols or the use of modified starches with altered gelatinization profiles.

7.2.2 Processing Technology Integration

Thermal processing parameters must be optimized according to the specific application and desired functional outcomes. For emulsion systems, pasteurization at 72–75 °C for 15–20 seconds provides adequate microbial safety while preserving protein functionality [41]. In high-temperature applications, rapid heating and cooling profiles minimize protein aggregation, with optimal results achieved when product temperature exceeds 85 °C for less than 3 minutes. The unique thermal stability of oat protein-β-glucan complexes allows for broader processing windows compared to many other plant proteins [8].

Extrusion technology applications require specific parameter optimization to leverage oat protein's texturization potential. Barrel temperature profiles should progress gradually from 70 to 140 °C along the extrusion length, with particular attention to moisture content management. Optimal results are achieved at moisture levels of 60–70%, with specific mechanical energy inputs maintained between 400 and 600 kJ/kg [8]. The screw configuration should balance between mixing efficiency and shear sensitivity, typically utilizing forward-conveying elements in the protein hydration zone followed by moderate-shear mixing elements for texturization.

High-pressure processing (HPP) and other alternative technologies offer promising approaches for functionality preservation. HPP treatments at 400–600 MPa effectively modify oat protein structure to enhance solubility while maintaining native functionality [42]. Cold plasma treatment represents another emerging technology, with exposure times of 2–5 minutes at medium power levels significantly improving protein solubility and surface activity without thermal degradation [43].

7.2.3 Clean Label

The development of clean-label products utilizing oat protein leverages its native functionality to replace synthetic additives. Emulsifier replacement represents one of the most significant applications, where oat protein's natural surface-active properties can substitute for chemical emulsifiers in numerous applications (Table 7.3). The key to successful replacement lies in optimizing homogenization parameters to ensure proper interface development.

Natural preservation strategies benefit from oat protein's antioxidant properties and water activity reduction capabilities. The protein's metal-chelating capacity and free-radical scavenging activity provide natural oxidation protection, particularly in lipid-containing systems. This allows for reduced usage of synthetic antioxidants while maintaining product shelf life. The water-binding capacity of oat protein additionally contributes to microbial stability by reducing water activity more effectively than many carbohydrate-based humectants.

Flavour system design for clean-label products must account for oat protein's minimal flavour impact while maximizing its compatibility with natural flavouring systems.

Table 7.3 Oat protein processing parameters for different applications.

Application	Optimal thermal treatment	Key equipment parameters	Critical control points
Beverage systems	75 °C for 20 s or 138 °C for 2s [45]	Homogenization –150200 bar	pH control, hydration time
Meat analogues [46]	Extrusion 140–160 °C	SME 400–600 kJ/kg	Moisture content, cooling rate
Bakery products	Baking 160–220 °C [47]	Dough development time	Hydration sequence, mixing intensity
Dairy alternatives	85–95 °C for 5–10 min [48]	High-shear mixing	Temperature ramp rate, holding time

The protein's neutral flavour profile enables simpler flavour systems with reduced masking requirements. However, careful selection of natural flavours is necessary, as certain terpene-based natural flavours may interact with oat protein's surface hydrophobic patches. Optimal compatibility is observed with yeast extracts and reaction flavours that complement oat's mild cereal notes [44].

The integration of these development strategies enables the creation of innovative food products that leverage oat protein's unique functional properties while meeting modern consumer demands for clean-label, nutritious options. The continued refinement of these approaches, combined with emerging processing technologies, promises to further expand oat protein's applications in the food industry.

7.3 Global Regulatory Framework

7.3.1 Safety Assessment and Approval Processes

The regulatory approval pathway for oat protein varies significantly across different jurisdictions, with three main approaches dominating the global landscape. In the United States, the generally recognized as safe (GRAS) determination process requires comprehensive scientific evidence, including toxicological studies, allergenicity assessments and intended use levels. The GRAS notification process typically involves submission of detailed dossiers to the FDA, with review periods extending 6–9 months. Key requirements include demonstration of safety under conditions of intended use, with particular attention to protein purity (typically requiring minimum 80% protein content) and absence of processing contaminants.

The European Union's Novel Food regulation (EU 2015/2283) presents a more structured approval pathway. OPI and concentrates fall under this regulation unless substantial history of consumption prior to 1997 can be demonstrated. The application process requires extensive scientific data, including 90-day rodent feeding studies, allergenicity assessments using established methodologies like EFSA's guidance, and detailed characterization of the production process. The average approval timeline extends 18–24 months, with specific attention to the extraction methods and solvent residues.

Health claim substantiation represents another critical regulatory hurdle. Under both FDA (21 CFR 101.14) and EFSA (Regulation EC 1924/2006) frameworks, protein content claims require minimum protein levels and specific protein quality assessments [49]. The protein digestibility-corrected amino acid score (PDCAAS) methodology remains the standard for protein quality evaluation, with oat protein typically achieving scores of 0.6-0.7, qualifying for 'good source of protein' claims but generally falling short of 'excellent source' requirements without amino acid supplementation [50].

7.3.2 Labelling Requirements

Nutritional labelling requirements for oat protein-containing products follow jurisdiction-specific rules with important nuances. In the United States, the FDA mandates declaration of protein content in grams per serving, with protein quality claims requiring PDCAAS documentation. The 'gluten-free' claim for oat protein requires rigorous testing to demonstrate gluten levels below 20 ppm, supported by ongoing monitoring using validated ELISA methods. The manufacturing process must ensure segregation from gluten-containing grains, with documented supply chain controls.

Allergen labelling presents particular challenges for oat protein. While oats are not among the major food allergens identified by the FDA, cross-contact with wheat during growing and processing necessitates careful consideration. The 'contains' statement must declare wheat if cross-contact cannot be ruled out, while processes achieving gluten levels below 20 ppm may qualify for 'gluten-free' labelling. In the European Union, oats must be declared when intentionally added, though they are not among the 14 major allergens requiring emphasized labelling [51].

Organic certification follows different standards across markets. USDA Organic certification requires that oat protein derivatives come from certified organic oats grown without prohibited pesticides, with processing aids limited to those included in the National List. The EU Organic regulation (EU 2018/848) imposes additional requirements regarding geographical origin and environmental impact, while the Canadian Organic Regime requires certification by accredited bodies following the Canadian Organic Standards [52].

7.3.3 Regional Regulatory Variations

North American regulations demonstrate both convergence and divergence between the United States and Canada. Health Canada's Natural and Non-prescription Health Products Directorate requires pre-market notification for novel oat protein products, with particular attention to amino acid composition and proposed health claims [27] (Table 7.4). The Canadian Food Inspection Agency enforces labelling requirements that align closely with US standards but with stricter bilingual (English/French) requirements and distinct serving size conventions [49].

The European Food Safety Authority standards emphasize the precautionary principle, requiring more extensive safety data than North American systems. Beyond novel food approval, oat protein products must comply with the EU's Farm to Fork strategy requirements regarding sustainability claims and environmental footprint declaration. The French Nutri-Score system, while voluntary, significantly impacts market access and formulation decisions, generally favouring plant proteins but penalizing certain processing methods (Table 7.4).

Asia-Pacific regulatory frameworks present the most diverse landscape. China's National Health Commission requires extensive safety review and approval for novel oat protein ingredients, with typical approval timelines extending 24–36 months [53]. Japan's Food for Specified Health Uses (FOSHU) system allows specific health claims but requires clinical trial evidence conducted in Japanese populations [54]. Australia and New Zealand follow the FSANZ code, which generally aligns with US approaches but with unique requirements for novel protein declaration and mandatory warning statements for potential allergens (Table 7.4).

The regulatory landscape for oat protein continues to evolve rapidly, with recent developments including increased emphasis on sustainable production methods, cleaner labelling requirements and harmonization efforts through international bodies like Codex Alimentarius. Successful market entry requires careful navigation of these complex and sometimes contradictory requirements, with particular attention to the interface between food and supplement regulations in different markets. The trend toward 'natural' claims

Table 7.4 Comparative regulatory requirements for oat protein products.

Region	Safety approval timeline (months)	Key documentation requirements	Special considerations
United States	6–9 (GRAS) [55]	Toxicology studies, usage level justification	GRAS notice voluntary but recommended
European Union	18–24 [56]	90-day feeding study, allergenicity assessment	Pre-market authorization mandatory
Canada	12–18 [57]	Novel food notification, labelling review	Bilingual requirements strict
China	24–36 [58]	Extensive safety portfolio, clinical data	Raw material traceability critical
Japan	18–24 [59]	Clinical trials in Japanese population	FOSHU claims require local studies
Australia/NZ	12–18 [60]	Novel food application, allergen assessment	Warning statements mandatory

and sustainable sourcing documentation represents an emerging challenge that crosses multiple regulatory domains.

7.4 Commercialization and Market Implementation

7.4.1 Scale-up Challenges

The transition from laboratory-scale production to industrial manufacturing of oat protein introduces significant challenges in preserving functional quality and batch-to-batch consistency. Key hurdles include inherent variability in protein content and functionality, which arise from differences in raw material composition and the sensitivity of protein structures to processing conditions.

Maintaining consistent protein functionality at commercial scale requires robust process control strategies. The implementation of process analytical technology (PAT) is critical, enabling real-time monitoring of critical quality attributes such as protein solubility, structural integrity and particle size distribution [61]. These systems facilitate immediate adjustments to extraction and purification parameters, ensuring the final product meets specified functional requirements. Advanced quality management systems incorporating predictive algorithms can anticipate deviations in protein quality, allowing for pre-emptive process modifications. Furthermore, digital traceability systems enhance supply chain transparency, providing comprehensive documentation of processing history and quality parameters from raw material to finished product.

Achieving economic viability in oat protein production demands integrated optimization of resource utilization and process efficiency. Energy-intensive unit operations, particularly extraction and drying, represent substantial portions of production costs. Implementation of advanced heat recovery systems and energy-efficient membrane filtration technologies can significantly reduce thermal and electrical energy consumption. Process intensification through continuous manufacturing systems offers advantages in yield improvement and resource conservation compared to batch processes. Additionally, the adoption of integrated biorefinery concepts enables valorization of co-streams, improving overall plant economics while minimizing waste generation.

Effective supply chain management must address the unique characteristics of oat protein production. Raw material strategies require careful consideration of varietal differences and agricultural practices that influence protein content and functionality. Sophisticated inventory management approaches, informed by predictive analytics, help balance the seasonality of agricultural production with year-round manufacturing needs. Specialized logistics protocols are essential to preserve protein functionality during transportation and storage, requiring controlled environmental conditions to prevent denaturation and maintain solubility characteristics.

The successful commercialization of oat protein relies on integrated solutions that address technical, economic and supply chain challenges simultaneously. Advanced process control methodologies, combined with continuous improvement practices and digital technologies, enable manufacturers to achieve scalable production while maintaining product quality and functional performance.

7.4.2 Consumer Acceptance and Market Positioning

The successful market implementation of oat protein hinges on a deep understanding of the drivers of consumer acceptance and the development of strategic positioning that leverages its inherent strengths. This requires a multifaceted approach integrating sensory science, consumer psychology and market intelligence.

Sensory Experience and Consumer Perception: Consumer acceptance is fundamentally guided by the product's sensory profile. For oat protein, key attributes include its texture, flavour neutrality and visual appeal. A smooth texture, free from grittiness, is paramount for consumer satisfaction across most application categories. The inherent mildness and neutral flavour profile of oat protein present a significant advantage over other plant proteins, which often carry strong, undesirable notes. This allows for cleaner flavour systems and reduces the need for extensive flavour masking. Consumer preference patterns vary across geographic regions and application categories, necessitating targeted product optimization. Long-term consumer loyalty is built on consistent delivery of these positive sensory experiences, underscoring the importance of stringent quality control from raw material selection through final processing.

Marketing Claims and Strategies: Effective communication is critical for market penetration. Marketing claims should be scientifically substantiated and strategically tailored to different consumer segments. Nutritional messaging, such as highlighting protein quality or specific health benefits, can significantly influence purchasing decisions, particularly when backed by credible scientific evidence. Sustainability narratives are increasingly important but require careful framing; overly technical metrics are often less effective than relatable stories about farming practices or ingredient origin. Educational initiatives that demonstrate product usage and explain nutritional advantages play a vital role in building consumer familiarity and trust. Partnerships with health professionals and the creation of transparent sourcing stories can enhance brand credibility and support a premium market position.

Competitive Positioning in the Plant Protein Market: Oat protein occupies a distinct niche within the competitive plant protein landscape. Its superior emulsification properties and neutral taste profile make it particularly well-suited for dairy alternatives and creamy applications, differentiating it from legumes and cereal-based competitors. In specific segments like sports nutrition, its combination of good functionality and digestive comfort allows for strategic positioning as an effective yet gentle alternative. From an economic perspective, the potential for integrated processing of the whole oat grain can offer cost-structure advantages at scale. This supports flexible pricing strategies, enabling competitive positioning in mass markets while also justifying premium pricing in segments where its functional benefits and sustainability credentials are most valued.

In summary, the successful market positioning of oat protein relies on an integrated strategy that optimizes its sensory attributes, communicates its benefits through credible and resonant messaging, and strategically leverages its unique functional and potential economic advantages within the diverse plant protein market. Continuous consumer insight and market adaptation are essential for maintaining relevance and competitive advantage.

7.5 Case Studies in Product Development

7.5.1 Successful Commercial Products Analysis

Oat-based Beverages: The remarkable market success of commercial oat-based beverages offers profound insights into effective product development methodologies. Industry leaders have established comprehensive development protocols beginning with meticulous raw material selection. Specific oat varieties are chosen based on their balanced nutritional composition, with particular attention to native protein and soluble fibre content [40]. These foundational choices directly influence the final product's sensory characteristics and nutritional profile.

Manufacturing processes typically employ enzymatic treatment protocols designed to optimize texture and flavour development while preserving nutritional value. The development of proprietary emulsion systems represents a critical technological advancement, combining oat protein with specific plant-based lipids and emulsifiers. These systems achieve exceptional stability while maintaining clean-label credentials, addressing consumer demand for recognizable ingredients.

Processing parameters are carefully controlled throughout production, with particular attention to homogenization and thermal treatment conditions. These controlled processes ensure product stability throughout the intended shelf life while maintaining protein integrity and functionality. The success of these products demonstrates the effective integration of ingredient science with processing technology.

Meat Analogue Products: The successful integration of oat protein in meat analogue formulations illustrates the importance of strategic ingredient combining. Industry formulations typically utilize oat protein in complementary systems with other plant proteins, leveraging their respective functional advantages. This approach maximizes texture development while enhancing moisture management and eating quality [62].

Processing technologies, particularly high-moisture extrusion, have been specifically adapted for oat-protein-containing systems [63]. The parameters are carefully optimized to account for oat protein's unique thermal and hydration properties. The inclusion of oat protein contributes significantly to the sensory experience, particularly in improving texture and preventing the dryness often associated with plant-based meat alternatives.

Flavour system development requires specialized approaches to complement oat's inherent cereal notes. Successful products incorporate flavour compounds that enhance umami characteristics while maintaining clean-label standards. The development process involves multiple iterations to achieve the optimal balance between meat-like flavour and oat's natural flavour profile.

Nutritional Supplement Formulations: Oat protein's application in nutritional supplements demonstrates its advantages in specialized nutrition markets. Successful products typically utilize specially processed OPI with enhanced functional properties. Advanced processing methods improve key characteristics, including solubility and digestibility, making the protein suitable for demanding applications like sports nutrition and clinical products.

Manufacturing processes employ controlled drying conditions designed to preserve protein functionality while ensuring microbial safety. The resulting ingredients demonstrate excellent performance in powder-based applications, with rapid dispersion and smooth texture. These characteristics are particularly important for consumer acceptance in the competitive supplement market.

Formulation strategies address the challenge of flavour compatibility through systematic ingredient selection and flavour masking technologies. Successful products combine oat protein with complementary flavour systems and functional ingredients that enhance both sensory and nutritional profiles. The development process emphasizes achieving a balance between nutritional efficacy and sensory appeal.

7.5.2 Development Process Documentation

From Laboratory to Pilot to Commercial Scale: The transition from concept to commercial product follows a structured development pathway with clearly defined evaluation criteria at each stage. Initial laboratory development focuses on establishing fundamental functional relationships and identifying critical parameters that influence product performance. This phase serves to validate core concepts and identify potential technical challenges.

Scale-up to pilot production represents a crucial transition where process parameters are refined and equipment compatibility is assessed. This stage often reveals unexpected interactions between ingredients and processing conditions that were not apparent at smaller scales. Successful navigation of this phase requires careful adjustment of operational parameters to maintain product quality while adapting to different equipment configurations.

Commercial implementation focuses on achieving consistent quality at manufacturing scale while maintaining economic viability. This phase involves implementing robust control systems and refining operational procedures to ensure reproducible results. The transition often involves significant adjustments to process parameters and may require modifications to initial formulation approaches to accommodate scale-related factors.

Formulation Iteration and Optimization: The formulation development process employs systematic approaches to balance multiple competing quality attributes. Development teams utilize structured experimental designs to understand interactions between key formulation variables and their impact on final product characteristics. This methodology enables efficient identification of optimal ingredient combinations and concentrations.

Consumer feedback is integrated throughout the development process through multiple rounds of sensory evaluation. Initial screening tests progress to increasingly sophisticated consumer research as formulations mature. This iterative process ensures that final products meet consumer expectations for sensory characteristics while delivering required functional performance.

The optimization process should balance technical feasibility with consumer preferences and economic considerations. Successful development requires careful consideration of how formulation changes affect manufacturing processes, shelf life and overall product economics. This holistic approach ensures that optimized formulations are viable for commercial production.

Quality by Designed Approaches: Implementation of quality begins with comprehensive identification of critical quality attributes through systematic risk assessment. These attributes are linked to specific process parameters through controlled experimentation, establishing defined relationships between formulation inputs and product outcomes.

The establishment of proven acceptable ranges for process parameters represents a fundamental outcome of the QbD approach [64]. This knowledge base enables flexible manufacturing within defined boundaries while ensuring consistent product quality. Understanding these parameter interactions is particularly important for oat protein applications due to the ingredient's unique functional characteristics.

Control strategy implementation combines procedural controls with technological monitoring systems. Standardized procedures ensure consistent raw material quality and process execution, while modern analytical technologies provide real-time quality verification. This integrated approach enables proactive quality management and reduces reliance on traditional end-product testing.

The documented development experiences across these product categories demonstrate that successful oat protein applications require methodical approaches that integrate fundamental science with practical manufacturing considerations. The accumulated knowledge provides valuable guidance for future development initiatives while highlighting the importance of systematic, stage-appropriate development methodologies.

7.6 Future Trends and Innovation Opportunities

7.6.1 Emerging Applications

3D Food Printing Applications: Oat protein is emerging as a promising material for 3D food printing applications due to its unique rheological properties and compatibility with additive manufacturing technologies. The protein's ability to form viscoelastic gels under specific conditions makes it suitable for creating complex structures with precise dimensional stability [65]. Research focuses on developing specialized printing formulations that maintain structural integrity during deposition while achieving desired texture profiles in the final product.

The printing process utilizes oat protein's thermal gelation properties to create self-supporting structures. By carefully controlling protein concentration and incorporating complementary hydrocolloids, manufacturers can achieve precise control over extrusion characteristics and layer adhesion. Post-printing treatments, including controlled humidity curing and mild thermal processing, enhance the structural stability of printed constructs while preserving nutritional quality.

Current development efforts address challenges related to printing resolution and production speed. Advanced printing systems incorporate multi-material capabilities, allowing for the integration of oat protein with other functional ingredients to create products with graded textures and targeted nutrient delivery. The compatibility of oat protein with various food-grade printing platforms enables the creation of customized products ranging from artistic culinary presentations to specialized nutritional products for populations with specific swallowing or dietary requirements.

Personalized Nutrition Platforms: The integration of oat protein into personalized nutrition platforms represents a significant innovation opportunity. The protein's neutral flavour profile, excellent digestibility and hypoallergenic characteristics make it an ideal base for tailored nutritional products. Advanced manufacturing technologies enable the production of customized formulations that respond to individual nutritional requirements, genetic profiles and health objectives.

Digital platforms combine user-specific data with algorithm-driven formulation systems to create personalized oat protein products. These systems consider factors including metabolic health indicators, physical activity levels and personal taste preferences to generate optimized nutritional solutions. The development of rapid assessment technologies allows for real-time formulation adjustments based on changing individual needs and preferences.

The convergence of oat protein technology with digital health monitoring creates new opportunities for dynamic nutrition management. Connected systems can adjust protein intake recommendations based on physiological data collected through wearable devices and digital health platforms. This approach supports precision nutrition strategies that optimize health outcomes through individually tailored oat protein formulations that evolve with changing nutritional requirements.

Sustainable Packaging Interactions: Oat protein's functional properties show significant potential for sustainable packaging applications, particularly in the development of biodegradable and edible packaging materials. Research focuses on creating protein-based films and coatings that extend product shelf life while reducing environmental impact. The inherent barrier properties of oat protein, particularly against oxygen and lipid migration, make it valuable for food protection applications.

The development of composite materials combining oat protein with natural polysaccharides creates packaging solutions with enhanced mechanical properties and functionality [66]. These materials can be engineered to provide specific barrier characteristics while maintaining full biodegradability. Advanced processing techniques, including electrospinning and solvent casting, enable the production of packaging materials with tailored thickness, transparency and mechanical strength.

Innovative applications include intelligent packaging systems that incorporate oat protein-based sensors for quality monitoring. These systems can detect changes in product freshness and provide visual indicators of quality status. The compatibility of oat protein with active compounds enables the development of packaging materials that release preservatives or nutrients in response to specific environmental triggers, creating dynamic protection systems that extend product shelf life while maintaining sustainability credentials [67].

The exploration of these emerging application areas demonstrates oat protein's versatility and potential to contribute to innovative solutions across multiple sectors. The successful development of these applications requires interdisciplinary approaches that combine materials science, nutrition research and digital technologies to create novel products that address evolving consumer needs and sustainability challenges.

7.6.2 Technological Advancements

Precision Fermentation Hybrids: The emergence of precision fermentation technologies offers innovative pathways for enhancing oat protein functionality and sustainability. This approach utilizes engineered microorganisms to produce specific protein components that can be combined with native oat proteins to create hybrid systems with superior functional properties. These hybrid proteins are designed to overcome inherent limitations of plant-based proteins while maintaining clean-label credentials.

The development process involves identifying specific protein sequences that can enhance particular functional characteristics, such as solubility or gelation properties. Microorganisms are then programmed to produce these protein components through controlled fermentation processes. The resulting protein ingredients are carefully integrated with oat protein extracts to create tailored functionality for specific applications. This technology enables the creation of protein systems with precisely controlled molecular structures and predictable performance characteristics [68].

Precision fermentation also supports sustainability objectives by reducing land and water requirements compared to traditional agriculture. The controlled production environment minimizes variations in protein quality and functionality while ensuring consistent supply [44]. This approach opens new possibilities for creating oat protein derivatives with enhanced nutritional profiles and functional properties that are difficult to achieve through conventional extraction methods alone.

Smart Processing Technologies: Advanced processing technologies incorporating artificial intelligence and machine learning are revolutionizing oat protein production. These smart systems continuously monitor and adjust process parameters in real time to optimize protein functionality and production efficiency [69]. Sensor networks collect vast amounts of data throughout the manufacturing process, enabling predictive adjustments that maintain optimal processing conditions.

The implementation of digital twin technology creates virtual replicas of production systems, allowing for simulation and optimization without disrupting actual production. These digital models can predict how changes in raw material characteristics or process parameters will affect final product quality, enabling proactive adjustments to maintain consistency. The integration of Internet of Things devices throughout the production chain provides unprecedented visibility into process performance and product quality.

Machine learning algorithms analyze historical production data to identify patterns and relationships that human operators might miss. These systems can predict potential quality issues before they occur and recommend preventive adjustments. The continuous learning capability of these systems means they become more effective over time, constantly refining processing parameters to improve product quality and production efficiency.

Bioavailability Enhancement: Innovative approaches to improving oat protein bioavailability focus on both processing technologies and formulation strategies. Advanced enzymatic hydrolysis methods are being developed to create specific peptide profiles that enhance absorption and utilization [70]. These controlled hydrolysis processes break down protein structures into more readily absorbable forms while preserving nutritional quality and minimizing bitter taste development.

Novel delivery systems, including microencapsulation and nanoemulsion technologies, protect protein molecules during digestion and enhance their delivery to absorption sites. These systems can be designed to control the release of amino acids, supporting sustained muscle protein synthesis and improving metabolic utilization. The combination of oat protein with specific absorption enhancers, such as certain plant compounds, further improves bioavailability through complementary mechanisms.

Research into protein–polyphenol complexes has shown promise for enhancing both the functional properties and biological efficacy of oat protein. These complexes can improve protein stability during processing and digestion while providing additional health benefits. The development of specialized processing methods that optimize protein structure for enhanced digestibility represents another important direction in bioavailability enhancement, particularly for applications in clinical nutrition and sports performance [71].

These technological advancements demonstrate the dynamic nature of oat protein research and development. The integration of biotechnology, digital technologies and advanced processing methods continues to expand the potential applications and improve the performance of oat protein in various food systems. These innovations support the development of next-generation oat protein ingredients with enhanced functionality, improved sustainability and superior nutritional efficacy.

7.6.3 Market Evolution and Growth Projections

Regional Market Development Patterns: The global market for oat protein exhibits distinct developmental trajectories across different geographical regions, shaped by varying consumer preferences, regulatory environments and agricultural infrastructures. In North American markets, growth is primarily driven by the robust expansion of plant-based dairy and meat alternative sectors, with oat protein establishing a strong position as a premium ingredient choice [39]. The market development reflects a sophisticated consumer base that values both functional performance and sustainability credentials, leading to rapid adoption across multiple product categories.

European markets demonstrate a more regulated but equally promising growth pattern, with particular strength in nutritional products and functional foods [72]. The development is characterized by stringent quality standards and a strong emphasis on scientific substantiation of health claims. Northern European countries show early adoption of innovative oat protein applications, while Mediterranean markets exhibit growing interest in traditional food products reformulated with oat protein to enhance their nutritional profiles.

Asia-Pacific regions present diverse development patterns, with mature markets like Japan and South Korea focusing on specialized nutritional and healthcare applications, while emerging economies prioritize basic nutrition and cost-effective protein solutions [73]. The development across these markets reflects varying stages of economic development, dietary traditions and regulatory frameworks, creating multiple distinct opportunities for market penetration and growth.

Ingredient Innovation Pipeline: The innovation pipeline for oat protein ingredients reflects ongoing research and development efforts across multiple dimensions. Current initiatives focus on enhancing fundamental functional properties through advanced processing technologies and modification methods. These efforts aim to address existing limitations while expanding the range of potential applications through tailored functionality development.

Significant resources are being directed towards sustainability innovations, including the development of more efficient extraction methods and the utilization of co-products from oat processing. These initiatives not only improve the environmental footprint of oat protein production but also contribute to better economic viability through increased value recovery from raw materials.

The pipeline also includes substantial work on nutritional enhancement, particularly regarding protein digestibility and amino acid profile optimization. Advanced breeding programs and biotechnological approaches are being employed to develop oat varieties with improved protein characteristics, while processing innovations focus on enhancing the bioavailability and functional performance of the resulting protein ingredients.

Consumer Trend Adaptation: The evolution of oat protein markets reflects ongoing adaptation to changing consumer preferences and lifestyle patterns. The strong alignment with plant-based dietary trends continues to drive market growth, with oat protein particularly well positioned due to its perceived naturalness and compatibility with clean label preferences. This alignment supports continued market expansion as consumer interest in plant-based nutrition maintains its upward trajectory.

Sustainability considerations are increasingly influencing market development, with consumers showing growing interest in the environmental attributes of protein sources. Oat protein's favourable sustainability profile compared to many alternative protein sources represents a significant advantage in this evolving landscape. Market players are responding by enhancing transparency in sourcing and production while developing more sophisticated communication strategies around environmental benefits.

The adaptation to health and wellness trends involves continuous innovation in product formulations and positioning strategies. The development of specialized products targeting specific health concerns and lifestyle needs reflects the market's maturation beyond basic nutritional supplementation. This trend is driving diversification across product categories and creating new opportunities for value-added applications of oat protein ingredients.

The convergence of these factors, regional market evolution, ongoing ingredient innovation and responsive adaptation to consumer trends, supports positive growth projections for oat protein markets. The continued expansion is expected to be driven by technological advancements that enhance functionality, growing consumer awareness of sustainability issues, and the development of increasingly sophisticated applications across food, beverage and nutritional product categories. The ability of market participants to anticipate and respond to these evolving patterns will be crucial for capturing growth opportunities in this dynamic market environment.

References

1 W. Ma et al., 'Role of particle size and roasted degree modulating the stability of oat milk', *Food Res. Int.*, vol. 221, p. 117391, 2025.

2 D. Lu, D. Roy, A. Acevedo-Fani, H. Singh, M. Waterland, and A. Ye, 'Physical properties and microstructure of hybrid processed cheeses formulated with plant protein and milk protein ingredients', *Food Hydrocoll.*, vol. 170, p. 111688, 2026.

3 M. Brückner-Gühmann, A. Benthin, and S. Drusch, 'Enrichment of yoghurt with oat protein fractions: structure formation, textural properties and sensory evaluation', *Food Hydrocoll.*, vol. 86, pp. 146–153, 2019.

4 G. Eazhumalai, G. T. K. Ranjitha, and U. S. Annapure, 'Cold plasma enhanced gelation and thermal properties of oat protein and its application in a selected model food system', *Sustain. Food Technol.*, vol. 3, no. 4, pp. 1203–1217, 2025.

5 S. Stajić et al., 'Tomato pomace powder as a functional ingredient in minced meat products—influence on technological and sensory properties of traditional serbian minced meat product ćevapi', *Processes*, vol. 12, no. 7, p. 1330, 2024.

6 S. M. Gaber, T. Dessev, D. Knezevic, G. Haustveit, and S. H. Knutsen, 'A feasibility study on oat concentrates as a single source of protein for production of meat analogues', *LWT*, vol. 222, p. 117626, 2025.

7 J. J. Ball, R. P. Wyatt, M. M. Coursen, B. D. Lambert, and J. T. Sawyer, 'Meat substitution with oat protein can improve ground beef patty characteristics', *Foods*, vol. 10, no. 12, p. 3071, 2021.

8 M. Immonen, A. Chandrakusuma, J. Sibakov, M. Poikelispää, and T. Sontag-Strohm, 'Texturization of a blend of pea and destarched oat protein using high-moisture extrusion', *Foods*, vol. 10, no. 7, p. 1517, 2021.

9 J. McLauchlan, A. I. I. Tyler, B. Chakrabarti, C. Orfila, and A. Sarkar, 'Oat protein: review of structure-function synergies with other plant proteins', *Food Hydrocoll.*, vol. 154, p. 110139, 2024.

10 L. Flander, U. Holopainen, K. Kruus, and J. Buchert, 'Effects of tyrosinase and laccase on oat proteins and quality parameters of gluten-free oat breads', *J. Agric. Food Chem.*, vol. 59, no. 15, pp. 8385–8390, 2011.

11 W. Wu et al., 'Leguminous proteins as beneficial baking emulsifiers: a comparative study with traditional sucrose ester', *Int. J. Biol. Macromol.*, vol.306, no. Pt 4, p. 141438, 2025.

12 V. R. Harwalkar and C. Y. Ma, 'Study of thermal properties of oat globulin by differential scanning calorimetry', *J. Food Sci.*, vol. 52, no. 2, pp. 394–398, 1987.

13 C. Yang et al., 'Ca2 induced irregular spherical oat protein-shellac nanoparticles as Pickering emulsions stabilizer to improve emulsion storage stability', *Food Chem.*, vol. 480, p. 143975, 2025.

14 M. E. Walters, C. C. Udenigwe, and A. Tsopmo, 'Structural characterization and functional properties of proteins from oat milling fractions', *J. Am. Oil Chem. Soc.*, vol. 95, no. 8, pp. 991–1000, 2018.

15 I. Aprodu, E. A. Badiu, and I. Banu, 'Influence of protein and water addition on gluten-free dough properties and bread quality', *Int. J. Food Eng.*, vol. 12, no. 4, pp. 355–363, 2016.

16 Z. Šmídová and J. Rysová, 'Gluten-free bread and bakery products technology', *Foods*, vol. 11, no. 3, p. 480, 2022.

17 J. Zhao, D. Ni, B. Bhandari, C. Gaiani, and S. Prakash, 'Impacts of oat flour fortification on the rheological, microstructural, digestibility, and sensory characteristics of low-fat, high-protein almond-based gels', *Food Hydrocoll.*, vol. 151, p. 109849, 2024.

18 C. Alsado, L. Lopez-Aldana, L. Chen, and W. Wismer, 'Consumer perception and sensory drivers of liking of fortified oat milks', *Foods*, vol. 12, no. 22, p. 4097, 2023.

19 Technical regulations of the customs union TR CU 021/2011. [2025-11-06], https://eacgroupcompany.com/en/regulations/trcu021-2011.

20 K. Kosová, L. Leišová-Svobodová, and V. Dvořáček, 'Oats as a safe alternative to triticeae cereals for people suffering from celiac disease? A review', *Plant Foods Hum. Nutr.*, vol. 75, no. 2, pp. 131–141, 2020.

21 R. Li and Y. L. Xiong, 'Sensitivity of oat protein solubility to changing ionic strength and pH', *J. Food Sci.*, vol. 86, no. 1, pp. 78–85, 2021.

22 L. Kumar, R. Sehrawat, and Y. Kong, 'Oat proteins: a perspective on functional properties', *LWT*, vol. 152, p. 112307, 2021.

23 R. Li, A. D. True, L. Sha, and Y. L. Xiong, 'Structural modification of oat protein by thermosonication combined with high pressure for O/W emulsion and model salad dressing production', *Int. J. Biol. Macromol.*, vol. 255, p. 128109, 2024.

24 A. L. Grosso, G. Cestonaro, M. Scampicchio, G. Ferrentino, and E. Costanzo, 'Development of a protein-enriched oat beverage: enhancing antioxidant activity, functional properties and stability with soy protein hydrolysates', *LWT*, vol. 222, p. 117644, 2025.

25 M. Pawlos, K. Szajnar, and A. Znamirowska-Piotrowska, 'Probiotic milk and oat beverages with increased protein content: survival of probiotic bacteria under simulated in vitro digestion conditions', *Nutrients*, vol. 16, no. 21, p. 3673, 2024.

26 J. E. Cluskey, Y. V. Wu, G. E. Inglett, and J. S. Wall, 'Oat protein concentrates for beverage fortification', *J. Food Sci.*, vol. 41, no. 4, pp. 799–804, 1976.

27 B. E. Enriquez Fernandez, P. Klassen, V. Mazurak, L. Chen, C. M. Prado, and W. V. Wismer, 'Acceptance of oat-based beverages tailored for patients with cancer', *J. Food Sci.*, vol. 86, no. 6, pp. 2671–2683, 2021.

28 C. Wang, S. Liang, H. Wang, and M. Guo, 'Physiochemical properties and probiotic survivability of symbiotic oat-based beverage', *Food Sci. Biotechnol.*, vol. 27, no. 3, pp. 735–743, 2017.

29 J. Metri-Ojeda, M. Ramírez-Rodrigues, L. Rosas-Ordoñez, and D. Baigts-Allende, 'Development and characterization of a low-fat mayonnaise salad dressing based on arthrospira platensis protein concentrate and sodium alginate', *Appl. Sci.*, vol. 12, no. 15, p. 7456, 2022.

30 E. Avci, A. Akcicek, Z. H. T. Cakmak, M. Z. Kasapoglu, O. Sagdic, and S. Karasu, 'Isolation of protein and fiber from hot pepper seed oil byproduct to enhance rheology, emulsion, and oxidative stability of low-fat salad dressing', *ACS Omega*, vol. 9, no. 9, pp. 10243–10252, 2024.

31 H. Mooliani and M. Nouri 'Optimization of oxidative, physical stability and microbial characteristics of salad dressing emulsions based on avocado and whey protein combined with mint (*Mentha spicata* L) extract', *J. Food Meas. Charact.*, vol. 15, no. 6, pp. 5713–5724, 2021.

32 S. L. Turgeon, C. Sanchez, S. F. Gauthier, and P. Paquin, 'Stability and rheological properties of salad dressing containing peptidic fractions of whey proteins', *Int. Dairy J.*, vol. 6, no. 6, pp. 645–658, 1996.

33 L. Chauvet, E. Charton, M. Lemaire, I. Le Huërou-Luron, and A. Deglaire, 'Human milk vs. cow-milk based infant formula proteins: structure, digestion and physiological impacts', *Front. nutr.*, vol. 12, p. 1635919, 2025.

34 Q. Ren et al., 'The association of formula protein content and growth in early infancy: a systematic review and meta-analysis', *Nutrients*, vol. 14, no. 11, p. 2255, 2022.

35 T. Bohn et al., 'Nutritional safety and suitability of a specific protein hydrolysate manufactured by fonterra co-operative group ltd derived from a whey protein concentrate and used in infant formula and follow-on formula', *EFSA J.*, vol. 23, no. 1, p. e9160, 2025.

36 H. Rafique et al., 'Dietary-nutraceutical properties of oat protein and peptides', *Front. nutr.*, vol. 9, p. 950400, 2022.

37 X. Li, L. Zhou, Y. Yu, J. Zhang, J. Wang, and B. Sun, 'The potential functions and mechanisms of oat on cancer prevention: a review', *J. Agric. Food Chem.*, vol. 70, no. 46, pp. 14588–14599, 2022.

38 P. Fric, D. Gabrovska, and J. Nevoral, 'Celiac disease, gluten-free diet, and oats', *Nutr. Rev.*, vol. 69, no. 2, pp. 107–115, 2011.

39 M. Immonen, J. Myllyviita, T. Sontag-Strohm, and P. Myllärinen, 'Oat protein concentrates with improved solubility produced by an enzyme-aided ultrafiltration extraction method', *Foods*, vol. 10, no. 12, p. 3050, 2021.

40 M. M. L. Grundy, D. J. McClements, S. Ballance, and P. J. Wilde, 'Influence of oat components on lipid digestion using an in vitro model: impact of viscosity and depletion flocculation mechanism', *Food Hydrocoll.*, vol. 83, pp. 253–264, 2018.

41 J. Haas, B. J. Kim, Z. Atamer, C. Wu, and D. C. Dallas, 'Effects of high-temperature, short-time pasteurization on milk and whey during commercial whey protein concentrate production', *J. Dairy Sci.*, vol. 108, no. 1, pp. 257–271, 2025.

42 S. Braspaiboon and T. Laokuldilok, 'High hydrostatic pressure: influences on allergenicity, bioactivities, and structural and functional properties of proteins from diverse food sources', *Foods*, vol. 13, no. 6, p. 922, 2024.

43 B. Li et al., 'Insights into cold plasma treatment on the cereal and legume proteins modification: principle, mechanism, and application', *Foods*, vol. 13, no. 10, p. 1522, 2024.

44 S. M. Tapia et al., 'Butter aroma compounds in plant-based milk alternatives through fermentation: screening of potential starter cultures and enhanced production in oat milk with *Lactococcus cremoris*', *LWT*, vol. 223, p. 117754, 2025.

45 E. G. Vasquez Orejarena, 'Development of a Functional Shelf Stable High Protein Dairy Beverage with Oat-Beta-Glucan', The Ohio State University, 2016.

46 S. H. V. Cornet, S. J. E. Snel, F. K. G. Schreuders, R. G. M. van der Sman, M. Beyrer, and A. J. van der Goot, 'Thermo-mechanical processing of plant proteins using shear cell and high-moisture extrusion cooking', *Crit. Rev. Food Sci. Nutr.*, vol. 62, no. 12, pp. 3264–3280, 2022.

47 E. Pyanikova, A. Kovaleva, O. Evdokimova, and A. Ryazantseva, 'Development of a semi-finished biscuit recipe for vegans', *E3S Web Conf.*, vol. 548, p. 02015, 2024. EDP Sciences.

48 R. McCarron, L. Methven, S. Grahl, R. Elliott, and S. Lignou, 'Fortification of pea and potato protein isolates in oat-based milk alternatives; effects on the sensory and volatile profile', *Foods*, vol. 13, no. 13, p. 2075, 2024.

49 Regulation (EC) No 1924/2006 of the European Parliament and of the Council of 20 December 2006 on nutrition and health claims made on foods, *OJ L*, vol. 404, 2006.

50 U. Holopainen-Mantila, S. Vanhatalo, P. Lehtinen, P. Lehtinen, and N. Sozer, 'Oats as a source of nutritious alternative protein', *J. Cereal Sci.*, vol. 116, p. 103862, 2024.

51 Regulation (EU) No 1169/2011 of the European Parliament and of the Council of 25 October 2011 on the provision of food information to consumers, amending Regulations (EC) No 1924/2006 and (EC) No 1925/2006 of the European Parliament and of the Council, and repealing Commission Directive 87/250/EEC, Council Directive 90/496/EEC, Commission Directive 1999/10/EC, Directive 2000/13/EC of the European Parliament and of the Council, Commission Directives 2002/67/EC and 2008/5/EC and Commission Regulation (EC) No 608/2004 Text with EEA relevance, *OJ L*, vol. 304, 2011.

52 Regulation - 2018/848 - EN - EUR-lex. [2025-11-05], https://eur-lex.europa.eu/eli/reg/2018/848/oj.

53 Safe food for Canadians regulations. [2025-11-05], https://laws-lois.justice.gc.ca/eng/regulations/SOR-2018-108/FullText.html.

54 R. Li, A. D. True, L. Sha, and Y. L. Xiong, 'Structure–functionality relationship and modification strategies of oat protein: challenges and opportunities', *Compr. Rev. Food Sci. Food Saf.*, vol. 24, no. 1, p. e70091, 2025.

55 Center for Veterinary Medicine. Human Foods Program. Center for Veterinary Medicine Human Foods Program. (2016-10) [2025-11-05], https://www.fda.gov/media/101042/download.

56 Regulation (EU) 2015/2283 of the European Parliament and of the Council of 25 November 2015 on novel foods, amending Regulation (EU) No 1169/2011 of the European Parliament and of the Council and repealing Regulation (EC) No 258/97 of the European Parliament and of the Council and Commission Regulation (EC) No 1852/2001 (Text with EEA relevance), *OJ L*, vol. 327, 2015.

57 Guidelines for the safety assessment of novel foods - canada.ca. [2025-11-05], https://www.canada.ca/en/health-canada/services/food-nutrition/legislation-guidelines/guidance-documents/guidelines-safety-assessment-novel-foods-2006.html.

58 Regulations on the Safety Review and Management of New Food Ingredients National Health Commission China Government Network. [2025-11-05], https://www.gov.cn/zhengce/2013-05/31/content_5713799.htm.

59 Risk Assessment | Food Safety Commission - Science of Food Safety. [2025-11-05], https://www.fsc.go.jp/hyouka/.

60 Food standards code legislation food standards Australia New Zealand. [2025-11-05], https://www.foodstandards.gov.au/food-standards-code/legislation.

61 D. P. Salem et al., 'Characterization of protein aggregation using hydrogel-encapsulated nIR fluorescent nanoparticle sensors', *ACS Sens.*, vol. 5, no. 2, pp. 327–337, 2020.

62 A. Knaapila, K. Kantanen, J. M. Ramos-Diaz, V. Piironen, M. Sandell, and K. Jouppila, 'Sensory and physical properties of fibrous meat analogs made from faba bean, pea, and oat using high-moisture extrusion', *Foods*, vol. 13, no. 10, p. 1444, 2024.

63 C. González-Galeana, A. Castañeda-Salazar, M. del C. Cortez-Trejo, M. Gaytán-Martínez, R. Campos-Vega, and S. Mendoza, 'Structural and functional properties of a high moisture extruded mixture of pea proteins (*Pisum sativum*), amaranth flour (*Amaranthus hypochondriacus*), and oat flour (*Avena sativa*)', *Food Chem.*, vol. 463, no. Pt 1, p. 141042, 2025.

64 D. J. Kalal and V. K. Redasani, 'Stability-indicating RP-HPLC method development and validation for estimation of mupirocin calcium in bulk and in pharmaceutical formulation', *Futur. J. Pharm. Sci.*, vol. 8, no. 1, 2022.

65 J. Zhang, Q. Chen, D. L. Kaplan, and Q. Wang, 'High-moisture extruded protein fiber formation toward plant-based meat substitutes applications: science, technology, and prospect', *Trends Food Sci. Technol.*, vol. 128, pp. 202–216, 2022.

66 L. Kang et al., 'Insights into ultrasonic treatment on the properties of pullulan/oat protein /nisin composite film: mechanical, structural and physicochemical properties', *Food Chem.*, vol. 402, p. 134237, 2023.

67 T. Song, S. Qian, T. Lan, Y. Wu, J. Liu, and H. Zhang, 'Recent advances in bio-based smart active packaging materials', *Foods*, vol. 11, no. 15, p. 2228, 2022.

68 M. A. Augustin, C. J. Hartley, G. Maloney, and S. Tyndall, 'Innovation in precision fermentation for food ingredients', *Crit. Rev. Food Sci. Nutr.*, vol. 64, no. 18, pp. 6218–6238, 2023.

69 M. S. Le, C. Hermansen, and Q. V. Vuong 'Oat milk by-product: a review of nutrition, processing and applications of oat pulp', *Food Rev. Int.*, vol. 41, no. 5, pp. 1538–1575, 2025.

70 H. Rafique et al., 'Ultrasound-assisted modification of oat protein isolates: structural and functional enhancements', *Ultrason. Sonochem.*, vol. 112, p. 112107204, 2024.

71 M. Chen et al., 'Self-assembled cinnamon essential oil-coffee polyphenol colloidal dispersion integrated into oat milk: effects on stability and digestive characteristics', *Food Res. Int.*, vol. 211, p. 116429, 2025.

72 L. Serra-Majem et al., 'Updating the Mediterranean diet pyramid towards sustainability: focus on environmental concerns', *Int. J. Environ. Res. Public Health*, vol. 17, no. 23, p. 8758, 2020.

73 A. K. Omer, S. Khorshidi, N. Mortazavi, and H. S. Rahman, 'A review on the antiviral activity of functional foods against COVID-19 and viral respiratory tract infections', *Int. J. Gen. Med.*, vol. 15, pp. 4817–4835, 2022.

8

Nutritional and Health Aspects of Oat Proteins

8.1 Introduction

Except for the β-glucan in oats, recent studies emphasise the importance of its protein content in contributing to notable nutritional and health benefits [1]. Oats are notable for their balanced amino acid composition, particularly their high lysine content, which is typically limited in cereals [2]. Additionally, they can generate various bioactive peptides with specific health-protective properties when subjected to enzymatic treatment under controlled conditions [3]. The unique characteristics of oat protein position it as an excellent source of plant-based nutrition and a promising functional ingredient relevant for disease prevention and human health. The potential health benefits of oat proteins and peptides are evident across various physiological systems [4]. These compounds have been shown to function as antioxidants and anti-inflammatory agents, crucial for safeguarding the human body against damage caused by free radicals, oxidative stress and inflammatory biomarkers [5], which are recognized as significant contributors to the development of nearly all chronic diseases. Oat proteins and peptides have the potential to mitigate cardiovascular disorders primarily by lowering low-density lipoprotein (LDL) cholesterol levels and preventing blood pressure-related damage, thereby contributing to blood pressure regulation [6, 7].

Oat proteins and peptides exhibit various effects on metabolic health, primarily associated with blood sugar regulation, insulin sensitivity and lipid metabolism. These characteristics underscore the significance of oat protein in the dietary management of type 2 diabetes and other metabolic syndromes [8]. The role of oat protein and peptides is increasingly recognized in immune modulation, as they enhance host defence while simultaneously suppressing the overactivation of inflammation-related pathways [9]. Recent studies indicate that oat peptides may have neuroprotective effects that contribute to cognitive health. This occurs through the enhancement of neurotransmitters, the prevention of oxidative damage in neural tissues and the interaction with various pathways of the gut–brain axis, potentially aiding in the protection against cognitive decline and neurodegeneration, such as symptoms associated with Alzheimer's disease [10, 11]. Furthermore, oats are notably recognized in relation to gluten-related disorders. Oat protein, a naturally gluten-free ingredient, is typically well tolerated by individuals exhibiting gluten sensitivity or symptoms akin to coeliac disease [12]. This attribute of oat protein renders it a suitable and safe option for gluten-free diets, offering nutritional and functional benefits while ensuring safety.

The growing global demand for plant-based proteins is driven by evolving dietary preferences, health awareness and sustainability concerns. Oat protein, characterized by a mild flavour and favourable consumer acceptance, offers potential as a sustainable alternative to animal proteins. In Europe, cereals contribute nearly 70% of plant protein intake, and replacing a portion of animal proteins with oat protein-based foods has been shown to maintain adequate protein intake while reducing environmental impact. These attributes position oat protein as a promising component in advancing the transition towards nutritionally adequate and environmentally sustainable plant-based diets. Beyond its nutritional value, oat protein underscores its significance as a unique dietary ingredient with broad applications in wellness and disease prevention. This chapter will present detailed information on each aspect, supported by scientific evidence regarding health benefits, underlying mechanisms and potential applications in functional foods, nutraceutical and clinical nutrition: merge and make better arrangements and sequence.

8.2 Potential of Oat Protein as a Part of Daily Nutrition

The nutritional benefits of oat protein are largely attributed to its balanced amino acid composition, relatively high content of essential amino acids, compatibility with gluten-free diets and low allergenic potential. Although the overall protein quality of oats is lower than that of soybean and pea, the amino acid score of oat protein ranges from 0.66 to 0.75, which is slightly lower than that of soy but substantially higher than that of wheat [13]. Oat protein has been shown to support physical performance and recovery, and a range of bioactive peptides derived from oat protein have demonstrated beneficial activities [14]. Protein is determined by both amino acid composition and its digestibility. Oat is classified as having 'no quality claim' as its digestible indispensable amino acid score (DIASS) is below 75 when evaluated against the reference pattern for children aged 0.3–3 years, with lysine identified as the limiting amino acid. Nevertheless, the DIAAS of oat protein exceeds that of hemp, rice, wheat and fava bean; although, it remains inferior to that of pea, potato, rapeseed, lupin, and animal-derived proteins. The protein digestibility corrected amino acid score (PDCAAS) of raw oat samples is approximately 69, decreasing to around 60 following cooking. These values are generally lower than those reported for soy protein, which range from 59 to 75 for raw samples and approximately 73 for cooked samples, but remain higher than those for wheat, which typically ranges from 40 and 42 in raw form and from 39 to 40 after cooking [13]. Thermal processing has been shown to reduce both DIAAS and PDCAAS values of oats protein, indicating that heat treatment alters amino acids accessibility. Kilning and stirring roasting, in particular, have been reported to decrease the amino acid score of oat proteins. While heat treatment can enhance protein digestibility through denaturation, which increases the accessibility of concealed peptide bonds to digestive enzyme.

The growing global demand for plant-based foods is driven by changes in dietary patterns, rising incomes and population growth [15]. Over two-thirds of consumers identify as omnivores, while the remainder follow vegetarian, vegan, or pescetarian. Flexitarian diets, primarily plant-based with occasional meat inclusion, are increasingly common and will influence a transition in dietary preferences shaped by social, cultural, environmental, traditional factors and income levels. Meat consumption in Europe is decreasing, with numerous consumers intending to embrace a flexitarian diet. The principal barriers to increased consumption of plant-based foods in Europe include cost, insufficient information and limited availability in food service settings, and insufficient consumer information. In contrast, the taste preferences and price remain the primary obstacles in United States.

In Europe, average protein intake is estimated at 102.7 g per capita per day, of which 58.3 g are derived from animal sources and 44.4 g from plant sources [16]. Cereals account for approximately 70% of plant-derived proteins intake both in Europe and globally. Consumer acceptance of mild-flavoured oat protein is significantly higher than that of other plant-based proteins, including soy and pea [14]. The global intake of oat protein is 0.1 g per capita per day, increasing to 0.8 g per capita per day in Nordic countries [16].

Average consumption of meat, eggs and seafood estimated at 117 g per capita per day, while intake of milk, yogurt and cheese is recorded at 97 g per capita per day, with substantial regional variation [17]. The Planetary Health Diet provides a framework for achieving dietary patterns that support both human health and environmental sustainability. According to the Eat-Lancet report, a diet designed to provide 2500 kcal per day should include approximately 232 g of whole grains, while limiting the combined intake of meat, fish and eggs to 84 g per day, and limiting dairy foods, including whole milk and dairy products, to 250 g per day. There is ongoing discussion regarding the ideal ratio of animal-based foods and whether this should be adjusted to guarantee sufficient intake of vitamin B12, calcium, iron and zinc. A transition towards plant-based diets would necessitate a substantial increase in whole grain consumption, alongside a reduced reliance on animal-derived foods. Recent studies have explored the feasibility of substituting animal proteins with cereal-based proteins, particularly oat protein [16, 18]. In Europe, it has been estimated that approximately 20% (11.6 g) of the current animal protein intake of 58 g per capita per day could be replaced by cereal proteins and other plant-based sources. In practical terms, this substitution could be achieved by consuming large portion of oat porridge, 400–500 mL of an oat-based yogurt or milk alternative, or approximately 29 g of an oat-based meat substitute. A recent study [18] examined the potential of utilising foods with oat protein concentrate as substitutes for conventional food items such as wheat bread, pasta and yogurt. Their calculations indicated that it is feasible to eliminate all beef from the diet while still achieving the same protein intake of 57 g per capita per day as found in the original Danish diet, by replacing traditional food products with those containing oat protein concentrate. Alternatively, it is feasible to decrease the consumption of beef from 26 to 16 g by substituting just 15% of the conventional food products with oat protein alternatives. This highlights the significance of foods rich in oat protein in facilitating the shift from animal-based to plant-based diets.

8.3 Role in Chronic Disease Prevention

This section provides a comprehensive discussion on the health-protecting functions of oat proteins and peptides (Figure 8.1). A short overview of oat protein-derived bioactive components with their enzymes and activities is given in Table 8.1.

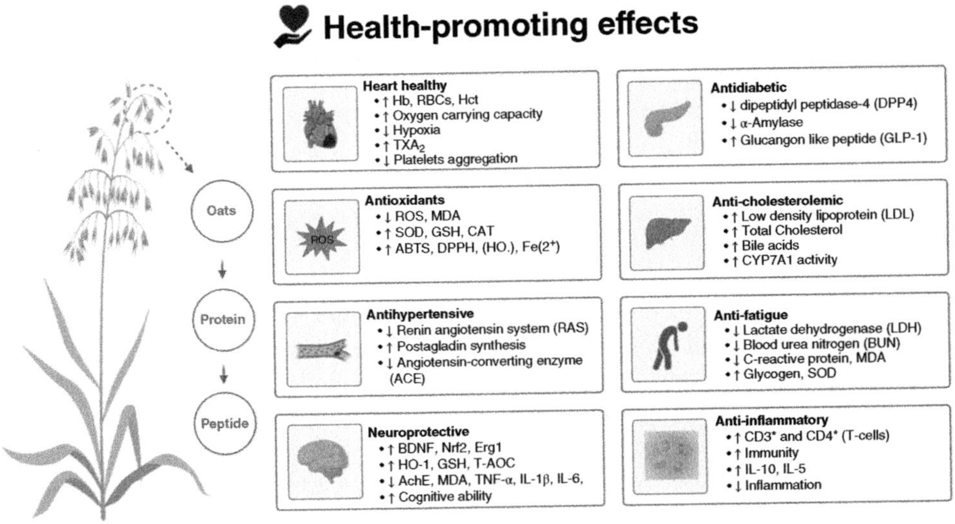

Figure 8.1 Health protecting functions of oat proteins and peptides.

Table 8.1 Oat protein-derived components and their bioactivity.

Protein fraction	Enzyme used	Product	Bioactivity	References
Total protein	Alcalase, Papain, Flavourzyme, Protamex	Hydrolysates	In vitro antioxidant	[19]
Globulin	Alcalase	IRIPIL, FLKPMT, NSKNFPTL, LIGRPIIY, FNDILRRGQLL	In vitro antioxidant	[20]
Total protein	Synthetic peptides	FNDRLRQGQLL, GLVYIL, GQTV, GQTVFNDRLRQGQLL, YHNAP, YHNAPGLVYIL, DVNNNANQLEPR	Cell line antioxidant	[21]
Total protein	Flavourzyme, Papain, Alcalase	Hydrolysates	In vitro antioxidant	[22]
Total protein	Alcalase, Papain, Flavourzyme, Protamex	Hydrolysates, pretreated with cellulose-degrading enzymes	Cell line antioxidant	[23]
Oat bran	—	Oat peptide-ferrous (OP-Fe+2) chelate	Antioxidant in mice model	[24]
Oat bran extract	—	Oat peptide	Antioxidant enzymes in human dermal fibroblast	[25]

Protein fraction	Enzyme used	Product	Bioactivity	References
Total protein	Papain	YFDEQNEQFR, GQLLIVPQ, SPFWNINAH, NINAHSVVY, RALPIDVL	In vitro anti-diabetic	[26]
Globulin	Trypsin	Hydrolysates, LQAFEPLR and EFLLAGNNK	Cell line antidiabetic	[27]
Total protein	Flavourzyme, Papain, Alcalase	Hydrolysates	Cell line antidiabetic	[28]
Total protein	Chemically synthesized	Protein, FFG, IFFFL, PFL, WCY, YPIL, CPA, FLLA and FEPL	In vitro anti-hypertensive	[29]
Globulin	Alcalase, Flavourzyme, Pepsin, Trypsin	SSYYPFK selected based on in silico analysis	In vitro anti-hypertensive	[30]
Total protein	Multiple proteases	Mixture of Oligopeptides	Immunomodulatory, anti-inflammatory, anti-cancer in mice model	[31]
Total protein	—	Oligopeptides	Anti-hypoxia in mice model	[32]
Total protein	—	Oatmeal, protein isolates	Anti-fatigue in mice model	[33]
Total protein	—	protein isolates	Anti-fatigue in clinical trial	[34]
Total and globulin protein	Pepsin Pancreatin and trypsin	Hydrolysates and Peptides	In vitro anti-thrombotic	[35]
Total protein	—	Protein isolates	Anti-cholesterolaemic in mice model	[36]
Total protein		Lunasin peptide,	Anti-cancer	[37]
Total protein	Alcalase	Hydrolysates and Peptides HL-8, RW-9, DF-10	In vitro and cell line neuroprotection	[10]

8.3.1 Oat Protein in Prevention of Oxidative Stress

Oxidative stress contributes to the development of diabetes, obesity and diabetes-related microvascular complications, such as diabetic retinopathy, end-stage renal disease, atherosclerosis and cardiovascular diseases [38–41]. Oxidative stress arises from the excessive accumulation of reactive free radicals within cells, including reactive oxygen species (ROS) and reactive nitrogen species (RNS). ROS and RNS play a crucial role in normal cellular function and the host defence system against invading bacteria; however, their excessive levels can lead to the onset and worsening of various pathologies, including neurological diseases and diabetes [42–45]. Cellular antioxidants, including glutathione, and antioxidant enzymes, such as superoxide dismutase (SOD), catalase (CAT) and glutathione peroxidase (GPx), sequester reactive oxygen species (ROS) and reactive nitrogen species (RNS) to sustain an optimal balance of cellular redox status [46, 47]. The disparity between the generation and elimination of ROS and RNS leads to their excessive accumulation. ROS and RNS function as signalling molecules at physiological concentrations; however, under oxidative conditions, elevated levels of ROS and RNS cause cellular damage through harmful interactions with proteins, lipids and DNA. This damage contributes to the development of various diseases associated with oxidative stress, including diabetes, obesity and neurological disorders such as Alzheimer's disease and Parkinson's disease [48–50].

Oats provide a significant supply of antioxidants, such as phytic acid, phenolic compounds, vitamin E and avenanthramides, which help mitigate oxidative stress [51]. The antioxidant defence system regulates the balance of ROS via the function of superoxide dismutase (SOD), glutathione peroxidase (GPx), catalase (CAT), as well as vitamins, minerals and co-factors, thereby preventing cellular oxidative stress. The antioxidant compounds exhibited radical scavenging activities via a single electron transfer process [52]. Oat proteins are increasingly recognized for their antioxidant potential, which may contribute to the prevention and management of oxidation-related disorders, delay oxidative deterioration in food systems and support overall health and quality of life [53]. Oat protein isolates and hydrolysates have demonstrated substantial antioxidant activity in assay targeting 2,2′ Azino-Bis-Ethylbenzoline-6-Sulfonic acid (ABTS), hydroxyl radicals (HO), superoxide anions (O.2) and Fe(2+) chelating assays [19]. Bioactive peptides (IRIPIL, FLKPMT, FNDILRRGQLL, LIGRPIIY and NSKNFPTL) derived from globulin fraction had the most significant scavenging activity for 2,2-diphenyl-1-picryl-hydrazyl-hydrate (DPPH) (IC50 $= 4.11 \pm 0.07$ mg/mL) and hydroxyl radicals (IC50 $= 1.83 \pm 0.03$ mg/mL) [20]. Another study revealed that oat peptides (GLVYIL, YHNAP and GQTV) exhibit cytoprotective properties and peroxyl radical scavenging abilities, demonstrating notable oxygen radical absorbance capacity (ORAC) values of 0.67 ± 0.02, 0.61 ± 0.04 and 0.52 ± 0.01 Trolox equivalent (TE)/μM, respectively. The cytoprotective efficacy of the peptides GLVYIL, YHNAP and GQTV correlated with their hydrophobicity but not with their ORAC values [21].

Oat protein hydrolysates have been shown to protect HepG2 cells from AAPH-induced oxidative stress by significantly enhancing the activities of antioxidant enzyme, including GPx, CAT and SOD, while simultaneously decreasing ROS levels [23]. Furthermore, peptides such as NINAHSVVY, YFDEQNEQFR and SPFWNINAH significantly inhibited lipid peroxidation and linolenic acid peroxidation by 52, 35 and 16%, respectively [26]. The incorporation of tyrosine at the N- or C-terminal and histidine inside a peptide sequence increased their activity, since both amino acids had strong electron- or proton-donating properties. Hydrophobicity is a crucial factor in lipid interactions [26]. A recent improvement to alleviate anaemia and oxidative stress involves using oat antioxidant peptide as a carrier to create a unique oat peptide-ferrous (OP-Fe+2) chelate. OP-Fe+2 has shown efficacy in mitigating anaemia and enhancing the activities of antioxidant enzymes, such as GSH and SOD, while reducing malondialdehyde (MDA) levels in the liver of an iron-deficient anaemic rat model [24]. Moreover, oat peptides effectively reduced H_2O_2-induced apoptosis and oxidative stress in human dermal fibroblasts via regulating cellular antioxidant enzymes [25]. These studies together suggested that peptides generated from oats may alleviate oxidative stress and related disorders, thereby facilitating the development of nutraceuticals or functional foods.

8.3.2 Oat Protein in Prevention of Diabetes

Diabetes is one of the most prevalent disorders worldwide, characterized by elevated blood glucose levels and associated with several serious health risks, including blindness, kidney failure, cardiovascular disease and multi-organ damage. An important factor in glucose regulation is dipeptidyl peptidase-4 (DPP4), also known as T-cell activation antigen CD26, which plays a critical role in both glucose metabolism and immune function. Consequently, inhibition of DPP4 has been recognized as a promising therapeutic strategy for diabetes management. In this context, plant-based natural and sustainable DPP4 inhibitors have attracted significant global attention as potential treatment option (Figure 8.2) [54]. It has been previously proven that oat peptides may inhibit dipeptidyl peptidase-4 (DPP4) and α-amylase while facilitating the release of glucagon-like peptide-1 (GLP-1). Diverse dietary bioactive peptides serve as antidiabetic drugs by modulating insulin resistance and energy metabolism [55]. Oat globulin peptides exhibited DPP4 inhibitory action in vitro, with half-maximal inhibitory concentration (IC50) values of 100.4 μg/mL for peptide LQAFEPLR and 2.04 mg/mL for oat tryptic hydrolysates. Oat peptides showed enhanced DPP4 inhibition relative to fish peptides, with 42.5% inhibition at a dosage of 5 mg/mL, while milk peptides had an IC50 range of 0.60–2.14 mg/mL [21, 26, 28]. Oat peptides suppressed

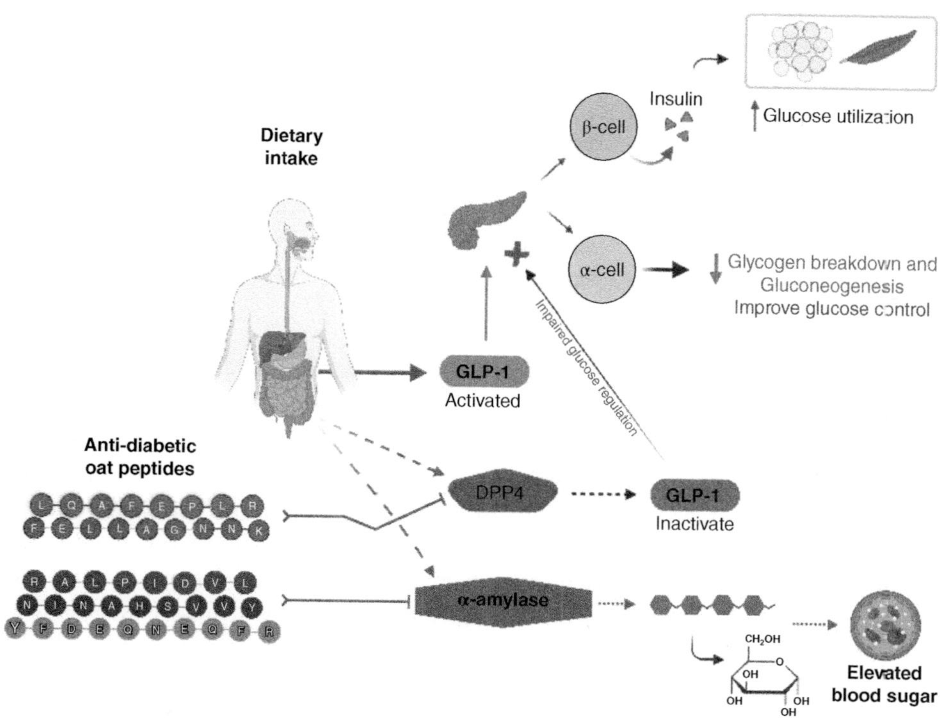

Figure 8.2 Anti-diabetic activity of oat peptides through inhibiting DPP4 and α-amylase pathways.

DPP4 activity by binding to its active site with low binding energy and reduced protein expression in Caco-2 cells. Moreover, oat globulin peptides demonstrated α-glucosidase inhibition, with IC50 values of 35.67 μg/mL for LQAFEPLR and 113.8 μg/mL for hydrolysates [27]. Walters et al. [22] investigated the antidiabetic potential of oat hydrolysates in NCI-H716 cells. The results indicate a significant suppression of DPP4 (30.6–53.6%) and α-amylase (18–32%), along with increased insulin secretion and glucose metabolism. The mechanism of inhibition is not well understood. A previous study [56] demonstrated that the inhibition of α-amylase by food-derived peptides generally occurs via competitive binding between polysaccharides and peptides, mostly involving their aromatic amino acids. GLP-1 promotes insulin production and suppresses glucagon release by acting as an incretin hormone, therefore regulating postprandial glucose levels. The release of glucagon-like peptide (GLP-1) in NCI-H716 cells increased, varying from 20.85 to 39.25 pM (picomoles) [22]. Studies demonstrate that food-derived peptides affect gene expression, stimulate bile acids and engage with calcium receptors [57]. Consequently, the peptidomics profile of hydrolysates is crucial for validating their possible role in activity.

Another study indicated that the peptides YFDEQNEQFR, NINAHSVVY and RALPIDVL exhibited potential inhibition of α-amylase in vitro, with IC50 values of 37.5, 67.3 and 72.8 μM, respectively. The peptide (YFDEQNEQFR), characterized by its acidic properties and the presence of tyrosine (Y) and arginine (R) amino acids, exhibited the highest α-amylase inhibitory activity, measured at 57. Oat peptides have demonstrated efficacy in alleviating symptoms of polydipsia, weight loss and polyphagia, thereby aiding in the regulation of blood glucose levels through enhanced insulin sensitivity and increased glycogen synthesis [58]. Oat grains and their bioactive compounds have been thoroughly investigated for their antidiabetic effects in human populations. Consistent consumption of oats over a period of 23 weeks can enhance fasting blood glucose levels and insulin concentrations by as much as 20%. Additionally, supplementation with beta-glucans has been shown to positively affect blood glucose, insulin, GLP-1, HbA1c and appetite-regulating hormones in individuals with type 2 diabetes [59, 60]. Current research on the antidiabetic potential of oat peptides is primarily confined to in vitro studies. Therefore, comprehensive in vivo investigations are necessary to elucidate the molecular mechanisms underlying the antidiabetic properties of oat bioactive peptides.

8.3.3 Oat Protein in Prevention of Hypertension

High blood pressure, or hypertension, is one of the leading causes of morbidity and mortality associated with cardiovascular disease worldwide [61]. In developed countries, including the United States, hypertension ranks among the most significant non-communicable disorders contributing to cardiovascular disease, heart failure and stroke [62]. Many young adults with hypertension rely on medications to reduce the risk of cardiovascular complications and mortality. However, hypertension remains one of the most consequential threats to individual and public health [63, 64]. Although antihypertensive medications lower the risk of cardiovascular disease and mortality, they do not fully reverse the condition [65]. Consequently, natural and sustainable alternatives, particularly those derived from plant-based bioactive compounds, have gained recognition for their potential role in hypertension management without adverse effects on consumers. Oat proteins and peptides are among these promising sustainable options, with potential to aid in the prevention and management of hypertension. The bioactive peptides derived from oats have demonstrated antihypertensive effects by influencing the renin–angiotensin system (RAS) (Figure 8.3).

Oat protein isolates revealed significant renin inhibitory action, with values between 40.50 and 70.5%, but the synthesized peptides showed comparatively lesser inhibition than the protein isolates. The attributes of renin inhibitory peptides are not as well defined as those of angiotensin-converting enzyme (ACE) inhibitory peptides [66]. Among the peptides, IFFFL mostly engaged in renin inhibition owing to the presence of bulky amino acids at the N-terminal. The increased renin inhibitory effect of protein isolates may also be ascribed to the inclusion of additional bioactive chemicals in the protein, such as phenolic compounds [29]. Oat protein isolates and peptides had a significant inhibitory impact on ACE, with inhibition rates for protein isolates ranging from 86.6 to 96.5%. The protein's maximal ACE inhibition value is similar to that of the positive control (captopril), which exhibited an ACE inhibition of 97.7%. The synthesized peptides WCY, FLLA and WWK exhibited substantial ACE inhibition, attaining rates of 97.8, 97 and 95.3%, respectively. The peptide FEPL demonstrated the minimal ACE inhibition value of 48.9% [29]. The diminished ACE inhibition capacity of FEPL is attributable to proline, which has been shown to reduce the binding affinity of the peptide for ACE [29].

The oat globulin peptide (SSYYPFK) exhibited a decrease in both systolic and diastolic blood pressure in a hypertensive rat model and shown significant ACE inhibitory action (IC50 : 91.82 μM). The peptide SSYYPFK exhibited a suppression of renin activity between 28.6 and 45.59%, concurrently decreasing intracellular endothelin-1 (ET-1) synthesis by 13.19–27.88% [30]. The excessive production of ET-1 functions as an intrinsic mediator in cardiovascular conditions, such as hypertension and atherosclerosis. ET-1 and nitric oxide are essential components in blood pressure control, and the peptide SSYYPFK may have antihypertensive effects via modulating both systems [67]. Clinical research has been undertaken on the antihypertensive characteristics of oatmeal, beta-glucan, dietary

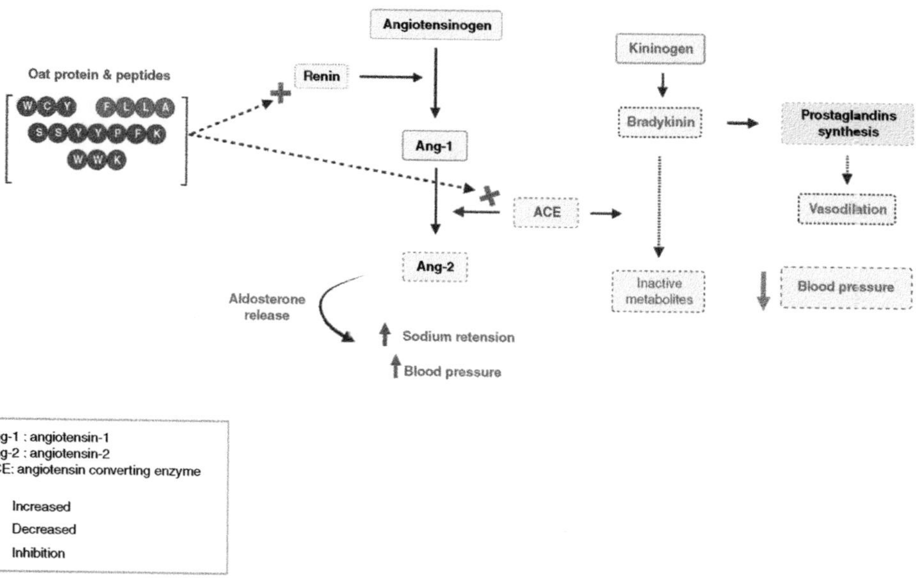

Figure 8.3 Antihypertensive activity of oat peptides by targeting RAS.

fibres, avenanthramides (AVA) and related supplementary derivatives. Most of these human intervention trials assessed the positive effects of oats and their active components on systolic or diastolic blood pressure in both hypertensive and normotensive persons [68]. The aforementioned study findings indicate that peptides generated from oat protein may efficiently suppress ACE and renin by engaging their respective pathways. These results indicate that these peptides may act as a functional component for the prevention of hypertension and associated diseases, subject to more intervention studies.

8.3.4 Oat Protein in Immune Function

Oat peptides exhibited immunomodulatory effects by augmenting both innate and adaptive immunity. Oat oligopeptides (OOPs) linked to significant elevations in interleukin IL, serum interferon (IFN)-γ, tumor necrosis factor (TNF)-α, percentages of T and Th cells, immunoglobulin IgA and IgG production and secretions of granulocyte macrophage colony-stimulating factors (GM-CSF). The research revealed that post-OOP treatment, the percentages of $CD3^+$ and $CD4^+$ T cells increased, signifying a rise in T cell number, which subsequently facilitates the cytokine release and mediates the cellular immune response [31].

CD4-T cells include T helper-1 (Th1) cells, which facilitate a cell-mediated immune response via the secretion of IL-2, TNF-α and INF-γ. Moreover, T-helper 2 (Th2) cells and GM-CSF promote humoral responses via the secretion of IL-4, IL-5 and IL-10 cytokines [69]. A previous study suggested that oat gluten protein and peptides may significantly enhance ConA-induced splenic lymphocyte transformation and delayed-type hypersensitivity. Moreover, a combination of oat peptides and American ginseng peptides has shown a significant improvement in the immunity of mice [70]. Oat bioactive peptides may enhance immunity; nevertheless, the exact processes by which food-derived bioactive peptides influence the immune system remain inadequately known.

8.3.5 Oat Protein in Hypoxia

The capacity of bioactive peptides sourced from animals and plants to mitigate hypoxia and several metabolic disorders has garnered significant attention [71–73]. OOPs can markedly elevate haemoglobin (Hb), red blood cell (RBC) and haematocrit (Hct) levels, hence improving the blood's oxygen transport capacity and utilisation rate [32]. The quantity of red blood cells and the haematocrit, which reflect the volume ratio of RBCs to total blood, are direct indicators of the blood t oxygen carrying-capacity ability. Haemoglobin (Hb) binds with oxygen to facilitate its transfer from regions of higher concentration to those of lower concentration, where it is required, with oxygen attached to an iron atom and distributed throughout the circulation [68, 70].

Furthermore, OOPs decreased lactate concentration and increased lactate dehydrogenase (LDH) activity, therefore augmenting the brain's resilience to lactic acidosis. The brain's inadequate antioxidant system and lipid membrane make it more vulnerable to oxidation. The failure of mitochondrial oxidase to fully convert oxygen to water in under hypoxic conditions causes a buildup of reduced equivalents in the respiratory chain, eventually leading to the production of ROS. These compounds induce lipid peroxidation in the brain, leading to the production of alkanes, epoxy fatty acids, alkanals, alkenals and aldehydes, including MDA [74–77]. Research revealed that OOPs decrease the brain's MDA levels, resulting in less lipid peroxidation and enhanced angiogenesis, thereby improving the hypoxic response [32].

8.3.6 Oat Protein in Fatigue Prevention

Oat bioactive peptides may mitigate exercise-induced tiredness by improving muscular strength [78]. Lactic acid buildup and acidosis are acknowledged as contributors to elevated hydrogen ion concentration, leading to reduced action potential, impaired sarcoplasmic reticulum absorption and calcium ion release [79]. Oat peptides exhibited a significant increase in LDH levels while simultaneously suppressing lactic acid generation. Additionally, oat peptides were shown to decrease blood urea nitrogen levels while increasing glycogen concentrations in the liver and muscles [78]. A separate investigation indicated that oat protein isolates significantly improve the physiological state of mice.

This improvement includes an increase in liver glycogen levels by 19.64%, a 20.27% enhancement in SOD activity in blood and an 81.32% increase in muscles, as well as a 13.58% rise in LDH levels. Additionally, there was a decrease in malondialdehyde (MDA) levels by 3.45% in blood and 53.12% in muscles, along with an 18.25% reduction in blood urea nitrogen (BUN) levels [33]. Hepatic glycogen typically serves a crucial function in supporting blood glucose utilisation and ensuring its levels remain within the physiological range. During intensive exercise, the depletion of glycogen significantly restricts energy availability and optimal power output. As a result, fatigue may occur when the majority of glycogen is depleted from the liver [80, 81].

Urea is synthesized as the ultimate result of protein metabolism in the liver, and blood urea nitrogen (BUN) acts as a sensitive marker of weariness, markedly increasing after strenuous activity [82–84]. A decreased concentration of LDH functions as a biomarker for muscular injury. This enzyme is essential in the glycolytic pathway and depends on NAD+ for the interconversion of pyruvate and lactate [85].

A clinical study indicated that oat protein supplementation for 14 days before and 4 days after exercise significantly reduced exercise-induced fatigue by alleviating physical discomfort and lowering the increase of plasma biomarkers, including creatine kinase, IL-6, C-reactive protein and myoglobin levels. Moreover, oat protein significantly alleviated the decline in joint range of motion, jump performance and muscular strength, while facilitating the healing of injured muscles after exercise in healthy people [34]. Scientific studies have shown that oat protein may significantly reduce exercise-induced weariness.

8.3.7 Oat Protein in Anti-thrombotic Function

The arachidonic acid (AA) pathway is essential for platelet aggregation, since AA directly affects the COX1–TXA2 synthase pathway to produce TXA2. COX1 is an essential enzyme in this pathway, associated with the metabolism of AA to promote TXA2 synthesis [86, 87]. Ultimately, TXA2 produces morphological changes in platelets and activates fibrinogen receptors, hence promoting platelet aggregation [88, 89]. Hydrolysates obtained from oats, barley and buckwheat are said to substantially inhibit platelet aggregation. Oat hydrolysates had considerable antiplatelet activity, with an IC50 value of 0.282 mg/mL [35]. Furthermore, oat globulin fractions of small, medium and large sizes significantly decreased AA-induced platelet aggregation by 67.69, 17.98 and 14.33%, respectively, while increasing the inhibitory rates to 73.11, 75.37 and 69.23%. These findings closely resemble the inhibitory rate of ASA (88.3%), which serves as a medical standard. The small-sized oat fraction had more activity than the mid- and large-sized fractions [35]. The results suggest that oat-derived bioactive peptides/hydrolysates might diminish platelet aggregation by successfully targeting the COX1-TXA2 synthase pathway, thereby aiding in the treatment of thrombosis and related chronic diseases.

8.3.8 Oat Protein in Cholesterol Management

Hyperlipidaemia arises from disturbances in lipid metabolism, leading to abnormally elevated plasma lipid levels. It is typically characterized by increased concentrations of total cholesterol (TC), triglycerides (TG) and low-density lipoprotein cholesterol (LDL-c), or by reduced levels of high-density lipoprotein cholesterol (HDL-c) [90]. The global burden of hyperlipidaemia has grown substantially in recent decades [90]. In 2008, the World Health Organization (WHO) estimated that 39% of adults worldwide had elevated plasma total cholesterol. More recently, over three million adults in the United States and Europe were reported to be diagnosed with hyperlipidaemia in 2023 [91]. The condition is largely associated with factors such as high-fat diets, pharmacological interventions and sedentary lifestyles. Although several pharmacotherapies, including statins, beta-blockers and ezetimibe, are widely prescribed, their use is often limited by adverse effects such as muscle pain, gastrointestinal disturbances and skin flushing [92]. This has prompted increasing interest in safe, non-pharmacological approaches for the management of hyperlipidaemia. In this context, food-derived proteins and bioactive peptides have gained considerable attention as promising agents in lipid regulation [93]. Among them, oat protein has demonstrated notable potential in mitigating hypercholesterolaemia.

The cholesterol-lowering effect of oats is primarily associated with its ability to reduce cholesterol absorption in the intestine or to impede the enterohepatic circulation of bile acids by facilitating the transport of cholesterol and bile acids to the colon, thus promoting their excretion via faeces. Oats possess many bioactive substances that modulate cholesterol metabolism in animals [94]. The hypocholesterolaemic effect of oats is markedly affected by their protein content. A pertinent investigation revealed a significant decrease in liver and plasma cholesterol levels in rats subjected to a hypercholesterolaemic diet, ascribed to enhanced faecal bile acid excretion [95]. Oat protein significantly reduced plasma low-density lipoprotein (LDL-C) and total cholesterol levels in the liver via promoting bile acid excretion and regulating liver CYP7A1 activity in an animal model [36]. The control of certain genes and enzymes, such as LDLR, HMG CoA reductase, HYP3A4 and CYP7A1, is essential for cholesterol homeostasis, as it enables the conversion of cholesterol to bile acids and its transport to hepatic cells, in addition to its function in bile acid metabolism [96].

A clinical trial revealed a significant decrease in triglycerides and total cholesterol in 268 hypercholesterolaemic individuals after consuming whole oat grain and β-glucan fortified products [97]. Oat bran containing β-glucan has shown substantial benefits in hypercholesterolaemic people, decreasing cholesterol levels by 23% while preserving high-density lipoprotein (HDL) levels in the bloodstream [98]. A clinical study demonstrated that the consumption of 6 g of oat β-glucan over eight consecutive weeks significantly reduced plasma LDL and total cholesterol levels (from 167.9 to 120.9 mg/dL and 231.8 to 194.2 mg/dL, respectively) while elevating plasma HDL from 39.4 to 49.5 mg/dL in overweight individuals with mild hypercholesterolaemia [99]. However, there is a scarcity of studies about the hypocholesterolaemic effects of oat protein and peptides.

8.3.9 Oat Protein in Preventing Cancer

Cancer remains one of the leading causes of morbidity and mortality worldwide and represents the second most prominent cause of death among individuals under the age of 70 in most countries. According to the 2020 Global Cancer Report, approximately 19.3 million new cases and 10 million deaths were reported across 36 types of cancers in 185 countries [100]. Ageing is considered one of the most significant risk factors, with the global rise in the elderly population further amplifying cancer incidence. In 2018, an estimated 2.3 million new cancer cases were diagnosed among adults aged 80 years or older, accounting for 13.3% of all new cases. This number is projected to increase to nearly 6.9 million by 2050 [101]. In terms of prevalence, breast cancer (11.7%), lung cancer (11.4%), prostate cancer (7.3%), nonmelanoma skin cancer (6.2%), colorectal cancer (6.0%), stomach cancer (5.6%), liver cancer (4.7%), rectal cancer (3.8%), cervical cancer (3.1%) and oesophageal cancer (3.1%) were the most frequently diagnosed cancers in 2020 [100]. Over recent years, a growing body of evidence has demonstrated significant associations between dietary habits, cancer development, prevention and adjuvant therapy [102, 103]. Whole grains, in particular, play an essential role in reducing the risk of cancer and other metabolic disorders [104]. Oats, as a prominent whole grain, have received increasing attention due to their potential chemopreventive effects, particularly against lung and colon cancers [105–107].

Among bioactive compounds, proteins, peptides and amino acids are notable for their anticancer activities through the regulation of angiogenesis and apoptosis—two critical processes in cancer prevention [108, 109]. One such peptide is lunasin, a 43-amino acid sequence originally identified in soy, which contains a cell adhesion motif (arginyl-glycyl-aspartic acid, RGD) and a poly-asparagine tail composed of nine residues [110]. Lunasin has also been detected in several cereals, including rye, barley, wheat and oats, with concentrations in oats ranging from 0.034 to 0.197 mg/g, depending on genotype [37]. The proposed anticancer mechanism of lunasin involves the induction of apoptosis by disrupting the balance of histone acetylation and deacetylation. Furthermore, oxidative stress and chronic inflammation are closely associated with cancer initiation and progression [111]. Studies have shown that hydrolyzed oat proteins exert cancer-preventive effects primarily through antioxidant and anti-inflammatory mechanisms. For instance, in a hepatocellular carcinoma (HepG2) cell model, seven peptides derived from hydrolyzed oat proteins were compared for their radical-scavenging activities. Among them, GLVYI (Gly-Leu-Val-Tyr-Ile) and YHNAP (Tyr-His-Asn-Ala-Pro) demonstrated the strongest antioxidant capacity [21]. In addition, administration of hydrolyzed OOPs (0.25–2.0 g/kg body weight) in BALB/C mice enhanced immune responses by stimulating natural killer (NK) cell activity and macrophage phagocytosis, while significantly increasing the levels of the anti-inflammatory cytokine interleukin-10 (IL-10) [31]. In conclusion, peptides derived from hydrolyzed oat proteins exhibit significant cancer-preventive potential through multiple mechanisms, including modulation of oxidative stress, enhancement of immune function and promotion of cancer cell apoptosis.

8.3.10 Oat Protein in Neuroprotective Function

Neurodegenerative illnesses, such as Parkinson's disease, Alzheimer's disease (AD), and multiple sclerosis, exert significant societal and family responsibilities. These disorders are linked to several clinical characteristics, including cholinergic system impairment, heightened oxidative stress, inflammatory responses, neurofibrillary tangles and amyloid plaque accumulation. The preservation of cholinergic neurons, their neurotransmitters and receptor systems is crucial for efficient synaptic transmission in the central nervous system. Deficiencies in this system hinder neuronal transmission, leading to diminished learning and memory capabilities [112]. Furthermore, ongoing oxidative stress during disease development exacerbates cholinergic imbalance [113].

For instance, lipid peroxidation has been shown to elevate acetylcholinesterase activity [114]. The strong interplay between oxidative stress and inflammation is also well established. Elevated ROS production not only drives inflammation but also accelerates neurodegenerative processes [115–117]. ROS-mediated activation of inflammatory genes promotes excessive release of pro-inflammatory mediators, fuelling neuroinflammation [118] and, in turn, amplifying ROS generation. In this context, natural antioxidant compounds have gained significant attention for managing neurodegenerative disorders, partly due to safety concerns associated with synthetic antioxidants [119–122]. Bioactive peptides derived from dietary proteins of animal, marine, insect and plant origin represent particularly promising candidates owing to their favourable digestion, absorption and excretion profiles, coupled with a lack of adverse side effects [123–127].

Oat protein hydrolysates and their isolated peptides (DF-10, HL-8 and RW-9) have demonstrated neuroprotective efficacy in scopolamine-induced zebrafish models. These peptides improved behavioural performance, reduced acetylcholinesterase activity, mitigated oxidative stress and lowered brain levels of pro-inflammatory cytokines, including TNF-α, IL-6 and IL-1β. These peptides enhanced the expression of neurotrophic-related (Bdnf), antioxidant-related (Nrf2) and neural activity-related (Erg1) genes [10]. Furthermore, study in a scopolamine-induced mice model showed that RW-9 attenuates AD-like symptoms via modulation of the gut–serum–brain axis, regulating hippocampal signaling pathways, neurotransmitters and gut microbiota composition. Together, these findings highlight coordinated gut–brain axis regulation as a central mechanism of peptide-mediated neuroprotection [11].

8.3.11 Role of Oat Protein in Coeliac Disease

Coeliac disease is triggered by the ingestion of gluten in individuals with gluten intolerance. Gluten, an alcohol-soluble complex protein, is predominantly present in wheat and related cereals such as barley and rye. In genetically predisposed individuals, gluten consumption induces an inappropriate immune response in the small intestine, leading to villous atrophy and crypt hyperplasia [128, 129]. This pathological response results in malabsorption of proteins, fats, carbohydrates, fat-soluble vitamins, folate and essential minerals, particularly iron and calcium. At present, strict lifelong exclusion of gluten from the diet is the only effective therapy. Oats are nutritionally favourable, providing a more balanced composition compared to other cereals. However, their safety in the diet of coeliac patients has been the subject of ongoing debate [130]. Earlier studies [131, 132] recommended the complete avoidance of oats, whereas later investigations [133] supported their inclusion in a gluten-free diet.

The suitability of oats for coeliac patients depends largely on their protein fractions, namely globulins, albumins, prolamins (avenins) and glutelins. Prolamins and glutelins represent the storage proteins of the grain endosperm, constituting approximately 60–70% of total cereal proteins. Among these, prolamins are less susceptible to hydrolysis and therefore more difficult to digest. Notably, oats contain a comparatively low proportion of prolamins (10–15% of total protein) compared to wheat (40–50%), rye (30–50%) and barley (35–45%). It has been suggested that oat prolamins may only exert toxic effects in coeliac patients when consumed in excessive quantities, in contrast to rye and barley, which are more toxic even in moderate amounts [134]. Furthermore, the prolamin content in oats varies with species, variety and cultivation condition, highlighting potential risks in their dietary use. Nonetheless, the European Commission Regulation (EC) No. 41/2009 has permitted the inclusion of oats in gluten-free products, provided that the gluten content does not exceed 20 ppm (mg/kg). Although oats are naturally gluten-free, contamination can occur during transportation, storage, milling or other processing when they come into contact with gluten-containing cereals [135]. Such contamination increases the risk of adverse reactions in individuals with coeliac disease, and therefore oats were historically excluded from the list of gluten-free foods. However, subsequent clinical studies have demonstrated that oats' consumption, not only in moderate but also in relatively large amounts, is also safe for the majority of adults with coeliac disease. Several studies have further recommended the inclusion of oats in the diets of children with coeliac disease [136–138]. Consequently, a variety of oat-based gluten-free products, such as biscuits, pasta and snacks, have been developed for coeliac patients [130]. More recently, a clinical trial using purified oat avenin protein reported that only approximately 3% of coeliac patients experienced acute allergic-like reactions resembling wheat allergy, whereas 97% of patients showed no adverse response following consumption [139]. These findings provide strong evidence supporting the safe inclusion of oats in the diet of most individuals with coeliac disease, with only a small subset of patients requiring oat avoidance.

Summary

Oat protein offers notable nutritional advantages owing to its well-balanced amino acid composition, high content of essential amino acids, suitability for gluten-free diets and low allergenic potential. The rising global demand for plant-derived foods is driven by shifting dietary preferences, increasing income levels, and population growth. However, barriers such as cost, limited awareness and restricted availability in food service outlets hinder the broader adoption of plant-based diets. In this context, oat protein-rich foods represent a valuable means of supporting the transition from animal to plant-based nutrition. Beyond their nutritional value, oat protein and peptides exhibit significant health-promoting properties, with oat-derived peptides demonstrating diverse biological activities through modulation of specific molecular pathways associated with chronic diseases. Nonetheless, further investigation is required to clarify their bioavailability, interactions with other dietary components and effects on human physiology. Advancing strategies to optimize and validate the nutritional and functional properties of oat protein and peptides will be essential for their effective integration into nutraceutical applications and the development of innovative functional food products.

References

1 S. Liu, H. Rafique, L. Zou, and X. Hu, "Therapeutic effects and mechanism of oat β-glucan plus montmorillonite powder on diarrhea in young rats," *Food Hydrocoll. Heal.*, vol. 4, no. 620, p. 100169, 2023, https://doi.org/10.1016/j.fhfh.2023.100169.

2 H. Rafique et al., "Ultrasound-assisted modification of oat protein isolates: structural and functional enhancements," *Ultrason. Sonochem.*, vol. 112, p. 107204, 2025, https://doi.org/10.1016/j.ultsonch.2024.107204.

3 L. Litson, W. Cai, J. Yang, C. M. Prado, and L. Chen, "Identifying peptides from oat protein with potential hypocholesterolemic and satiety effects," *J. Funct. Foods*, vol. 128, p. 106793, 2025, https://doi.org/10.1016/j.jff.2025.106793.

4 U. Holopainen-Mantila, S. Vanhatalo, P. Lehtinen, and N. Sozer, "Oats as a source of nutritious alternative protein," *J. Cereal Sci.*, vol. 116, p. 103862, 2024, https://doi.org/10.1016/j.jcs.2024.103862.

5 Y.-F. Chu et al., "In vitro antioxidant capacity and anti-inflammatory activity of seven common oats," *Food Chem.*, vol. 139, no. 1–4, pp. 426–431, 2013, https://doi.org/10.1016/j.foodchem.2013.01.104.

6 P. Raj et al., "Oat-protein-based diet lowers blood pressure and prevents cardiac remodeling and dysfunction in spontaneously hypertensive rats," *Nutrients*, vol. 16, no. 22, p. 3870, 2024, https://doi.org/10.3390/nu16223870.

7 J. Bouchard et al., "Oat protein modulates cholesterol metabolism and improves cardiac systolic function in high fat, high sucrose fed rats," *Appl. Physiol. Nutr. Metab.*, vol. 49, no. 6, pp. 738–750, 2024, https://doi.org/10.1139/apnm-2023-0440.

8 L. Ramírez Fuentes, C. Richard, and L. Chen, "Sequential alcalase and flavourzyme treatment for preparation of α-amylase, α-glucosidase, and dipeptidyl peptidase (DPP)-IV inhibitory peptides from oat protein," *J. Funct. Foods*, vol. 87, p. 104829, 2021, https://doi.org/10.1016/j.jff.2021.104829.

9 O. Chen et al., "The role of oat nutrients in the immune system: a narrative review," *Nutrients*, vol. 13, no. 4, p. 1048, 2021, https://doi.org/10.3390/nu13041048.

10 H. Rafique et al. "Characterization and exploration of the neuroprotective potential of oat-protein-derived peptides in PC12 cells and scopolamine-treated zebrafish," *Nutrients*, vol. 16, p. 117, 2024.

11 Hamad Rafique et al. "Oat peptide ameliorates cognitive impairment via mediating gut-brain axis in mice: A multi-omics approach," *Journal of Agriculture and Food Research*, vol. 24, no. 102394, 2025, https://doi.org/10.1016/j.jafr.2025.102394.

12 X. Huang et al. "A global view of oat immunogenicity for celiac disease, from genes to cellular response," *J. Cereal Sci.*, vol. 119, p. 103994, 2024, https://doi.org/10.1016/j.jcs.2024.103994.

13 M. G. Nosworthy et al. "Effect of cooking on the in vitro and in vivo protein quality of soy, oat and wheat varieties," *Cereal Chem.*, vol. 100, no. 2, pp. 460–472, 2023, https://doi.org/10.1002/cche.10623.

14 F. Boukid, "Oat proteins as emerging ingredients for food formulation: where we stand?," *Eur. Food Res. Technol.*, vol. 247, pp. 535–544, 2021.

15 J. Szenderák, D. Fróna, and M. Rákos, "Consumer acceptance of plant-based meat substitutes: a narrative review," *Foods*, vol. 11, no. 9, p. 1274, 2022, https://doi.org/10.3390/foods11091274.

16 K. S. Poutanen et al. "Grains – a major source of sustainable protein for health," *Nutr. Rev.*, vol. 80, no. 6, pp. 1648–1663, 2022, https://doi.org/10.1093/nutrit/nuab084.
17 V. Miller et al. "Global, regional, and national consumption of animal-source foods between 1990 and 2018: findings from the Global Dietary Database," *Lancet Planet. Heal.*, vol. 6, no. 3, pp. e243–e256, 2022, https://doi.org/10.1016/S2542-5196(21)00352-1.
18 L. Mogensen et al. "Potential to reduce GHG emissions and land use by substituting animal-based proteins by foods containing oat protein concentrate," *J. Clean. Prod.*, vol. 274, p. 122914, 2020, https://doi.org/10.1016/J.JCLEPRO.2020.122914.
19 R. Esfandi, W. G. Willmore, and A. Tsopmo, "Peptidomic analysis of hydrolyzed oat bran proteins, and their in vitro antioxidant and metal chelating properties," *Food Chem.*, vol. 279, pp. 49–57, 2019, https://doi.org/10.1016/j.foodchem.2018.11.110.
20 S. Ma, M. Zhang, X. Bao, and Y. Fu, "Preparation of antioxidant peptides from oat globulin," *CyTA J. Food*, vol. 18, no. 1, pp. 108–115, 2020.
21 Y. Du, R. Esfandi, W. G. Willmore, and A. Tsopmo, "Antioxidant activity of oat proteins derived peptides in stressed hepatic HepG2 cells," *Antioxidants*, vol. 5, no. 4, p. 39, 2016.
22 M. E. Walters, W. G. Willmore, and A. Tsopmo, "Antioxidant, physicochemical, and cellular secretion of glucagon-like peptide-1 properties of oat bran protein hydrolysates," *Antioxidants*, vol. 9, no. 6, p. 557, 2020.
23 R. Esfandi, W. G. Willmore, and A. Tsopmo, "Antioxidant and anti-apoptotic properties of oat bran protein hydrolysates in stressed hepatic cells," *Foods*, vol. 8, no. 5, p. 160, 2019.
24 H. Yuanqing et al. "The preparation, antioxidant activity evaluation, and iron-deficient anemic improvement of oat (*Avena sativa* L.) peptides–ferrous chelate," *Front. Nutr.*, vol. 8, p. 348, 2021.
25 B. Feng, L. Ma, J. Yao, Y. Fang, Y. Mei, and S. Wei, "Protective effect of oat bran extracts on human dermal fibroblast injury induced by hydrogen peroxide," *J. Zhejiang Univ. Sci. B*, vol. 14, no. 2, pp. 97–105, 2013, https://doi.org/10.1631/jzus.B1200159.
26 R. Esfandi, I. Seidu, W. Willmore, and A. Tsopmo, "Antioxidant, pancreatic lipase, and α-amylase inhibitory properties of oat bran hydrolyzed proteins and peptides," *J. Food Biochem.*, vol. 46, p. e13762, 2022.
27 F. Wang et al. "Oat globulin peptides regulate antidiabetic drug targets and glucose transporters in Caco-2 cells," *J. Funct. Foods*, vol. 42, pp. 12–20, 2018.
28 T.-Y. Wang, C.-H. Hsieh, C.-C. Hung, C.-L. Jao, M.-C. Chen, and K.-C. Hsu, "Fish skin gelatin hydrolysates as dipeptidyl peptidase IV inhibitors and glucagon-like peptide-1 stimulators improve glycaemic control in diabetic rats: a comparison between warm-and cold-water fish," *J. Funct. Foods*, vol. 19, pp. 330–340, 2015.
29 S. Bleakley, M. Hayes, N. O'Shea, E. Gallagher, and T. Lafarga, "Predicted release and analysis of novel ACE-I, renin, and DPP-IV inhibitory peptides from common oat (*Avena sativa*) protein hydrolysates using in silico analysis," *Foods*, vol. 6, no. 12, p. 108, 2017.
30 Y. Zheng et al. "Isolation of novel ACE-inhibitory peptide from naked oat globulin hydrolysates in silico approach: molecular docking, in vivo antihypertension and effects on renin and intracellular endothelin-1," *J. Food Sci.*, vol. 85, no. 4, pp. 1328–1337, 2020.
31 R. Mao, L. Wu, N. Zhu, X. Liu, R. Liu, and Y. Li, "Naked oat (*Avena nuda* L.) oligopeptides: immunomodulatory effects on innate and adaptive immunity in mice via cytokine secretion, antibody production, and Th cells stimulation," *Nutrients*, vol. 11, no. 4, p. 927, 2019.

32 J. R. Di Li, Q. Du, P. Liu, and Y. Li, "The anti-hypoxic effects of oat (*Avena sativa* L.) oligopeptides in mice," *Am. J. Transl. Res.*, vol. 13, no. 3, p. 1657, 2021.

33 C. Xu, J. Lv, S. You, Q. Zhao, X. Chen, and X. Hu, "Supplementation with oat protein ameliorates exercise-induced fatigue in mice," *Food Funct.*, vol. 4, no. 2, pp. 303–309, 2013.

34 Z. Xia et al. "Effects of oat protein supplementation on skeletal muscle damage, inflammation and performance recovery following downhill running in untrained collegiate men," *Food Funct.*, vol. 9, no. 9, pp. 4720–4729, 2018.

35 G. Yu, F. Wang, B. Zhang, and J. Fan, "In vitro inhibition of platelet aggregation by peptides derived from oat (*Avena sativa* L.), highland barley (*Hordeum vulgare* Linn. var. nudum Hook. f.), and buckwheat (*Fagopyrum esculentum* Moench) proteins," *Food Chem.*, vol. 194, pp. 577–586, 2016.

36 L. Tong et al. "Effects of dietary oat proteins on cholesterol metabolism of hypercholesterolaemic hamsters," *J. Sci. Food Agric.*, vol. 96, no. 4, pp. 1396–1401, 2016.

37 I. Nakurte et al. "Detection of the lunasin peptide in oats (*Avena sativa* L)," *J. Cereal Sci.*, vol. 57, no. 3, pp. 319–324, 2013, https://doi.org/10.1016/j.jcs.2012.12.008.

38 M. Brownlee, "Biochemistry and molecular cell biology of diabetic complications," *Nature*, vol. 414, no. 6865, pp. 813–820, 2001, https://doi.org/10.1038/414813a.

39 V. P. Reddy, X. Zhu, G. Perry, and M. A. Smith, "Oxidative stress in diabetes and Alzheimer's disease," *J. Alzheimer's Dis.*, vol. 16, no. 4, pp. 763–774, 2009, https://doi.org/10.3233/JAD-2009-1013.

40 V. P. Reddy and A. Beyaz, "Inhibitors of the Maillard reaction and AGE breakers as therapeutics for multiple diseases," *Drug Discov. Today*, vol. 11, no. 13–14, pp. 646–654, 2006, https://doi.org/10.1016/j.drudis.2006.05.016.

41 S. Furukawa et al. "Increased oxidative stress in obesity and its impact on metabolic syndrome," *J. Clin. Invest.*, vol. 114, no. 12, pp. 1752–1761, 2004, https://doi.org/10.1172/JCI21625.

42 Y. Xu et al. "Microenvironment-responsive metal-phenolic nanozyme release platform with antibacterial, ROS Scavenging, and osteogenesis for periodontitis," *ACS Nano*, vol. 17, no. 19, pp. 18732–18746, 2023, https://doi.org/10.1021/acsnano.3c01940.

43 S. Kaur et al. "The role of mitophagy in various neurological diseases as a therapeutic approach," *Cell. Mol. Neurobiol.*, vol. 43, no. 5, pp. 1849–1865, 2023, https://doi.org/10.1007/s10571-022-01302-8.

44 G. Gao, L. You, J. Zhang, Y.-Z. Chang, and P. Yu, "Brain iron metabolism, redox balance and neurological diseases," *Antioxidants*, vol. 12, no. 6, p. 1289, 2023, https://doi.org/10.3390/antiox12061289.

45 R. Waseem, A. Shamsi, S. N. Kazim, and A. Islam, "An insight into mitochondrial dysfunction and its implications in neurological diseases," *Curr. Drug Targets*, vol. 22, no. 14, pp. 1585–1595, 2021, https://doi.org/10.2174/1389450121999201230204050.

46 J. M. MatÉs, C. Pérez-Gómez, and I. N. De Castro, "Antioxidant enzymes and human diseases," *Clin. Biochem.*, vol. 32, no. 8, pp. 595–603, 1999, https://doi.org/10.1016/S0009-9120(99)00075-2.

47 T. Ji et al., "The thioesterase APT1 is a bidirectional-adjustment redox sensor," *Nat. Commun.*, vol. 14, no. 1, p. 2807, 2023, https://doi.org/10.1038/s41467-023-38464-y.

48 M. Valko, D. Leibfritz, J. Moncol, M. T. D. Cronin, M. Mazur, and J. Telser, "Free radicals and antioxidants in normal physiological functions and human disease," *Int. J. Biochem. Cell Biol.*, vol. 39, no. 1, pp. 44–84, 2007, https://doi.org/10.1016/j.biocel.2006.07.001.

49 J. Zhang, J. Hu, W. Sang, J. Wang, and Q. Yan, "Peroxynitrite (ONOO–) redox signaling molecule-responsive polymersomes," *ACS Macro Lett.*, vol. 5, no. 8, pp. 919–924, 2016, https://doi.org/10.1021/acsmacrolett.6b00474.

50 L. Fialkow, Y. Wang, and G. P. Downey, "Reactive oxygen and nitrogen species as signaling molecules regulating neutrophil function," *Free Radic. Biol. Med.*, vol. 42, no. 2, pp. 153–164, 2007, https://doi.org/10.1016/j.freeradbiomed.2006.09.030.

51 S. Bryngelsson, L. H. Dimberg, and A. Kamal-Eldin, "Effects of commercial processing on levels of antioxidants in oats (*Avena sativa* L.)," *J. Agric. Food Chem.*, vol. 50, no. 7, pp. 1890–1896, 2002, https://doi.org/10.1021/jf011222z.

52 J. Chen, Y. Hu, J. Wang, H. Hu, and H. Cui, "Combined effect of ozone treatment and modified atmosphere packaging on antioxidant defense system of fresh-cut green peppers," *J. Food Process. Preserv.*, vol. 40, no. 5, pp. 1145–1150, 2016.

53 M. M. Baakdah and A. Tsopmo, "Identification of peptides, metal binding and lipid peroxidation activities of HPLC fractions of hydrolyzed oat bran proteins," *J. Food Sci. Technol.*, vol. 53, no. 9, pp. 3593–3601, 2016.

54 A. Hossain et al. "Characterization of plant-derived natural inhibitors of dipeptidyl peptidase-4 as potential antidiabetic agents: a computational study," *Pharmaceutics*, vol. 16, no. 4, p. 483, 2024, https://doi.org/10.3390/pharmaceutics16040483.

55 S. Chakrabarti, F. Jahandideh, S. T. Davidge, and J. Wu, "Milk-derived tripeptides IPP (Ile-Pro-Pro) and VPP (Val-Pro-Pro) enhance insulin sensitivity and prevent insulin resistance in 3T3-F442A preadipocytes," *J. Agric. Food Chem.*, vol. 66, no. 39, pp. 10179–10187, 2018.

56 F. Payan, "Structural basis for the inhibition of mammalian and insect α-amylases by plant protein inhibitors," *Biochim. Biophys. Acta*, vol. 1696, no. 2, pp. 171–180, 2004.

57 K. Kim, M. Park, Y. M. Lee, M. R. Rhyu, and H. Y. Kim, "Ginsenoside metabolite compound K stimulates glucagon-like peptide-1 secretion in NCI-H716 cells via bile acid receptor activation," *Arch. Pharm. Res.*, vol. 37, no. 9, pp. 1193–1200, 2014.

58 J. Wang et al. "Hypoglycemic effects of oat oligopeptides in high-calorie diet/STZ-induced diabetic rats," *Molecules*, vol. 24, no. 3, p. 558, 2019, https://doi.org/10.3390/molecules24030558.

59 E. Rytter et al. "Changes in plasma insulin, enterostatin, and lipoprotein levels during an energy-restricted dietary regimen including a new oat-based liquid food," *Ann. Nutr. Metab.*, vol. 40, no. 4, pp. 212–220, 1996.

60 J. L. Pino, V. Mujica, and M. Arredondo, "Effect of dietary supplementation with oat β-glucan for 3 months in subjects with type 2 diabetes: a randomized, double-blind, controlled clinical trial," *J. Funct. Foods*, vol. 77, p. 104311, 2021.

61 G. A. Roth et al. "Global burden of cardiovascular diseases and risk factors, 1990–2019," *J. Am. Coll. Cardiol.*, vol. 76, no. 25, pp. 2982–3021, 2020, https://doi.org/10.1016/j.jacc.2020.11.010.

62 M. J. Pencina et al. "Quantifying importance of major risk factors for coronary heart disease," *Circulation*, vol. 139, no. 13, pp. 1603–1611, 2019, https://doi.org/10.1161/CIRCULATIONAHA.117.031855.

63 D. Ettehad et al. "Blood pressure lowering for prevention of cardiovascular disease and death: a systematic review and meta-analysis," *Lancet*, vol. 387, no. 10022, pp. 957–967, 2016, https://doi.org/10.1016/S0140-6736(15)01225-8.

64 J. D. Bundy et al. "Systolic blood pressure reduction and risk of cardiovascular disease and mortality," *JAMA Cardiol.*, vol. 2, no. 7, p. 775, 2017, https://doi.org/10.1001/jamacardio.2017.1421.

65 R. M. Carey, P. Muntner, H. B. Bosworth, and P. K. Whelton, "Prevention and control of hypertension," *J. Am. Coll. Cardiol.*, vol. 72, no. 11, pp. 1278–1293, 2018, https://doi.org/10.1016/j.jacc.2018.07.008.

66 N. D. L. Fisher and N. K. Hollenberg, "Renin inhibition: what are the therapeutic opportunities?," *J. Am. Soc. Nephrol.*, vol. 16, no. 3, pp. 592–599, 2005.

67 Y.-Q. Zhao, L. Zhang, J. Tao, C.-F. Chi, and B. Wang, "Eight antihypertensive peptides from the protein hydrolysate of Antarctic krill (Euphausia superba): isolation, identification, and activity evaluation on human umbilical vein endothelial cells (HUVECs)," *Food Res. Int.*, vol. 121, pp. 197–204, 2019.

68 J. Bouchard et al. "Impact of oats in the prevention/management of hypertension," *Food Chem.*, vol. 381, p. 132198, 2022.

69 S. L. Constant and K. Bottomly, "Induction of Th1 and Th2 CD4+ T cell responses: the alternative approaches," *Annu. Rev. Immunol.*, vol. 15, no. 1, pp. 297–322, 1997.

70 Y. Tang et al. "Bioactive components and health functions of oat," *Food Rev. Int.*, vol. 39, no. 7, pp. 4545–4564, 2023, https://doi.org/10.1080/87559129.2022.2029477.

71 X. Gao et al. "PEDF and PEDF-derived peptide 44mer protect cardiomyocytes against hypoxia-induced apoptosis and necroptosis via anti-oxidative effect," *Sci. Rep.*, vol. 4, no. 1, pp. 1–7, 2014.

72 C. S. Lee, E. Y. Choi, S. C. Lee, H. J. Koh, J. H. Lee, and J. H. Chung, "Resveratrol inhibits hypoxia-induced vascular endothelial growth factor expression and pathological neovascularization," *Yonsei Med. J.*, vol. 56, no. 6, pp. 1678–1685, 2015.

73 J. Wang et al. "Investigations on the antifatigue and antihypoxic effects of Paecilomyces hepiali extract," *Mol. Med. Rep.*, vol. 13, no. 2, pp. 1861–1868, 2016.

74 J. P. Kehrer and L. G. Lund, "Cellular reducing equivalents and oxidative stress," *Free Radic. Biol. Med.*, vol. 17, no. 1, pp. 65–75, 1994.

75 E. Shohami, E. Beit-Yannai, M. Horowitz, and R. Kohen, "Oxidative stress in closed-head injury: brain antioxidant capacity as an indicator of functional outcome," *J. Cereb. Blood Flow Metab.*, vol. 17, no. 10, pp. 1007–1019, 1997.

76 B. Halliwell, "Role of free radicals in the neurodegenerative diseases," *Drugs Aging*, vol. 18, no. 9, pp. 685–716, 2001.

77 H. Rauchova, M. Vokurkova, and J. Koudelova, "Hypoxia-induced lipid peroxidation in the brain during postnatal ontogenesis," *Physiol. Res.*, vol. 61, p. S89, 2012.

78 Z. H. U. Na, R. MAO, and L. I. U. Rui, "Anti-fatigue effect of oat peptide in mice: an experimental study," 中国公共卫生, vol. 34, no. 9, pp. 1242–1245, 2018.

79 O. Surenkok, A. Kin-Isler, A. Aytar, and Z. Gültekin, "Effect of trunk-muscle fatigue and lactic acid accumulation on balance in healthy subjects," *J. Sport Rehabil.*, vol. 17, no. 4, pp. 380–386, 2008.

80 K. Sahlin, E. K. Sallstedt, D. Bishop, and M. Tonkonogi, "Turning down lipid oxidation during heavy exercise—what is the mechanism," *J. Physiol. Pharmacol.*, vol. 59, no. Suppl 7, pp. 19–30, 2008.

81 J. M. Jia and C. F. Wu, "Antifatigue activity of tissue culture extracts of *Saussurea involucrata*.," *Pharm. Biol.*, vol. 46, no. 6, pp. 433–436, 2008.

82 L. You, M. Zhao, J. M. Regenstein, and J. Ren, "In vitro antioxidant activity and in vivo anti-fatigue effect of loach (*Misgurnus anguillicaudatus*) peptides prepared by papain digestion," *Food Chem.*, vol. 124, no. 1, pp. 188–194, 2011, https://doi.org/10.1016/J.FOODCHEM.2010.06.007.

83 J.-F. Ding, Y.-Y. Li, J.-J. Xu, X.-R. Su, X. Gao, and F.-P. Yue, "Study on effect of jellyfish collagen hydrolysate on anti-fatigue and anti-oxidation," *Food Hydrocoll.*, vol. 25, no. 5, pp. 1350–1353, 2011.

84 Y. Zhang, X. Yao, B. Bao, and Y. Zhang, "Anti-fatigue activity of a triterpenoid-rich extract from Chinese bamboo shavings (*Caulis bamfusae* in taeniam)," *Phytother. Res.*, vol. 20, no. 10, pp. 872–876, 2006.

85 J. S. Coombes and L. S. McNaughton, "Effects of branched-chain amino acid supplementation on serum creatine kinase and lactate dehydrogenase after prolonged exercise," *J. Sports Med. Phys. Fitness*, vol. 40, no. 3, p. 240, 2000.

86 S. P. Jackson and S. M. Schoenwaelder, "Antiplatelet therapy: in search of the 'magic bullet'," *Nat. Rev. Drug Discov.*, vol. 2, no. 10, pp. 775–789, 2003.

87 X.-H. Wang et al. "Cyclooxygenase inhibitors in some dietary vegetables inhibit platelet aggregation function induced by arachidonic acid," *Zhongguo shi yan xue ye xue za zhi*, vol. 19, no. 5, pp. 1260–1263, 2011.

88 D.-H. Lee et al. "Inhibitory effects of epigallocatechin-3-gallate on microsomal cyclooxygenase-1 activity in platelets," *Biomol. Ther. (Seoul).*, vol. 21, no. 1, p. 54, 2013.

89 E. Oder, M. K. Safo, O. Abdulmalik, and G. J. Kato, "New developments in anti-sickling agents: can drugs directly prevent the polymerization of sickle haemoglobin in vivo?," *Br. J. Haematol.*, vol. 175, no. 1, pp. 24–30, 2016.

90 A. Pirillo, M. Casula, E. Olmastroni, G. D. Norata, and A. L. Catapano, "Global epidemiology of dyslipidaemias," *Nat. Rev. Cardiol.*, vol. 18, no. 10, pp. 689–700, 2021, https://doi.org/10.1038/s41569-021-00541-4.

91 L. Wei, H. Wu, X. Wang, L. Wen, B. Cui, and Y. Cheng, "Comprehensive review of plant-derived anti-hyperlipidemia peptides: production, anti-hyperlipidemia mechanism, and structure-activity relationship study," *Food Chem.*, vol. 461, p. 140715, 2024, https://doi.org/10.1016/j.foodchem.2024.140715.

92 D. Rozman and K. Monostory, "Perspectives of the non-statin hypolipidemic agents," *Pharmacol. Ther.*, vol. 127, no. 1, pp. 19–40, 2010, https://doi.org/10.1016/j.pharmthera.2010.03.007.

93 A. Howard and C. C. Udenigwe, "Mechanisms and prospects of foodprotein hydrolysates and peptide-induced hypolipidaemia," *Food Funct.*, vol. 4, no. 1, pp. 40–51, 2013, https://doi.org/10.1039/C2FO30216K.

94 M. L. Connolly, X. Tzounis, K. M. Tuohy, and J. A. Lovegrove, "Hypocholesterolemic and prebiotic effects of a whole-grain oat-based granola breakfast cereal in a cardio-metabolic 'at risk' population," *Front. Microbiol.*, vol. 7, p. 1675, 2016.

95 L. Guo, L.-T. Tong, L. Liu, K. Zhong, J. Qiu, and S. Zhou, "The cholesterol-lowering effects of oat varieties based on their difference in the composition of proteins and lipids," *Lipids Health Dis.*, vol. 13, no. 1, pp. 1–10, 2014.

96 C. Daou and H. Zhang, "Oat beta-glucan: its role in health promotion and prevention of diseases," *Compr. Rev. food Sci. food Saf.*, vol. 11, no. 4, pp. 355–365, 2012.

97 K. C. Maki et al. "Food products containing free tall oil-based phytosterols and oat β-glucan lower serum total and LDL cholesterol in hypercholesterolemic adults," *J. Nutr.*, vol. 133, no. 3, pp. 808–813, 2003.

98 J. W. Anderson et al. "Lipid responses of hypercholesterolemia men to oat-bran and wheat-bran intake," *Am. J. Clin. Nutr.*, vol. 54, no. 4, pp. 678–683, 1991.

99 N. Reyna-Villasmil et al. "Oat-derived β-glucan significantly improves HDLC and diminishes LDLC and non-HDL cholesterol in overweight individuals with mild hypercholesterolemia," *Am. J. Ther.*, vol. 14, no. 2, pp. 203–212, 2007.

100 H. Sung et al. "Global cancer statistics 2020: GLOBOCAN estimates of incidence and mortality worldwide for 36 cancers in 185 countries," *CA. Cancer J. Clin.*, vol. 71, no. 3, pp. 209–249, 2021, https://doi.org/10.3322/caac.21660.

101 S. Pilleron et al. "Estimated global cancer incidence in the oldest adults in 2018 and projections to 2050," *Int. J. Cancer*, vol. 148, no. 3, pp. 601–608, 2021, https://doi.org/10.1002/ijc.33232.

102 S. D. Mittelman, "The role of diet in cancer prevention and chemotherapy efficacy," *Annu. Rev. Nutr.*, vol. 40, no. 1, pp. 273–297, 2020, https://doi.org/10.1146/annurev-nutr-013120-041149.

103 T. J. Key, K. E. Bradbury, A. Perez-Cornago, R. Sinha, K. K. Tsilidis, and S. Tsugane, "Diet, nutrition, and cancer risk: what do we know and what is the way forward?," *BMJ*, p. m511, 2020, https://doi.org/10.1136/bmj.m511.

104 D. Aune et al. "Whole grain consumption and risk of cardiovascular disease, cancer, and all cause and cause specific mortality: systematic review and dose-response meta-analysis of prospective studies," *BMJ*, p. i2716, 2016, https://doi.org/10.1136/bmj.i2716.

105 D. Paudel, B. Dhungana, M. Caffe, and P. Krishnan, "A review of health-beneficial properties of oats," *Foods*, vol. 10, no. 11, p. 2591, 2021, https://doi.org/10.3390/foods10112591.

106 M. Damazo-Lima et al., "Chemopreventive effect of the germinated oat and its phenolic-AVA extract in azoxymethane/dextran sulfate sodium (AOM/DSS) model of colon carcinogenesis in mice," *Foods*, vol. 9, no. 2, p. 169, 2020, https://doi.org/10.3390/foods9020169.

107 W. Guo et al. "Avenanthramides inhibit proliferation of human colon cancer cell lines in vitro," *Nutr. Cancer*, vol. 62, no. 8, pp. 1007–1016, 2010, https://doi.org/10.1080/01635581.2010.492090.

108 E. G. de Mejia and V. P. Dia, "The role of nutraceutical proteins and peptides in apoptosis, angiogenesis, and metastasis of cancer cells," *Cancer Metastasis Rev.*, vol. 29, no. 3, pp. 511–528, 2010, https://doi.org/10.1007/s10555-010-9241-4.

109 B. H. Sarmadi and A. Ismail, "Antioxidative peptides from food proteins: a review," *Peptides*, vol. 31, no. 10, pp. 1949–1956, 2010.

110 B. O. de Lumen, "Lunasin: a cancer-preventive soy peptide," *Nutr. Rev.*, vol. 63, no. 1, pp. 16–21, 2005, https://doi.org/10.1301/nr.2004.janr.16-21.

111 S. Reuter, S. C. Gupta, M. M. Chaturvedi, and B. B. Aggarwal, "Oxidative stress, inflammation, and cancer: how are they linked?," *Free Radic. Biol. Med.*, vol. 49, no. 11, pp. 1603–1616, 2010, https://doi.org/10.1016/j.freeradbiomed.2010.09.006.

112 Q. Huang, C. Liao, F. Ge, J. Ao, and T. Liu, "Acetylcholine bidirectionally regulates learning and memory," *J. Neurorestoratology*, vol. 10, no. 2, p. 100002, 2022, https://doi.org/10.1016/j.jnrt.2022.100002.

113 A. Singh, R. Kukreti, and L. Saso, "Oxidative stress : a key modulator in neurodegenerative diseases," *Molecules*, vol. 24, pp. 1–20, 2019.

114 J. M. Kim et al. "Ginsenoside Re ameliorates brain insulin resistance and cognitive dysfunction in high fat diet-induced C57BL/6 mice," *J. Agric. Food Chem.*, vol. 65, no. 13, pp. 2719–2729, 2017, https://doi.org/10.1021/acs.jafc.7b00297.

115 M. K. Foret et al. "Effect of antioxidant supplements on lipid peroxidation levels in primary cortical neuron cultures," *Free Radic. Biol. Med.*, vol. 130, pp. 471–477, 2019, https://doi.org/10.1016/J.FREERADBIOMED.2018.11.019.

116 A. M. Giudetti, M. Salzet, and T. Cassano, "Oxidative stress in aging brain: nutritional and pharmacological interventions for neurodegenerative disorders," *Oxid. Med. Cell. Longev.*, vol. 2018, p. 3416028, 2018, https://doi.org/10.1155/2018/3416028.

117 J. Yuan, P. Amin, and D. Ofengeim, "Necroptosis and RIPK1-mediated neuroinflammation in CNS diseases," *Nat. Rev. Neurosci.*, vol. 20, no. 1, pp. 19–33, 2019, https://doi.org/10.1038/s41583-018-0093-1.

118 D. S. A. Simpson, "ROS generation in microglia: understanding oxidative stress and inflammation in neurodegenerative disease," *Antioxidants*, vol. 9, pp. 1–27, 2020.

119 I. K. Bae, K. J. Kim, J. S. Choi, Y. Il Choi, and J. H. Ha, "Quality properties and storage characteristics of pyeonyuk with different additional levels of turmeric powder," *Food Sci. Anim. Resour.*, vol. 39, no. 1, pp. 35–44, 2019, https://doi.org/10.5851/KOSFA.2019.E1.

120 J. Pokorný, "Are natural antioxidants better-and safer-than synthetic antioxidants?," *Eur. J. Lipid Sci. Technol.*, vol. 109, no. 6, pp. 629–642, 2007, https://doi.org/10.1002/ejlt.200700064.

121 M. M. A. Hussein and S. F. Gaafar, "Histidine-dipeptides in relation to diabetes and obesity," *Int. J. Vet. Sci.*, vol. 11, no. 2, pp. 221–228, 2022.

122 K. D. Kiliç, A. Gökhan, E. Y. Sözmen, and A. Uysal, "Liver histology and biochemistry of exposed newborn and infant rats with experimental aflatoxicosis," *Pak. Vet. J.*, vol. 42, no. 4, pp. 453–460, 2022.

123 M. Cai, B. Dou, J. E. Pugh, A. M. Lett, and G. S. Frost, "The impact of starchy food structure on postprandial glycemic response and appetite: a systematic review with meta-analysis of randomized crossover trials," *Am. J. Clin. Nutr.*, vol. 114, no. 2, pp. 472–487, 2021, https://doi.org/10.1093/ajcn/nqab098.

124 H. Chen et al. "Identification of antioxidative peptides from defatted walnut meal hydrolysate with potential for improving learning and memory," *Food Res. Int.*, vol. 78, pp. 216–223, 2015, https://doi.org/10.1016/J.FOODRES.2015.10.008.

125 E. K. Kim et al. "In vitro investigation on antioxidative effect of *Inonotus obliquus* extracts against oxidative stress on PC12 cells," *J. Appl. Biol. Chem.*, vol. 54, no. 1, pp. 112–117, 2011, https://doi.org/10.3839/jksabc.2011.016.

126 S. Sudhakar and R. A. Nazeer, "Structural characterization of an Indian squid antioxidant peptide and its protective effect against cellular reactive oxygen species," *J. Funct. Foods*, vol. 14, pp. 502–512, 2015, https://doi.org/10.1016/J.JFF.2015.02.028.

127 T. M. Asala et al. "The antioxidant and hematopoietic effects of the methanolic extract fractions of *Ocimum basilicum* in acetaminophen-induced albino rats," *Int. J. Vet. Sci.*, vol. 11, no. 3, pp. 289–294, 2022.

128 P. J. Wahab, B. J. A. Crusius, J. W. R. Meijer, and C. J. J. Mulder, "Gluten challenge in borderline gluten-sensitive enteropathy," *Am. J. Gastroenterol.*, vol. 96, no. 5, pp. 1464–1469, 2001, https://doi.org/10.1111/j.1572-0241.2001.03812.x.

129 A. Fasano and C. Catassi, "Current approaches to diagnosis and treatment of celiac disease: an evolving spectrum," *Gastroenterology*, vol. 120, no. 3, pp. 636–651, 2001, https://doi.org/10.1053/gast.2001.22123.

130 C. Ballabio et al. "Molecular characterisation of 36 oat varieties and in vitro assessment of their suitability for coeliacs' diet," *J. Cereal Sci.*, vol. 54, no. 1, pp. 110–115, 2011, https://doi.org/10.1016/j.jcs.2011.04.004.

131 W. K. Dicke, H. A. Weijers, and J. H. v. D. Kamer, "Coeliac disease the presence in wheat of a factor having a deleterious effect in cases of coeliac disease," *Acta Paediatr.*, vol. 42, no. 1, pp. 34–42, 1953, https://doi.org/10.1111/j.1651-2227.1953.tb05563.x.

132 P. G. Baker and A. E. Read, "Oats and barley toxicity in coeliac patients," *Postgrad. Med. J.*, vol. 52, no. 607, pp. 264–268, 1976, https://doi.org/10.1136/pgmj.52.607.264.

133 E. K. Janatuinen et al. "A comparison of diets with and without oats in adults with celiac disease," *N. Engl. J. Med.*, vol. 333, no. 16, pp. 1033–1037, 1995, https://doi.org/10.1056/NEJM199510193331602.

134 P. J. Kumar and M. G. J. Farthing, "Oats and celiac disease," *N. Engl. J. Med.*, vol. 333, no. 16, pp. 1075–1076, 1995, https://doi.org/10.1056/NEJM199510193331610.

135 P. M. Kanerva, T. S. Sontag-Strohm, P. H. Ryöppy, P. Alho-Lehto, and H. O. Salovaara, "Analysis of barley contamination in oats using R5 and ω-gliadin antibodies," *J. Cereal Sci.*, vol. 44, no. 3, pp. 347–352, 2006, https://doi.org/10.1016/j.jcs.2006.08.005.

136 E. J. Hoffenberg et al. "A trial of oats in children with newly diagnosed celiac disease," *J. Pediatr.*, vol. 137, no. 3, pp. 361–366, 2000, https://doi.org/10.1067/mpd.2000.109003.

137 L. Hogberg, "Oats to children with newly diagnosed coeliac disease: a randomised double blind study," *Gut*, vol. 53, no. 5, pp. 649–654, 2004, https://doi.org/10.1136/gut.2003.026948.

138 K. Holm et al. "Oats in the treatment of childhood coeliac disease: a 2-year controlled trial and a long-term clinical follow-up study," *Aliment. Pharmacol. Ther.*, vol. 23, no. 10, pp. 1463–1472, 2006, https://doi.org/10.1111/j.1365-2036.2006.02908.x.

139 M. Y. Hardy et al. "Purified oat protein can trigger acute symptoms linked to immune activation in coeliac disease patients but not histological deterioration," *Gut*, vol. 74, no. 6, pp. 906–917, 2025, https://doi.org/10.1136/gutjnl-2024-333589.

9

Future Perspective of Oat Protein

Oat protein exhibits distinctive nutritional and functional properties, including higher total protein content, superior amino acid composition, reduced allergenicity and potential health benefits such as mitigation of chronic disease risk, alleviation of fatigue and neuroprotective effects. It also demonstrates pronounced antioxidant, anti-inflammatory and immunomodulatory activities. In food processing applications, oat protein provides enhanced sensory attributes compared to legume and oilseed proteins. Products such as oat milk, bakery items, dietary supplements and other oat protein-enriched formulations are increasingly entering the consumer market. Despite these developments, the application of oat protein as a functional food ingredient remains at an early stage, and food companies are actively investing in technologies to produce high-quality oat protein products with improved functionality and consumer acceptability.

9.1 Sustainability: Carbon Footprint Comparison with Animal Proteins

Sustainable development is defined as development that meets the needs of the present without compromising the ability of future generations to satisfy their own needs, emphasizing the harmonious integration of economic, social and environmental dimensions [1, 2]. Sustainable agriculture, grounded in this paradigm, promotes green and low-carbon practices through emission reduction, carbon sequestration and systemic transformation [3]. Dietary structure adjustment plays a pivotal role in advancing agricultural sustainability, requiring a tripartite strategy: reducing emissions at the production stage, optimizing consumption patterns and coordinating the entire supply chain. At the production level, this entails implementing low-carbon technologies and ecological farming models, whereas at the consumption level, it involves promoting sustainable diets and minimizing food waste. Such dietary shifts can act as a catalyst for agricultural decarbonization, generating dual benefits for environmental sustainability and public health [4].

As of July 2025, the global population is estimated at 8.217 billion. Food is fundamental to human survival, with protein being essential for growth, maintenance and cellular function. Food proteins not only satisfy nutritional requirements but also shape food systems, as individual dietary choices impact personal health and collectively influence the future trajectory of agriculture and environmental sustainability. Protein deficiency remains a pressing global concern, affecting adults, children and infants worldwide [5, 6].

From a sustainability perspective, the development of plant- and animal-derived proteins must balance nutritional adequacy, environmental impact and social considerations. Animal protein production, particularly from livestock, is resource-intensive, requiring extensive land and generating substantial greenhouse gas emissions, including methane, which accounts for approximately 14.5% of global anthropogenic emissions. In contrast, producing equivalent quantities of plant protein generates only 5–10% of the carbon emissions and consumes markedly less water. Land-use efficiency also favours plant proteins; for example, soybeans yield roughly 20 times more protein per hectare than beef, thereby mitigating competition between human food and livestock feed [6, 7].

Health considerations further favour plant-based proteins. Excessive consumption of animal protein is associated with increased cardiovascular risk, whereas plant proteins—rich in dietary fibre and phytosterols—can contribute to cholesterol reduction. Combining complementary plant proteins, such as grains (deficient in lysine) and legumes (deficient in methionine), enhances overall protein digestibility. To align with carbon reduction targets, prioritizing plant proteins in diets, partially replacing animal proteins, can mitigate environmental pressures. This strategy involves improving plant protein utilization through food combinations (e.g., grain–legume blends) and fostering a sustainable dietary pattern that emphasizes plant proteins while incorporating animal proteins in moderation, thus balancing nutritional adequacy with ecological impact [6, 7].

Based on life cycle assessment (LCA) methodology, 58 households and 16 oat-processing enterprises in China's main oat-growing regions were surveyed to quantify the carbon footprint of oat production. During cultivation, the carbon footprint per unit area was 800.29 ± 263.77 kg $CO_2e \cdot h/m^2$, and the carbon footprint per unit yield was 0.380 ± 0.125 t CO_2e/t. Among them, large-scale oat growers exhibited a per-unit output carbon footprint of 0.380 ± 0.386 t CO_2e/t and per-unit area footprint of 801.93 ± 814.05 kg CO_2eh/m^2, close to the overall average. Smallholder (retail) oat producers had a per-unit area footprint of 648.54 ± 875.31 kg $CO_2e \cdot h/m^2$ (19% lower than average) and a per-unit output footprint of 0.422 ± 0.570 t CO_2e/t (11.1% lower than average). For oat processing, the carbon footprint per unit of product was 69.67 ± 5.77 kg CO_2e/t for oat flour, 130.62 ± 10.86 kg CO_2e/t for oat flakes and 50.76 ± 4.81 kg CO_2e/t for oat dehulled rice [8]. Considering the entire life cycle of oat wholemeal foods, the carbon footprint during the cultivation phase was substantially lower than that of three staple crops: maize (4052 kg $CO_2e \cdot h/m^2$, 0.48 t CO_2e/t), rice (11,881 kg $CO_2e \cdot h/m^2$, 1.60 t CO_2e/t) and wheat (5455 kg $CO_2e \cdot h/m^2$, 0.75 t CO_2e/t) [9]. Within oat cultivation, chemical fertilizer usage and irrigation-related electricity consumption were identified as primary carbon emission sources. Among processing steps, oatmeal production exhibited the largest carbon footprint, whereas oat flakes and dehulled oats required higher electricity consumption than wheat and rice processing. If oat is converted into pure oat protein, the estimated carbon footprint is approximately 5333 kg $CO_2 e \cdot h/m^2$ and 2.53 t CO_2e/t. For comparison, beef production generates $26.5 - 60.0$ t CO_2e/t, cotton $22.9 - 39.2$ t CO_2e/t, and pork $3.0 - 11.2$ t CO_2e/t, highlighting oat protein's substantially lower environmental impact [10].

By analyzing the carbon footprint across oat production and processing, this study provides a scientific basis for the sustainable development of the oat industry. Plant-based proteins, particularly oat protein, offer significant advantages over animal proteins—especially red meat—in terms of carbon reduction, resource efficiency, and health benefits [10, 11]. Through technological optimization and strategic dietary integration, the substitution potential of plant proteins can be further realized, promoting both environmental sustainability and nutritional adequacy.

9.2 Emerging Technologies

A review of the literature indicates that oat β-glucan has attracted considerably more research attention than oat protein. Most studies have focused on oat-based food processing, such as oat flour, oat milk, flakes, and bran, rather than on oat protein, its derived peptides, or globulin fractions. In terms of nutritional characterization, research on chemical composition predominates, whereas investigations into functional properties remain relatively limited (Figure 9.1).

A search of international patent databases using the keyword 'oat protein' identified 609 records from 2015 to 2025. Among these, 17 were international patents, and 592 were Chinese patents. Of these, only 23 patents were directly focused on oat protein, including: 4 on non-thermal processing techniques (chemical modification, enzymatic treatment, water extraction, ball milling), 6 on enzymatic production of peptides, 5 on oat protein product development and 8 on medical or non-food applications.

The limited number of patents suggests either technological immaturity or the existence of unpublished innovations. Enhancing protein extraction and processing methods

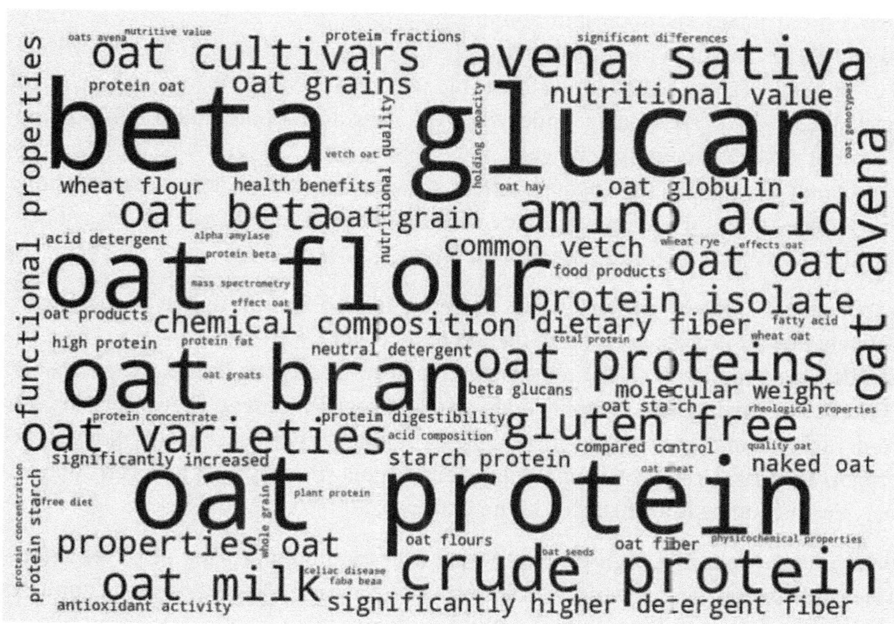

Figure 9.1 Oat protein literature reference survey results.

could improve the taste, texture, production cost, and overall consumer acceptability of oat protein products. Pure oat protein powder exhibits a distinct grainy odour and poor solubility, often leading to sedimentation in beverages. While enzymatic hydrolysis or fermentation can ameliorate flavour, these approaches increase production costs by approximately 20–30%. Compared to soy protein, consumer awareness of oat protein remains relatively low, with only 12% of surveyed individuals able to accurately distinguish between different types of plant proteins.

9.2.1 High-protein Oat Varieties Breeding

Protein content and amino acid composition are critical quality indicators of oats. While both genetic and environmental factors influence oat protein content, genotype represents the most decisive determinant. The high-protein trait in cultivated and wild oats is controlled by recessive alleles [12].

Cultivated oats generally exhibit protein contents ranging from 12.0 to 20.0%, with minor differences observed between *Avena sativa* and *Avena nuda*, though these variations are not significant for raw material processing [12]. Among oat species, tetraploid varieties, such as *Avena murphyi* Ladiz and *Avena Maroccana Gdgr.*, can reach protein levels of 25.26%, whereas hexaploid species, like *Avena Fatua L.* and *Avena. Sterilis L.*, also exceed 25% [12].

Chinese breeders have successfully developed high-protein varieties by crossing tetraploid *A. maroccana* (maternal parent) with cultivated naked oat varieties (e.g., Pin 16 and Pin 2), resulting in a new variety with 18% protein content [12]. Several high-protein naked oat cultivars have been developed, including Jinyan 9 (21.22%), Dingyou 6 (20.86%), Neinongdayou 2 (19.49%), Pinyan 1 (18.70%), Baiyan 1 (18.17%), Bayou 3 (16.80%) and Jizhangyou 1 (18.1%) [13].

Commercial oat flakes show protein content ranging from 11.32 to 13.70%, with the highest averages in Canadian samples (13.70%), followed by New Zealand (13.27%), China (13.04%), Denmark (12.99%), the United States (12.00%), Sweden (11.98%) and the United Kingdom (11.32%) [14]. These data underscore the substantial potential for improving protein content in cultivated oats.

Environmental conditions significantly affect oat growth and protein accumulation. Generally, longer growth duration correlates with higher protein content, whereas short-duration varieties display more variable protein levels.

1. **Temperature:** Optimal growth occurs between 10 and 35 °C; higher temperatures negatively impact protein accumulation and reduce yield.
2. **Rainfall:** Oats require ~300–400 mm during the growing season. Excess rainfall (>400 mm) increases lodging risk, lowering both yield and protein content. Conversely, dry- or semi-dry regions may produce lower grain yields but higher protein concentrations.
3. **Nitrogen Fertilization:** Protein content increases proportionally with nitrogen application, typically ranging from 10 to 100 kg/ha [12].

By crossing high-yield and high-protein parental lines and employing pedigree selection, it is feasible to develop oat varieties with protein content ≥20% and β-glucan content ≥5%. Cultivating these varieties in high-altitude regions (41°N–43°N, >1,200 m elevation) with long daylight hours (>2000 annual sunshine hours), cold temperatures (daily fluctuations >10 °C, ~2100 °C effective accumulated temperature), and extended growth cycles (130–150 days) can further enhance protein accumulation to 20%. Such strategies provide high-quality raw materials for oat protein food development [12].

9.2.2 Oat Protein Polymerization

From surveys of patent applications and research publications, extrusion technology, high-pressure technology, and biochemical/biological technologies have been demonstrated to modulate oat protein structure.

9.2.2.1 Oat Protein Form Polymers with Other Components During the Extrusion Process

High-moisture extrusion (HME), conducted at moisture contents ranging from 40 to 80% [15], is characterized by a temperature profile along the extrusion direction that follows a low–high–low gradient. In this process, water acts as a plasticizer, reducing the material's melting temperature and apparent viscosity. This facilitates more complete protein denaturation and molecular chain rearrangement under relatively mild shear conditions, promoting the formation of an ordered, dense fibrous structure [16–18]. The high-moisture environment also enhances protein–water interactions, providing favourable conditions for molecular chain mobility and directional alignment [15, 18]. Notably, HME is effectively performed only with twin-screw extruders. Compared to low-moisture extrusion, HME products exhibit a higher degree of texturization and superior elasticity.

During HME, oat protein undergoes a structural transformation progressing from an ordered to a disordered state, culminating in a re-ordered configuration. The process unfolds in three distinct stages:

1. **Initial Denaturation (30–90 °C):** Under the combined effects of shear and barrel heating, protein molecular chains unfold, as evidenced by a reduction in β-sheet content, an increase in random coil structures, and tertiary structure alterations. The microenvironment of tryptophan residues shifts from hydrophobic to hydrophilic, exposing hydrophobic and sulfhydryl groups—indicative of initial denaturation [19].
2. **Extensive Denaturation (Melting Zone):** In the high-temperature, high-pressure melting zone, proteins undergo extensive denaturation, with increased β-turn content. Through disulfide bond formation, hydrophobic interactions, hydrogen bonding, and other non-covalent forces, molecular rearrangement and cross-linking occur, forming protein aggregates [20, 21].
3. **Structural Reorganization (Cooling Die):** In the cooling die, molten proteins align along the extrusion axis under laminar flow, solidifying to form textured products with a meat-like fibrous structure.

9.2.2.2 High Pressure Can Change the Oat Protein Molecular Weight

Ultra-high-pressure processing (UHP; 100–1000 MPa), also called high hydrostatic pressure processing, is a physical, nonthermal food processing technique. By applying mechanical stress, UHP modulates the microstructure of food, causing unfolding and reorganization of oat globulin and exposing hydrophobic and sulfhydryl groups. This improves solubility and water-holding capacity while avoiding the nutritional losses associated with heat treatment [22]. Our research demonstrates that UHP (100–500 MPa) modifies the secondary and tertiary structures of oat proteins, disrupting ionic bonds, hydrogen bonds, hydrophobic interactions, and disulfide bonds [23].

During UHP, proteins denature and aggregate via hydrophobic hydration, increasing the content of soluble proteins [24]. Compared with normal pressure, UHP induces secondary structure changes in oat proteins: α-helices unfold, exposing buried hydrophobic amino acid side chains, and α-helices transform into more flexible β-turns [25, 26]. Consequently, β-sheets, random coils, and α-helices decrease, whereas β-turn content increases. Hydrophobic interactions and disulfide bond content initially rise with pressure but subsequently decline. Pressure disrupts hydrogen bonds, hydrophobic interactions, and other stabilizing forces, leading to denaturation, re-extension, rearrangement, and linkage of protein chains, resulting in new protein structures with exposed fluorescent groups [27–29]. The molecular size of oat proteins initially increases and then decreases with rising pressure. UHP promotes the formation of large-molecular-weight aggregates, where polymerization of smaller aggregates generates large-molecular-weight monomers via non-covalent interactions. At certain pressure levels, even non-covalent and covalent interactions can be disrupted [27, 30].

9.2.3 Enzymatic Hydrolysis Technology Can Increase the Protein Functions

Enzymatic hydrolysis of oat protein enables the production of bioactive oat peptides with diverse physiological functions, including immunomodulatory, neuroprotective, and antihypertensive activities. This provides an effective technological pathway for developing functionally targeted nutritional ingredients [31].

As a representative oat protein beverage, oat milk often faces challenges such as poor product stability and susceptibility to phase separation [32]. However, combined enzymatic treatment strategies can substantially enhance emulsifying properties and systemic stability.

Glutaminase hydrolyzes proteins into small peptides and free amino acids, improving solubility and modifying interfacial properties. This optimizes oil droplet size distribution, enhancing emulsion homogeneity, and long-term stability [33].

Amylases (e.g., α-amylase and glucoamylase) effectively reduce system viscosity by disrupting gel network structures and inhibiting starch retrogradation, thereby preventing sedimentation and phase separation during storage [34].

Cellulase degrades structural polysaccharides (e.g., β-1,4 glycosidic bonds), disrupting cell wall integrity and releasing more soluble dietary fiber (e.g., β-glucan) and intracellular components. This increases continuous-phase viscosity and hydration capacity, conferring improved suspension stability and textural uniformity [35].

Collectively, these enzymatic strategies address oat milk stability issues while leveraging the functional potential of oat protein-derived peptides.

9.2.4 Oat Protein Non-food Utilization

Plant proteins, predominantly globulins, demonstrate extensive potential in medical, tissue engineering, and cosmetic applications due to their biocompatibility, biodegradability and structural versatility.

Medical Applications: Cereal globulins can alleviate alcohol-induced liver oxidative stress and protect against acute alcoholic liver injury [36]. Diets rich in plant proteins benefit hepatitis B cirrhosis patients, improving malnutrition and low protein levels [37]. Soy globulin β-glycine regulates intestinal microbiota to generate short-chain fatty acids, mitigating stress-induced cardiac dysfunction and preserving cardiac function [38]. Plant-based diets are associated with reduced inflammation, improved muscle maintenance, and enhanced recovery in surgical or critical care patients [39].

Plant proteins (e.g., soy, corn) serve as biological scaffolds for cell growth and tissue regeneration, leveraging biocompatibility and degradability [40]. Recombinant human collagen derived from plant proteins, with programmable molecular structures and scalable production, has become a cornerstone of medical device innovation. For example, 3D bioprinting of plant-derived collagen can generate human skin-like models for drug testing. In 2024, Wuhan Heyuan Biotechnology Co., Ltd. submitted the world's first plant-based recombinant human albumin injection (HY1001, Aofumin) for marketing approval, targeting liver cirrhosis with hypoalbuminemia ($\leq$30g/L) [41].

Plant proteins exhibit high skin affinity, enhancing moisturization, while hydrolyzed plant proteins (e.g., soy peptides) further improve water retention. These proteins also condition hair, improving texture, shine, and protection. Among plant proteins, soy protein is particularly valued for its moisture absorption, antioxidant activity, and surface activity, making it pivotal in cosmetic formulations. Commercialized products include wheat protein firming lotions, keratin-based hair masks, and white tea shower gels [42–44].

9.3 Challenges in Scaling and Commercialization

Oat protein holds substantial potential in the context of the growing health-conscious consumption trend and rapid technological advancements. However, to fully unlock its market potential, it must address nutritional limitations and adapt to evolving distribution and consumption channels.

9.3.1 Raw Material Supply and Quality Control

The separation, fractionation, and preparation of oat protein still face challenges related to high processing costs and raw material limitations. Initially, oat protein was extracted from byproducts of oat food processing, but this approach suffered from high lipase activity, microbial contamination, and significant interference from impurities. Currently, oat bran serves as the primary raw material, leading to substantial improvements in protein purity, yield, solubility and overall quality compared to earlier methods.

Nevertheless, the oat protein industry remains constrained by factors such as: limited availability of high-protein oat varieties, environmental susceptibility, and the need to balance extraction efficiency with retention of protein bioactivity. For instance, enzymatic hydrolysis requires precise control of the degree of hydrolysis to prevent functional property degradation, while membrane filtration must preserve the target protein's molecular weight. Although advancements have been achieved in technologies combining oat β-glucan with proteins (e.g., ultrasonic-assisted subcritical extraction), large-scale production costs remain relatively high [45].

9.3.2 Processing Technology Bottleneck

Enzymatic extraction and membrane filtration are the primary separation methods for oat protein processing, though both present technical challenges. The enzymatic method, while highly efficient and mild, involves relatively high extraction costs, stringent process conditions and complex control requirements. Membrane filtration, in contrast, offers a more streamlined and scalable approach.

Membrane filtration employs semi-permeable membranes (e.g., ultrafiltration) to separate oat protein through a molecular sieving mechanism, retaining macromolecular proteins while allowing smaller molecules such as sugars and salts to pass. This technology offers four key advantages:

1. **High-purity Extraction:** Enables isolation of oat β-glucan, proteins and peptides from oat bran with purity exceeding 90%.
2. **High Extraction Efficiency:** Achieved using hollow fibre ultrafiltration membranes (e.g., MOF503) under optimized conditions (0.1–0.5 MPa, 15–40 °C), resulting in protein extraction rates up to 50%.
3. **Bioactivity Preservation:** The low-temperature operation helps maintain oat protein bioactivity, including immune-related properties of globulins.
4. **Enhanced Solubility:** Significantly improves protein solubility and product stability, facilitating industrial-scale production, enabling β-glucan fractionation by molecular weight and the recovery of high-value peptides [46].

Enzymatic extraction stands out as an efficient and mild technique that maximizes retention of nutritional value and biological activity. By employing cellulase to degrade cell walls and amylase to hydrolyze starch, this method reduces interference from impurities and enhances protein yield. Combined enzyme treatments have demonstrated extraction rates exceeding 58%. Compared to traditional alkaline methods, enzymatic extraction avoids amino acid damage (e.g., lysine racemization under strong alkali). The mild reaction conditions (pH 7–8, 37–50 °C) preserve protein physiological activity while improving product purity. Additionally, enzymatic hydrolysis enhances solubility, yields a lighter-coloured product, and generates bioactive peptides with higher bioavailability, making it particularly suitable for developing high-value oat protein products. However, further research is required to optimize continuous semi-solid enzymatic hydrolysis, aiming to reduce production costs and enable large-scale industrial application [47].

While membrane filtration excels in purity and scalability, enzymatic extraction offers superior bioactivity retention. The choice between these methods depends on specific application requirements. Future research directions should focus on: developing more cost-effective enzyme formulations, optimizing continuous processing systems, exploring hybrid approaches that combine the strengths of both methods.

9.3.3 Market and Brand Challenges

The oat protein market has experienced sustained growth, driven by increasing consumer demand for healthier dietary options. Government policies promoting whole-grain consumption, coupled with growing recognition of oat protein's nutritional benefits—including potential roles in glycaemic regulation and weight management—have significantly contributed to industry expansion.

Current market data indicate that oat protein is priced at approximately ¥80/kg on average, with mid-to-high-end products ranging from ¥120 to ¥200/kg and high-purity variants commanding ¥200–¥300/kg. Market projections suggest that the Chinese oat peptide product sector, including protein formulations, is expected to reach ¥1 billion by 2025, with a compound annual growth rate (CAGR) of 7–9%. If this trajectory continues, the market value could exceed ¥5 billion by 2030. Leading brands, such as Seamild, Beishi, Quaker, Ffit8 and Intelligence, have already secured substantial market share and influence.

Given this landscape, consumers are advised to prioritize products with high levels of essential nutrients, such as protein and dietary fibre, select formulations with minimal additives and choose package sizes aligned with specific consumption patterns—whether for breakfast, meal replacements or snacks [48].

9.3.4 Policy Requirement

The oat protein industry currently lacks standardized methods for accurately assessing both protein quality and quantity. To address this gap, a comprehensive standardization framework should be established across multiple dimensions, including protein content and quality standards, processing techniques, functional characteristics, certification systems and market promotion strategies. Implementing such a framework will enhance standardization, thereby promoting high-quality industry development [49].

1. **Establishing Protein Content and Quality Standards:** Clearly defined evaluation criteria for oat protein content and quality are fundamental for industrial development. This involves the implementation of standardized analytical methods for protein quantification (e.g., Kjeldahl nitrogen determination) and quality classification based on parameters such as essential amino acid composition and digestibility. These standards are essential for differentiating high-, medium- and low-protein products in the marketplace. Furthermore, advancing rapid detection technologies is crucial for efficient protein identification, helping to prevent the circulation of counterfeit or substandard products [50].
2. **Enhancing Processing Technique and Functional Property Standards:** The functional properties of oat protein, particularly solubility and emulsifying capacity, significantly influence its performance in food and health supplement applications. It is imperative to develop standardized testing protocols for these functional attributes (e.g., emulsifying activity, foaming capacity) to ensure consistent product quality and performance [50].
3. **Implementing Certification and Market Promotion Standards:** A robust certification and traceability system should be established, drawing inspiration from existing models such as 'gluten-free' certification. This system should encompass authenticity certification for oat protein products and implement a 'one product, one code' traceability mechanism to enhance market credibility and consumer trust [51].

9.4 Consumer Perception and Market Trend

From the perspectives of consumers and market dynamics, the future potential of oat protein is primarily driven by three key factors: health-driven demand, expansion of application scenarios and technological innovation.

Oats, rich in soluble dietary fibre, β-glucan and high-quality protein, have emerged as a preferred choice among health-conscious consumers seeking to manage blood sugar levels, reduce fat intake and support cardiovascular health. This trend aligns with the broader wellness-driven market movement, thereby fuelling growing demand for oat protein products.

Simultaneously, the application scope of oat protein has expanded beyond traditional breakfast cereals into diverse sectors such as baking, snack production and personal care, fostering a diversified application landscape.

Technological advancements, particularly in enzymatic hydrolysis and encapsulation technologies, are pivotal for enhancing the functional properties of oat protein. These innovations not only improve product performance but also elevate market competitiveness, ensuring sustained industry growth [52, 53].

9.4.1 Fitness and Athletic Populations

Oats serve as an excellent protein source for fitness enthusiasts, providing multiple benefits including energy provision, muscle recovery and weight management. Rich in branched-chain amino acids (BCAAs) such as leucine, isoleucine and valine, oats promote muscle protein synthesis and facilitate rapid physical recovery. The soluble dietary fibre in oats contributes to satiety, appetite regulation and delayed fat absorption, effectively supporting reductions in body fat percentage. These characteristics make oats particularly suitable for individuals in weight-loss or body composition optimization programs.

9.4.2 Chronic Disease Management

Oat protein exhibits significant potential in mitigating sub-health conditions in individuals with hypertension, hyperglycaemia, and hyperlipidaemia, primarily due to the synergistic effects of high-quality oat protein and β-glucan.

Oat protein provides essential amino acids that support metabolic demands, immune function and tissue repair in individuals with elevated blood pressure, blood sugar or cholesterol levels. Concurrently, oat β-glucan forms a viscous gel in the intestinal tract, which inhibits cholesterol absorption, enhances insulin sensitivity, and promotes bile acid excretion, collectively reducing low-density lipoprotein cholesterol (LDL-C) and total cholesterol and alleviating cardiovascular burden.

Furthermore, oats are rich in potassium and magnesium, which contribute to vascular elasticity and blood pressure stabilization. Scientific dietary incorporation of oats can thus improve metabolic indicators and overall health outcomes in populations with chronic metabolic conditions.

9.4.3 Metabolic Regulation and Wheat Protein Allergy Groups

Among grains, oats are distinguished by their high protein content, which serves as a nutritional substrate for the immune system and supports enhanced immune defence. Oat protein is primarily composed of globulins and lacks allergenic proteins such as gliadin and gluten, which are responsible for coeliac disease, making oats generally well-tolerated by individuals with wheat allergies. Additionally, oat β-glucan has been shown to strengthen intestinal barrier function and mitigate inflammation associated with food intolerances.

It should be noted, however, that oat protein allergies, though rare, do occur, and affected individuals should exercise caution when consuming oat-based products.

9.4.4 Special Physiological Stages

Oat protein and amino acids can enhance immune function in pregnant women, meet the increased nutritional demands during gestation and support overall body resilience. For children, oats are rich in high-quality protein, dietary fibre, B vitamins and essential minerals (including iron, calcium and magnesium), contributing to healthy growth and development. As a nutritionally balanced food, moderate oat consumption can significantly improve the health status of special populations, though consumption methods should be tailored to individual physiological conditions and dietary needs.

9.4.5 Cosmetic Applications

Oat protein and β-glucan exhibit notable efficacy in dermatological applications through multiple mechanisms. They contribute to skin barrier repair, improvement of elasticity and firmness, reduction of wrinkles and roughness and formation of a protective film. Additionally, these compounds inhibit melanin synthesis, brighten the complexion, delay skin ageing and alleviate redness, swelling and itching, including UV-induced irritation. They also enhance skin water retention and reduce transepidermal water loss, making them particularly beneficial for sensitive and dry skin. Due to its mild nature and low allergenic potential, oat protein is recognized as a safe and effective plant-based active ingredient, frequently incorporated into premium and hypoallergenic skincare formulations.

Beyond cosmetic applications, oats demonstrate exceptional agronomic resilience, including cold tolerance, adaptability to poor soils and drought resistance, rendering them well-suited to climate change and global warming conditions. Oat cultivation contributes to reduced carbon emissions and lower water consumption, while its carbon sequestration and water-saving characteristics offer innovative approaches for ecological agriculture.

As a 'plant gold' with dual nutritional and ecological value, oats possess significant potential across health, food innovation and sustainable development domains. Advanced processing techniques can further optimize protein utilization, enhancing both functional and nutritional properties. Rich in high-quality protein and soluble dietary fibre (β-glucan), oats provide synergistic benefits for blood sugar regulation and cholesterol reduction, aligning with global dietary guidelines advocating increased consumption of protein- and fibre-rich foods.

References

1 J. M. Zhou, "Dictionary of Soil Science," Beijing, China: Science Press, 2013. [In Chinese].

2 World Commission on Environment and Development, "Our Common Future," New York: Oxford University Press, 1987.

3 "Modern sustainable agriculture-the evolution of knowledge and practice in food systems," *China Network*, 2021-09-15, https://baijiahao.baidu.com/s?id=1711044867834528763&wfr=spider&for=pc [In Chinese].

4 P. Awasthi, "Socio-economic challenges and sustainable development in developing countries," *SMS Management Insight*, vol. 7, no. 2, pp. 56–63, 2011.

5 FAO, "The State of the World's Land and Water Resources for Food and Agriculture: Managing Systems at Risk," 2011.

6 R. N. Sudarshan, P. D. W. Janitha, and S. Laurie, "Sustainable Protein Sources," Academic Press, 2017.

7 J. Gelski, "Dialing into plant-based protein," *Food Business News*, 2015-04-09.

8 S. Y. Xu et al., "Oat carbon footprint research based on household survey," *J. Triticeae Crops*, vol. 32, no. 12, pp. 1459–1467, 2019.

9 D. Zhang, "Analysis of Carbon Footprint of China's Cereal Crops and Strategies for Emission Reduction," China Agricultural University, 2017. [In Chinese].

10 X. Wang and Y. Qi, "Greenhouse gases emission of food life circle in China," *China Popul. Resour. Environ.*, vol. 23, no. 07, pp. 70–76, 2013. [In Chinese].

11 A. Yang, "Screening and Identification of Excellent Germplasm Resources of Oat and Genome-wide Association Analysis of Protein Content," Inner Mongolia Agriculture University, 2024. [In Chinese].

12 Y. Y. Peng, "Oat Germplasm Resources and Cultivation Management of Oat in Southwest China," Beijing, China: China Agricultural University Press, 2009. [In Chinese].

13 C. Z. Ren and C. Yang, "Chinese Oat Variety Catalogue," Beijing: China Agricultural Press, 2018. [In Chinese].

14 X. Z. Hu, J. M. Zheng, X. P. Li, C. Xu, and Q. Zhao, "Chemical composition and sensory characteristics of oat flakes: a comparative study of naked oat flakes from China and hulled oat flakes from western countries," *J. Cereal Sci.*, vol. 60, no. 2, pp. 297–301, 2014.

15 Y. Q. Fang, Y. M. Wei, and B. Zhang, "Transformations of protein structure in extrusion," *J. Chin. Cereals Oils Assoc.*, vol. 28, no. 5, pp. 100–103, 2013. [In Chinese].

16 R. Osen, S. Toelstede, P. Eisner, and U. Schweiggert-Weisz, "Effect of high moisture extrusion cooking on protein–protein interactions of pea (*Pisum sativum* L.) protein isolates," *Int. J. Food Sci. Technol.*, vol. 50, no. 6, pp. 1390–1396, 2015.

17 Y. M. Zhang, "Texturized Properties of Oat Protein and Development of Textured Products," Shaanxi Normal University, Xian, China, 2025. [In Chinese].

18 C. J. R. Verbeek, S. C. P. Huchukwu, and J. M. Bier, "The role of extrusion conditions on the mechanical properties of thermoplastic protein," *Int. Polym. Process.*, vol. 33, no. 2, pp. 180–190, 2018.

19 M. J. L. Sandoval, R. Osen, S. Hiermaier, and G. Ganzenmüller, "Towards understanding the mechanism of fibrous texture formation during high-moisture extrusion of meat substitutes," *J. Food Eng.*, vol. 242, pp. 8–20, 2018.

20 J. Q. Song et al., "Research progress on the conformational regulation of pea protein by extrusion and its correlation with textural structure," *J. Chin. Cereals Oils Assoc.*, vol. 40, no. 3, pp. 200–208, 2025. [In Chinese].

21 T. He, J. Wang, and X. Hu, "Effect of heat treatment on the structure and digestion properties of oat globulin," *Cereal Chem.*, vol. 98, no. 3, pp. 740–748, 2021.

22 L. M. G. Castro, E. M. C. Alexandre, J. A. Saraiva, and M. Pintado, "Impact of high pressure on starch properties: a review," *Food Hydrocoll.*, vol. 106, p. 105877, 2020.

23 S. S. Jiang, "Study on the Mechanism of Ultra-high Pressure and Enzyme on the Processing Characteristics and Quality Control of High-content Oat Bread," Shaanxi Normal University, Xian, China, 2025. [In Chinese].

24 H. H. Liu and M. I. Kuo, "Ultra high pressure homogenization effect on the proteins in soy flour," *Food Hydrocoll.*, vol. 52, pp. 741–748, 2016.

25 G. Romuald et al., "Effect of ultra-high pressure homogenization on structural and techno-functional properties of egg yolk granule proteins," *LWT*, vol. 178, p. 114624, 2023.

26 M. F. Xu et al., "Ultra-high pressure improved gelation and digestive properties of Tai Lake whitebait myofibrillar protein," *Food Chem.: X*, vol. 21, p. 101061, 2024.

27 X. Yang, Y. Su, and L. Li, "Study of soybean gel induced by *Lactobacillus plantarum*: protein structure and intermolecular interaction," *LWT*, vol. 119, p. 108794, 2020.

28 Z. W. Guo, Y. N. Guo, B. L. Li, L. Z. Jiang, Z. J. Wang, and J. Liu, "Effects of high-pressure homogenization on structural and emulsifying properties of soybean protein thermal aggregates," *Trans. Chin. Soc. Agric. Mach.*, vol. 52, no. 4, pp. 351–358, 2021. [In Chinese].

29 I. Sonoo, B. F. Xiao, and H. Katsuyuki, "Behavior of protein aggregates via electrostatic interactions or hydrogen bonds during dough formation," *J. Cereal Sci.*, vol. 111, p. 103683, 2023.

30 H. Rafique et al., "Oat peptide ameliorates cognitive impairment via mediating gut-brain axis in mice: a multi-omics approach," *J. Agric. Food Res.*, vol. 24, p. 102394, 2025.

31 P. Peng, H. Rafique, J. D. Zhang, Q. Liu, and X. Z. Hu, "Analysis of the mechanism of starch gelatinization, disintegration and component interaction during roasting processing of Chinese traditional oat food," *Food Chem.*, vol. 492, no. 1, p. 145358, 2025.

32 T. T. L. Nguyen, R. G. Gilbert, M. J. Gidley, and G. P. Fox, "The contribution of β-glucan and starch fine structure to texture of oat-fortified wheat noodles," *Food Chem.*, vol. 324, p. 126858, 2020.

33 Z. Q. Jiang, T. S. Sontag-Strohm, H. Salovaara, J. Sibakov, P. Kanerva, and J. Loponen, "Oat protein solubility and emulsion properties improved by enzymatic deamidation," *J. Cereal Sci.*, vol. 64, pp. 126–132, 2015.

34 Q. Liang, W. H. Ma, B. H. Sun, and X. X. Wang, "Effect of enzymatic hydrolysis modes on the stability of oat milk," *J. Henan Univ. Technol.: Nat. Sci. Ed.*, vol. 45, no. 6, pp. 71–81, 2024. [In Chinese].

35 M. Zhang et al., "Enzymatic hydrolysis of oat core flour improves physiochemical and sensory behaviors for oat milk," *J. Cereal Sci.*, vol. 115, p. 103841, 2024.

36 J. H. Huang, A. M. Liao, Z. J. Wei, et al., Preparation method of plant functional protein and application of plant functional protein in protection of acute alcoholic liver injury, 2025, https://patentscope2.wipo.int/search/zh/detail.jsf?docId=CN331406360&_cid=JP2-MKC1GT-72797-1

37 M. Wu, D. Wang, Z. B. Zhu, and S. M. Yao, “Protein nutritional support therapy for patients with hepatitis B-related liver cirrhosis,” *Chin. Foreign Med. J.*, vol. 29, no. 16, p. 2, 2010. [In Chinese].

38 N. Furukawa et al., “Soy protein β-conglycinin ameliorates pressure overload-induced heart failure by increasing short-chain fatty acid (SCFA)-producing gut microbiota and intestinal SCFAs,” *Clin. Nutr.*, vol. 43, no. 12, pp. 124–137, 2024.

39 C. I. M. D. Sukawati, “Plant- vs. animal-based protein comparison in the aging process and its role in perioperative medicine and critical care: a narrative review,” *Clin. Nutr. ESPEN*, vol. 69, p. 932, 2025.

40 A. T. Guduru, S. Sankaran, and D. Bhatia, “Plant-based biodegradable and biocompatible polymers for tissue engineering applications,” *Carbohydr. Res.*, vol. 558, p. 109699, 2025.

41 C. L. Long et al., “Progress in application of recombinant collagen in medical devices,” *Chin. J. Med. Instrum.*, vol. 49, no. 6, pp. 640–646, 2025. [In Chinese].

42 Z. B. Zhang, G. Liu, H. G. Wang, and Y. M. Dong, “The application of plant protein in cosmetics,” *Flavour Fragrance Cosmetics*, vol. 4, p. 5, 2007. [In Chinese].

43 S. Q. Xu and B. Liu, “Plant protein in hair care cosmetics,” *China Surfactant Deterg. Cosmet.*, vol. 34, no. 2, p. 4, 2004. [In Chinese].

44 H. M. Chen and Y. F. Hua, “Application of soy protein in cosmetics,” *China Surfactant Deterg. Cosmet.*, vol. 30, no. 6, p. 3, 2000. [In Chinese].

45 X. Z. Hu and C. Z. Ren, “China Oat Industry Report (2016-2020),” Shaanxi Press, 2021. [In Chinese].

46 X. Z. Hu and C. Z. Ren, “Oat Processing and Function,” Beijing: Science Press, 2016. [In Chinese].

47 White book of China oat milk industry, 2023, https://ifnd.caas.cn/xwzx/kyjz/b25a427ad1004d85a472cd8bbba940bd.htm [In Chinese].

48 M. Annamalai, L. T. Lim, and A. Amanat, “Plant Protein Foods,” Springer, 2022.

49 H. Rafique et al., “Dietary-nutraceutical properties of oat protein and peptides,” *Front. Nutr.*, vol. 9, p. 950400, 2022.

50 C. Z. Ren and Y. G. Hu, “China Oat,” China Agriculture Press, 2013. [In Chinese].

51 Z. K. Zhou, “Modern Cereal Science and Nutrition,” Beijing: Scientific Press, 2025. [In Chinese].

52 J. Qiu and Z. G. Li, “Whole Grain Material,” Beijing: China Light Industry Press, 2024. [In Chinese].

53 China Cereals, Oils and Foodstuffs Association, “Eat Grains for Healthy,” China Light Industry Press, 2025. [In Chinese].

Index

a

acylation 83, *84*
advanced protein extraction methods 62–67
albumins 43
amino acids
  physiological functions of 38–41
  profile of oat protein 35–37, **36**, **37**
  regulatory functions of 38–41
animal-based proteins 3–5, **4**, 79, 88–90, **89**, 181–183
  environmental and resource implications 5
  functional characteristics 3–4
  nutritional characteristics 3–4
  plant-based and 3–5, **4**
  processing considerations 5
animal husbandry
  feeding effects on livestock 6–7
  health of oat for 6–7
  nutritional composition of oat grass 6
  oat hay benefits for Tibetan livestock 7
  oat silage advantages for dairy cows 7
  oat straw characteristics and limitations 7
anti-thrombotic function 167–168
Arginine (Arg) 40
Asian dominance in plant-based dairy market 3
aspartic acid 40–41
avenanthramides (AVNs) 17–19

b

bakery and confectionery applications 133–135
behavioural change
  health as key driver of 2
  sustainability as key driver of 2
benchmarking against competition 108–109
beverages 135–137, **138**
bioavailability enhancement 150
biological processing of protein 86–88
Biological Value (BV) 37
branched chain amino acids (BCAAs) 38–39
burger patties 131–132

c

cancer prevention 169
carbon footprint comparison 181–183
cereals
  comparison of protein and other components 20–22, **20**, **21**
  significance of oat protein over 17–27
chemical composition, of oat protein 35–49
chemical processing
  of oat protein 75–96
  of protein 81–86
China
  enduring tradition with plant-based proteins 3
  Han Dynasty 3, 6
  role in global oat production 7–8, **8**
cholesterol management 168–169
chronic disease
  management 190
  prevention 159–171, *160*, **160–161**
clean-label products 140–141, **140**

coeliac disease 170–171
cold atmospheric plasma processing (CAPP) 80
cold plasma processing 80, *81*
commercialization 143–145
commercial product 146
comparative analysis 117–118, **118**
confectionery applications 134, **134**
consumer acceptance 144–145
consumer choice
  health as key driver of 2
  sustainability as key driver of 2
consumer perception 144, 190–191
consumer trend adaptation 151
cosmetic and pharmaceutical uses 138–139, 191
cream products 129–130

d

D-aspartic acid (D-Asp) 40
deamidation 84–85
deep eutectic protein extraction 62–63
deep eutectic solvents (DES) 62–63
defatting, of oat flour 58
designed approaches 147
development process documentation 146–147
diabetes 163–164, *163*
digestibility 90
Digestible Indispensable Amino Acid Score (DIAAS) 20, 37
dry fractionation method 61–62
dynamic high-pressure fluidization 78–79

e

emulsification 112–115
  foaming characteristics 92–93
emulsions 135–137
environmental factors 122
enzymatic hydrolysis technology 186
enzymatic processing 86–87
enzyme-assisted extraction (EAE) 62, 64–66, *65*
essential amino acids (EAAs) 21–23, 35–38, 43
extraction and purification technologies, of oat protein 57–68
extraction with combined techniques 66–67
extrusion processing 79

f

fatigue prevention 167
fermentation processing 87–88
fitness and athletic populations 190
foaming agent 114–115, *115*
foaming behaviour 113–114, **113**
foaming capacity 112–115
foaming characteristics 92–93
food applications 107–109
  challenges of incorporating legume in 25–27
  challenges of incorporating pulses in 25–27
  importance of functionality in 107–109
food industry applications 129–139
food system 122–123
formulation
  design principles 139
  iteration and optimization 146–147
functional characteristics, of oat proteins 88–95
functionality
  benchmarking against competition 108–109
  defining functional properties 107–108
  importance in food applications 107–109
functional properties, of oat protein 107–124
future trends 147–151

g

gelation 116–119
global oat production 7–8, **8**
global regulatory framework 141–143
globulin-dominant plant proteins 90, 91
globulins 41–42, *42*
glutelin 43
gluten-containing grains 10–12
gluten-free bakery 133–134

gluten proteins 10–12
glycation 81–83
glycosylation 81–83
green chemistry 62
ground meat analogues 131–132
growth projections 150–151

h

Han Dynasty 3, 6
health benefits of oat, for human being 5
high hydrostatic pressure (HHP) 77–78
high lipase activity 94–95
high-moisture extrusion (HME) 79, 90, 185
high-pressure processing 77–79
high-protein oat varieties breeding 184–185
hulled and naked oats 17–19, **18**, **19**
human health, and plant-based proteins 1–3
hydrogen bond acceptors (HBAs) 62–63
hydrogen bond donors (HBDs) 62–63
hypertension 164–166, *165*
hypoxia 166–167

i

immune function 166
industrial applications 118–119
industrial scale protein extraction 68
infant formula and clinical nutrition 137–138
ingredient innovation pipeline 151
innovation opportunities 147–151
innovative products 6
interfacial activity, fundamental principles of 112

l

Lactiplantibacillus plantarum B-16 88
L-aspartic acid (L-Asp) 40
legumes
  challenges of incorporating in food applications 25–27
  comparison of oat protein with 23–25
  significance of oat protein over 17–27
liquid-assisted protein extraction 59–61
low-moisture extrusion 79

m

market and brand challenges 188–189
market evolution 150–151
market implementation 143–145
marketing claims and strategies 144
market positioning 144–145
market trend 190–191
meat analogue products 145–146
meat analogues 131–133
metabolic regulation 191
molecular and structural features, of oat protein 43–48

n

Net Protein Utilization (NPU) 37
neuroprotective function 170
non-essential amino acids (NEAAs) 35–38
nutritional labelling requirements 141–142
nutritional quality evaluation, of oat protein 37–38
nutritional supplement formulations 146

o

oat-based beverages 145
oat dough characteristics
  high hardness 91–92
  low elasticity 91–92
oat flour
  defatting of 58
  high-β-glucan 9
  roasted 5
oat milk 6, 129–130
oat protein concentrates (OPC) 79
oat protein gelation, molecular basis of 116
oat protein isolates (OPIs) 38, 46
oat protein non-food utilization 186–187
oat protein polymerization 185–186
oat proteins (OP) 1–14
  albumins 43
  amino acid profile of 35–37, **36**, **37**
  as an emulsifier 112–113
  in anti-thrombotic function 167–168
  benchmarking against competition 108–109

oat proteins (OP) (*Cont.*)
carbon footprint comparison with animal proteins 181–183
case studies in product development 145–147
chemical composition of 35–49
in cholesterol management 168–169
in chronic disease prevention 159–171, *160*, **160–161**
classification of 41–43
in coeliac disease 170–171
commercialization and market implementation 143–145
comparison with common pseudocereals 22–23
comparison with legumes 23–25
composition of 9–10
consumer perception 190–191
emerging technologies 183–187
emulsification 112–115
extraction and purification technologies of 57–68
in fatigue prevention 167
as a foaming agent 114–115, *115*
foaming behaviour 113–114, **113**
foaming capacity 112–115
foaming characteristics 92–93
food industry applications 129–139
functionality in food applications 107–109
functionality matters 108
functional properties of 107–124
fundamental role of solubility in 109–111
future perspective of 181–191
future trends 147–151
gelation 116–119
gel properties, factors influencing 116–117
global oat product classification 9
global regulatory framework 141–143
globulins 41–42, *42*
glutelin 43
health aspects of 157–171
high hardness 91–92
high lipase activity 94–95
historical and current significance of 5–12
historical significance of 5–6
in hypoxia 166–167
in immune function 166
industrial applications of 118–119
innovation opportunities 147–151
interfacial activity 112
low allergenicity to gluten-containing grains 10–12
low elasticity 91–92
market trend 190–191
modification strategies for enhanced solubility 111
molecular features of 43–48
in neuroprotective function 170
nutritional advantages of 9
nutritional aspects of 157–171
nutritional quality evaluation of 37–38
nutritional superiority of 10
oat dough characteristics 91–92
and other plant proteins 117–118, **118**
as part of daily nutrition 158–159
pH stability 109–112, *110*
physical and chemical processing of 75–96
polysaccharides 119–123
potential of 158–159
practical applications 115
in preventing cancer 169
in prevention of diabetes 163–164, *163*
in prevention of hypertension 164–166, *165*
in prevention of oxidative stress 161–163
primary structure of 43–45, **44**, *45*
processing and functional/physicochemical characteristics of 88–95
product development strategies 139–141
prolamins 42–43
protein conversion coefficient 93–94, **94**
quaternary structure of 47–48, *47*
rise of plant-based proteins 1–5
scaling and commercialization 187–189
secondary structure of 45–47, *46*, *47*

significance over cereal and legumes 17–27
solubility 109–112, *110*
stabilization mechanisms 113–114, **113**
strategic positioning of **124**
structural characteristics of 35–49
structural features of 43–48
sustainability 181–183
technical considerations 131, 133, 134–135, 136–137
tertiary structure of 45–47, *46*, *47*
texturization characteristics 88–90, 116–119
unique characteristic of 9–10
utilization of 7–9

oats
cultural and culinary context 6
global consumption patterns 6
health benefits for human being 5
historical significance of 5–6
medicinal and modern health benefits 5–6
nutritional and historical significance 5
oat milk and innovative products 6
protein content in 9
utilization of 7–9

oxidative stress 161–163

p

personalized nutrition platforms 148
pH shifting 85–86
pH stability 109–112, *110*
physical processing, of oat protein 75–96
physicochemical characteristics, of oat proteins 88–95
plant-based dairy alternatives 129–131
plant-based dairy market 3
plant-based proteins
and animal-based proteins 3–5, **4**
Chinese enduring tradition with 3
environmental and resource implications 5
functional characteristics 3–4
importance for human health 1–3
nutritional characteristics 3–4
processing considerations 5
rise of 1–5

plant protein market 145
plant proteins 75–78, 82–83, 88, **89**, 117–118, **118**
anti-nutritional compounds in 77
chemical modification of 83
fermentation of 88
globulin-dominant 90, 91
hydrophobicity of 83
texturization 88, 90

policy requirements 189
polysaccharides 119–123
applications in food system 122–123
environmental factors governing interaction behaviour 122
precision modulation of functional properties 120–122
unique synergistic effects 119–120

precision fermentation hybrids 149
precision modulation 120–122
primary structure, of oat protein 43–45, **44**, *45*
processing technology bottleneck 188
processing technology integration 139–140
product development strategies 139–141
prolamins 42–43
protein
acylation 83, *84*
biological processing of 86–88
chemical processing of 81–86
cold plasma processing 80, *81*
comparison with common cereals 20–22, **20**, **21**
deamidation 84–85
distribution in hulled and naked oats 17–19, **18**, **19**
enzymatic processing 86–87
extrusion processing 79
fermentation processing 87–88
glycation and glycosylation 81–83
high-pressure processing 77–79
pH shifting 85–86
physical processing of 75–81
thermal processing 76–77

protein conversion coefficient 93–94, **94**
Protein Digestibility-corrected Amino Acids Score (PDCAAS) 20–21, 37
Protein Efficiency Ratio (PER) 20, 37
protein-enriched baked products 134
protein extraction
  deep eutectic 62–63
  with dry fractionation method 61–62
  existing challenges in 67–68
  future perspective for industrial scale 68
  industrial scale 68
  liquid-assisted 59–61
  ultrasonic-assisted 63–64, *64*
protein extraction methods
  advanced 62–67
  advantages and disadvantages of **59**
  deep eutectic protein extraction 62–63
  enzyme-assisted extraction 64–65, *65*
  extraction with combined techniques 66–67
  pulsed electric field 65–66, *66*
  ultrasonic-assisted protein extraction 63–64, *64*
protein texturization 88
pseudocereals 22–23
pulsed electric field (PEF) 62, 65–67, *66*
pulses, in food applications 25–27
purification technologies, of oat protein 57–68

q
quality control 187
quaternary structure, of oat protein 47–48, *47*

r
raw material supply 187
ready-to-drink protein beverages 135–136
regional market development patterns 150–151
regional regulatory variations 142–143, **143**
regulatory and physiological functions, of amino acids 38–41
reverse micelles extraction (RME) 62

s
safety assessment and approval processes 141
salad dressing applications 136
scale-up challenges 143–144
scaling and commercialization, challenges in 187–189
seafood alternatives 132–133
secondary structure, of oat protein 45–47, *46*, *47*
sensory experience 144
smart processing technologies 149–150
solubility 109–112, *110*
  characterization techniques 112
  modification strategies for enhanced 111
  role of, in oat protein 109–111
special physiological stages 191
stabilization mechanisms 113–114, **113**
Streptoverticillium mobaraense 86
structural characteristics, of oat protein 35–49
structured products 131–133
subcritical water extraction (SWE) 62
successful commercial products analysis 145–146
sustainability 181–183
  as key driver of behavioural change 2
  as key driver of consumer choice 2
sustainable packaging interactions 148–149

t
technological advancements 149–150
tertiary structure, of oat protein 45–47, *46*, *47*
texturization characteristics 88–90, 116–119
thermal processing 76–77
3D food printing applications 147–148

u
ultra-high-pressure processing (UHP) 185–186
ultrasonic-assisted extraction (UAE) 62–64, 66

ultrasonic-assisted protein
extraction 63–64, *64*
unique synergistic effects 119–120

v

vegan cheese 130

w

wheat protein allergy groups 191
whole-muscle analogues 132

y

yogurt alternatives 130–131

Printed and bound by CPI Group (UK) Ltd, Croydon, CR0 4YY
17/09/2026
14964268-0001